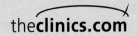

# ULTRASOUND CLINICS

## Abdominal Ultrasound

*Guest Editor*
LESLIE M. SCOUTT, MD

July 2007 • Volume 2 • Number 3

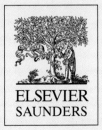

An imprint of Elsevier, Inc
PHILADELPHIA LONDON TORONTO MONTREAL SYDNEY TOKYO

**W.B. SAUNDERS COMPANY**

*A Division of Elsevier Inc.*

1600 John F. Kennedy Boulevard • Suite 1800 • Philadelphia, Pennsylvania 19103-2899

http://www.theclinics.com

**ULTRASOUND CLINICS Volume 2, Number 3**
**July 2007 ISSN 1556-858X, ISBN-13: 978-1-4160-5214-2, ISBN-10: 1-4160-5214-3**

*Editor:* Barton Dudlick

*Reprints:* For copies of 100 or more, of articles in this publication, please contact the Commercial Reprints Department, Elsevier Inc., 360 Park Avenue South, New York, New York 10010-1710. Tel.: (+1) 212-633-3813; Fax: (+1) 212-462-1935 E-mail: reprints@elsevier.com.

The ideas and opinions expressed in *Ultrasound Clinics* do not necessarily reflect those of the Publisher. The Publisher does not assume any responsibility for any injury and/or damage to persons or property arising out of or related to any use of the material contained in this periodical. The reader is advised to check the appropriate medical literature and the product information currently provided by the manufacturer of each drug to be administered to verify the dosage, the method and duration of administration, or contraindications. It is the responsibility of the treating physician or other health care professional, relying on independent experience and knowledge of the patient, to determine drug dosages and the best treatment for the patient. Mention of any product in this issue should not be construed as endorsement by the contributors, editors, or the Publisher of the product or manufacturers' claims.

*Ultrasound Clinics* (ISSN 1556-858X) is published quarterly by W.B. Saunders, 360 Park Avenue South, New York, NY 10010-1710. Months of publication are January, April, July, and October. Business and editorial offices: 1600 John F. Kennedy Boulevard, Suite 1800, Philadelphia, Pennsylvania 19103-2899. Accounting and circulation offices: 6277 Sea Harbor Drive, Orlando, FL 32887-4800. Periodicals postage paid at New York NY, and additional mailing offices. Subscription prices are USD 175 per year for US individuals, USD 245 per year for US institutions, USD 87 per year for US students and residents, USD 199 per year for Canadian individuals, USD 233 per year for Canadian institutions, USD 199 per year for international individuals, USD 268 per year for international institutions, and USD 99 per year for Canadian and foreign students/residents. To receive student/resident rate, orders must be accompanied by name of affiliated institution, date of term, and the signature of program/residency coordinator on institution letterhead. Orders will be billed at individual rate until proof of status is received. Foreign air speed delivery is included in all Clinics subscription prices. All prices are subject to change without notice. **POSTMASTER:** Send address changes to *Ultrasound Clinics*, Elsevier Periodicals Customer Service, 6277 Sea Harbor Drive, Orlando, FL 32887-4800. **Customer Service: 1-800-654-2452 (US). From outside of the US, call (+1) 407-345-4000.**

Printed in the United States of America.

# ABDOMINAL ULTRASOUND

## GUEST EDITOR

**LESLIE M. SCOUTT, MD**
Professor of Diagnostic Radiology, Chief, Section
of Ultrasound, Chief, Ultrasound Service,
Department of Diagnostic Radiology, Yale
University School of Medicine, New Haven,
Connecticut

## CONTRIBUTORS

**SUSAN J. ACKERMAN, MD**
Associate Professor of Radiology, Medical
University of South Carolina, Charleston, South
Carolina

**SHWETA BHATT, MD**
Instructor, Department of Imaging Sciences,
University of Rochester Medical Center, University
of Rochester School of Medicine, Rochester, New
York

**JAMAL BOKHARI, MD**
Associate Professor of Diagnostic Radiology,
Section Chief, Emergency Radiology, Department
of Diagnostic Radiology, Yale University School of
Medicine, New Haven, Connecticut

**ROBERT T. BRAMSON, MD**
Department of Radiology, Children's Hospital
Boston, Harvard Medical School, Boston,
Massachusetts

**CARLO BUONOMO, MD**
Associate Professor, Department of Radiology,
Children's Hospital Boston, Harvard Medical
School, Boston, Massachusetts

**VIKRAM S. DOGRA, MD**
Professor of Radiology, Urology and BME,
Associate Chair of Education and Research,
Director of Ultrasound, Department of Imaging
Sciences, University of Rochester Medical Center,
University of Rochester School of Medicine,
Rochester, New York

**HAMAD GHAZALE, MS, RDMS**
Associate Professor and Director, Diagnostic
Medical Sonography Program, Rochester Institute
of Technology, Rochester, New York

**ULRIKE M. HAMPER, MD, MBA**
Professor of Radiology and Urology, Director,
Division of Ultrasound, Johns Hopkins Medical
Institutes, Johns Hopkins University School of
Medicine, Baltimore, Maryland

**KEYANOOSH HOSSEINZADEH, MD**
Assistant Professor of Radiology, Department
of Radiology, Division of Abdominal Imaging,
University of Pittsburgh School of Medicine,
University of Pittsburgh Medical Center
(Presbyterian Campus), Pittsburgh, Pennsylvania

**ABID IRSHAD, MD**
Assistant Professor of Radiology, Medical
University of South Carolina, Charleston, South
Carolina

**HYUN-JUNG JANG, MD**
Assistant Professor, Department of Medical
Imaging, Toronto General Hospital, University
of Toronto, Toronto, Ontario, Canada

**TAE KYOUNG KIM, MD**
Associate Professor, Department of Medical
Imaging, Toronto General Hospital, University
of Toronto, Toronto, Ontario, Canada

**EDWARD Y. LEE, MD, MPH**
Assistant Professor, Department of Radiology,
Children's Hospital Boston, Harvard Medical
School, Boston, Massachusetts

**SARAH SARVIS MILLA, MD**
Assistant Professor, Department of Radiology,
New York University Medical Center, New York,
New York

**CINDY R. MILLER, MD**
Department of Diagnostic Radiology, Yale
University School of Medicine, New Haven,
Connecticut

**HICHAM MOUKADDAM, MD**
Staff Radiologist, Department of Diagnostic
Radiology, Yale New Haven Hospital, New Haven,
Connecticut

**JOHN S. PELLERITO, MD**
Associate Chairman, Chief, Division of US, CT
and MRI; Director, Peripheral Vascular Laboratory,
North Shore University Hospital, Manhasset;
Assistant Professor of Radiology, New York,
New York

**JEFFREY POLLAK, MD**
Professor of Diagnostic Radiology, Associate
Professor of Surgery, Co-Section Chief Vascular/
Interventional Radiology, Department of
Diagnostic Radiology, Yale University School
of Medicine, New Haven, Connecticut

**PHIL W. RALLS, MD**
Department of Radiology, Keck School
of Medicine, University of Southern California,
Los Angeles, California

**MARGARITA V. REVZIN, MD, MS**
Department of Radiology, North Shore University
Hospital, Manhasset, New York

**DEBORAH J. RUBENS, MD**
Professor of Imaging Sciences and Biomedical
Engineering, Department of Imaging Sciences,
University of Rochester Medical Center, Rochester,
New York

**STEVEN R. SAWYERS, MD**
Resident, Diagnostic Radiology, Yale University
School of Medicine, New Haven, Connecticut

**LESLIE M. SCOUTT, MD**
Professor of Diagnostic Radiology, Chief, Section
of Ultrasound, Chief, Ultrasound Service,
Department of Diagnostic Radiology, Yale
University School of Medicine, New Haven,
Connecticut

**SHEILA SHETH, MD**
Associate Professor of Radiology and Pathology,
Department of Radiology, School of Medicine,
Johns Hopkins University, Baltimore, Maryland

**JENNIFER SWART, MD**
Resident, Department of Radiology, School
of Medicine, Johns Hopkins University, Baltimore,
Maryland

**HISHAM TCHELEPI, MD**
Department of Radiologic Sciences, Wake-Forest
University School of Medicine, Medical Center
Boulevard, Winston-Salem, North Carolina

**STEPHANIE R. WILSON, MD**
Professor, Department of Medical Imaging,
Toronto General Hospital, University of Toronto,
Toronto, Ontario; Professor of Radiology,
University of Calgary, Calgary, Alberta, Canada

**JADE WONG-YOU-CHEONG, MD**
Associate Professor of Radiology, Department
of Radiology, Section of Abdominal Imaging,
University of Maryland School of Medicine,
University of Maryland Medical Center, Baltimore,
Maryland

# ABDOMINAL ULTRASOUND

Volume 2 • Number 3 • July 2007

# Contents

screening modality for evaluating the post-transplant liver and for the detection and follow-up of LT complications. This article reviews the role of sonography in LT.

Patients who have gallbladder or bile duct disease may present acutely with right upper quadrant pain, nausea or vomiting, midepigastric pain, or jaundice. The etiologies of biliary disease include inflammation with or without infection, noninflammatory disorders, and benign or malignant neoplasms of the gallbladder or ducts. Ultrasound has become the primary imaging modality for the initial work-up of suspected biliary disease. This article reviews the principal diseases of the biliary tract, strategies for imaging them with ultrasound, and specific imaging patterns that aid diagnosis.

Sonography is important in imaging patients with clinically suspected acute pancreatitis. All patients who present with acute pancreatitis for the first time should have sonography to evaluate the biliary tree for gallstones as a cause of pancreatitis. Sonography can also determine if bile duct dilatation, suggestive of obstruction, is present. However, the most sensitive prognostic indicator in patients with acute pancreatitis is quantification of pancreatic gland necrosis, which currently cannot be accurately assessed with ultrasound.

This article reviews the different types of pancreas allograft transplantation, including the various forms of duct management and venous drainage. Sonographic technique and common sonographic findings are described. The role of sonography in the effective diagnosis and treatment of allograft disorders is emphasized. Limitations of sonography in the workup of these patients are discussed, along with the incorporation of alternative and complementary imaging modalities.

Abdominal aortic aneurysm (AAA) is a disease of aging, and the prevalence is expected to increase as the population of elderly patients grows. AAAs are associated with high mortality, as rupture of an AAA is the tenth leading cause of death in the United States. This review describes the sonographic technique for evaluation of the abdominal aorta and associated pathologies of the abdominal aorta, including abdominal aortic aneurysm.

Hypertension affects up to 58.4 million people in the United States and is one of the most common diseases worldwide, with well known morbidity and mortality. The vast majority of patients who have hypertension, approximately 90% to 98%, have essential hypertension without structural lesions or other abnormalities identifiable by currently available imaging modalities. It is estimated that only 0.5% to less than 5% of all patients who have hypertension have true renovascular hypertension defined as hypertension secondary to renal artery stenosis. This article reviews the imaging of renal artery stenosis.

clinical and sonographic features of selected common abdominal masses in infants and children. The authors highlight the important clinical characteristics of these abdominal masses and specific sonographic imaging features that allow clinicians to differentiate among the common abdominal masses in pediatric patients.

## THE CLINICS ARE NOW AVAILABLE ONLINE!

Access your subscription at:
www.theclinics.com

## GOAL STATEMENT

The goal of the *Ultrasound Clinics* is to keep practicing radiologists and radiology residents up to date with current clinical practice in ultrasound by providing timely articles reviewing the state of the art in patient care.

## ACCREDITATION

The *Ultrasound Clinics* is planned and implemented in accordance with the Essential Areas and Policies of the Accreditation Council for Continuing Medical Education (ACCME) through the joint sponsorship of the University of Virginia School of Medicine and Elsevier. The University of Virginia School of Medicine is accredited by the ACCME to provide continuing medical education for physicians.

The University of Virginia School of Medicine designates this educational activity for a maximum of 15 *AMA PRA Category 1 Credits*™. Physicians should only claim credit commensurate with the extent of their participation in the activity.

The American Medical Association has determined that physicians not licensed in the US who participate in this CME activity are eligible for 15 *AMA PRA Category 1 Credits*™.

Credit can be earned by reading the text material, taking the CME examination online at http://www.theclinics.com/home/cme, and completing the evaluation. After taking the test, you will be required to review any and all incorrect answers. Following completion of the test and evaluation, your credit will be awarded and you may print your certificate.

## FACULTY DISCLOSURE/CONFLICT OF INTEREST

The University of Virginia School of Medicine, as an ACCME accredited provider, endorses and strives to comply with the Accreditation Council for Continuing Medical Education (ACCME) Standards of Commercial Support, Commonwealth of Virginia statutes, University of Virginia policies and procedures, and associated federal and private regulations and guidelines on the need for disclosure and monitoring of proprietary and financial interests that may affect the scientific integrity and balance of content delivered in continuing medical education activities under our auspices.

The University of Virginia School of Medicine requires that all CME activities accredited through this institution be developed independently and be scientifically rigorous, balanced and objective in the presentation/discussion of its content, theories and practices.

All authors/editors participating in an accredited CME activity are expected to disclose to the readers relevant financial relationships with commercial entities occurring within the past 12 months (such as grants or research support, employee, consultant, stock holder, member of speakers bureau, etc.). The University of Virginia School of Medicine will employ appropriate mechanisms to resolve potential conflicts of interest to maintain the standards of fair and balanced education to the reader. Questions about specific strategies can be directed to the Office of Continuing Medical Education, University of Virginia School of Medicine, Charlottesville, Virginia.

*The authors/editors listed below have identified no professional or financial affiliations for themselves or their spouse/partner:*
Susan J. Ackerman, MD; Shweta Bhatt, MD; Jamal Bokhari, MD; Robert T. Bramson, MD; Carlo Buonomo, MD; Vikram S. Dogra, MD; Barton Dudlick (Acquisitions Editor); Hamad Ghazale, MS, RDMS; Ulrike M. Hamper, MD, MBA; Keyanoosh Hosseinzadeh, MD; Abid Irshad, MD; Sarah Sarvis Milla, MD; Cindy R. Miller, MD; Hicham Moukaddam, MD; John S. Pellerito, MD; Jeffrey Pollak, MD; Phil W. Ralls, MD; Margarita Revzin, MD, MS; Deborah J. Rubens, MD; Steven R. Sawyers, MD; Leslie M. Scoutt, MD (Guest Editor); Sheila Sheth, MD; Jennifer Swart, MD; Hisham Tchelepi, MD; and, Jade Wong-You-Cheong, MD.

*The authors/editors listed below have identified the following professional or financial affiliations for themselves or their spouse/partner:*
**Hyun-Jung Jang, MD** is an agent for Bristol-Myers-Squibb.
**Tae Kyoung Kim, MD** is an agent for Bristol-Myers-Squibb.
**Edward Y. Lee, MD, MPH** has a research fellowship with GE/AUR.
**Stephanie R. Wilson, MD** is a consultant for Siemens US, an agent for Bristol Myers Squibb, and an agent for Philips.

*Disclosure of Discussion of non-FDA approved uses for pharmaceutical products and/or medical devices:*
The University of Virginia School of Medicine, as an ACCME provider, requires that all faculty presenters identify and disclose any "off label" uses for pharmaceutical and medical device products. The University of Virginia School of Medicine recommends that each physician fully review all the available data on new products or procedures prior to instituting them with patients.

## TO ENROLL

To enroll in the Ultrasound Clinics Continuing Medical Education program, call customer service at 1-800-654-2452 or visit us online at www.theclinics.com/home/cme. The CME program is available to subscribers for an additional fee of $205.00.

# ULTRASOUND CLINICS

Ultrasound Clin 2 (2007) xi–xii

# Preface

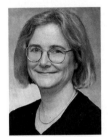

Leslie M. Scoutt, MD
*Section of Ultrasound*
*Department of Diagnostic Radiology*
*Yale University School of Medicine*
*333 Cedar Street, New Haven, CT 06520, USA*

*E-mail address:*
leslie.scoutt@yale.edu

Leslie M. Scoutt, MD
*Guest Editor*

This issue of the *Ultrasound Clinics* is dedicated to ultrasound imaging of the abdomen. Abdominal ultrasound is often the first-line imaging modality used to evaluate the kidneys, liver, gallbladder, pancreas, spleen, abdominal aorta, and other blood vessels in the abdomen, and as such can be extremely helpful in diagnosing a variety of conditions, including abdominal aortic aneurysms, gallstones, acute cholecystitis, renal calculi, complications of acute pancreatitis, and appendicitis. Hence, abdominal ultrasound plays an extremely important role in the work-up of the patient presenting with acute abdominal pain. Doppler ultrasound evaluation of the abdomen is also important in evaluation of potential organ transplant recipients as well as to assess for postoperative complications in organ transplant. Doppler ultrasound of the abdominal vessels is frequently used to diagnose arterial stenoses and arterial or venous thrombosis in patients suspected of portal or hepatic vein thrombosis, mesenteric ischemia, or renal artery stenosis. In many cases, the appropriate use of abdominal ultrasound imaging can avoid the necessity of performing more invasive and costly procedures.

We took great care to assemble a group of leading radiologists to provide up-to-date and clinically relevant information about a wide spectrum of abdominal disease entities. For example, we discuss abdominal aortic aneurysms and the Centers for Medicare and Medicaid Services recent approval for a one-time AAA screening for men between the ages of 65 and 75.

Our hope is that the discussions of techniques and concepts in abdominal ultrasound imaging presented in this issue will benefit readers who are new to the practice of ultrasound as well as imaging specialists and clinicians. We would like to hear from our readers with suggestions or comments and requests for future topics. This is our second year of publication, and as our popularity and readership grows, our goal will be to continue to provide easily comprehensible, clinically relevant information for our readers to enhance their practice of radiology.

I am honored to be the Guest Editor of this issue of the *Ultrasound Clinics*. I wish to express my

doi:10.1016/j.cult.2007.08.003

sincere thanks to Lisa M. Hribko, my administrative assistant, for her assistance in helping me to complete this issue on schedule. I would also like to thank Dr. Vikram Dogra for his support and insightful suggestions as well as all the authors for their excellent contributions. Finally, I am extremely grateful to Barton Dudlick at Elsevier for his administrative and editorial assistance.

# ULTRASOUND CLINICS

Ultrasound Clin 2 (2007) 333–354

# Hepatic Neoplasms: Features on Grayscale and Contrast Enhanced Ultrasound

Tae Kyoung Kim, MD, Hyun-Jung Jang, MD, Stephanie R. Wilson, MD*

## An overview

Liver masses may be incidentally detected on sonography or they may be seen on surveillance scans in high-risk or symptomatic patients. Once identified, it is necessary to determine which masses are significant, requiring confirmation of their diagnosis, and which masses are likely to be insignificant and benign, not requiring further evaluation to confirm their nature. On a sonographic study there is considerable overlap in the appearances of focal liver masses, but the excellent contrast and spatial resolution of state-of-the-art ultrasound equipment allows for the development of some guidelines for the initial management of patients once a liver mass is seen [1]. These include recognition of the following features:

- A hypoechoic halo identified around an echogenic or isoechoic liver mass is an ominous sonographic sign necessitating definitive diagnosis.

- A hypoechoic and solid liver mass is highly likely to be significant and also requires definitive diagnosis.
- Multiple solid liver masses may be significant and raise the possibility of metastatic or multifocal malignant liver disease. Hemangiomas, however, are also frequently multiple.
- Clinical history of malignancy, chronic liver disease or hepatitis, and symptoms referable to the liver are requisite pieces of information for interpretation of a focal liver lesion.

Traditionally confirmation of the nature of most sonographically detected solid masses with any concerning features has been performed with contrast-enhanced CT or more recently MR imaging scan. Today, however, ultrasound, augmented by contrast-enhanced ultrasound (CEUS), allows for excellent characterization and detection of most focal liver disease. Noninvasive characterization of focal liver lesions is largely based on their

Department of Medical Imaging, Toronto General Hospital, University of Toronto, 585 University Avenue, Toronto, Ontario, Canada M5G 2N2
* Corresponding author. Foothills Medical Centre, 1403 29 Street SW, Calgary, Alberta, T2N 2T9, Canada.
*E-mail address:* stephanie.wilson@uhn.on.ca (S.R. Wilson).

doi:10.1016/j.cult.2007.08.006

enhancement patterns on contrast-enhanced imaging. The use of microbubble contrast agents combined with specialized ultrasound techniques has significantly expanded the role of ultrasound in the diagnosis of focal liver lesions based on their vascularity and specific enhancement features [2,3]. Immediate characterization of benign lesions has huge clinical impact, reducing time to diagnosis, allaying the patient's anxiety, and reducing unnecessary costly further imaging. In malignant lesions, differentiation of metastasis from hepatocellular carcinoma (HCC) and multiple nodules in a cirrhotic liver is possible with dynamic real-time CEUS. Furthermore, with the advantage of real-time scanning, CEUS can evaluate small lesions, indeterminate on CT or MR imaging, because CEUS is far less affected by timing issues. This article describes the sonographic and CEUS features of commonly encountered benign and malignant lesions seen in the liver.

## Benign hepatic neoplasms

Hemangioma, focal nodular hyperplasia (FNH), and liver cell adenoma comprise the most commonly encountered benign liver masses seen in any sonography department, whereas hepatic lipoma and angiomyolipoma occur infrequently but can be diagnosed with great specificity even on baseline grayscale scan.

## *Cavernous hemangioma*

Cavernous hemangiomas are the most common benign tumors of the liver, occurring in approximately 4% of the population. They occur in all age groups but are more common in adults, particularly women. The vast majority of hemangiomas are small, asymptomatic, and discovered incidentally. Large lesions may rarely produce symptoms of acute abdominal pain caused by hemorrhage or thrombosis within the tumor. Traditional teaching suggested that once hemangiomas are identified in the adult, they usually have reached a stable size, and change in appearance or size is uncommon [4,5]. We now believe that this is not always true, and in the authors' own practice have documented substantial growth of some lesions over many years of follow-up [6]. Histologically, hemangiomas consist of multiple vascular channels that are lined by a single layer of endothelium and separated and supported by fibrous septae. The vascular spaces may contain thrombi.

The sonographic appearance of cavernous hemangioma varies. Typically the lesion is small, less than 3 cm in diameter, well defined, homogeneous, and hyperechoic (Fig. 1A) [7]. The increased echogenicity has been related to the numerous interfaces between the walls of the cavernous sinuses and the blood within them [8]. Inconsistently seen and a nonspecific finding, posterior acoustic enhancement has been correlated with hypervascularity on angiography [9]. It is

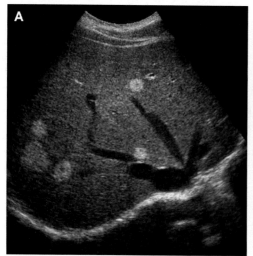 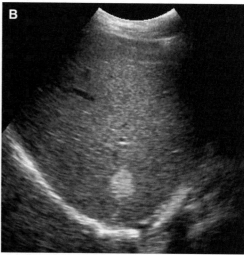

*Fig. 1.* Small homogeneous echogenic nodules in the liver: two different diagnoses. (*A*) Transverse ultrasound image in a 46-year-old woman shows multiple well-defined homogeneous echogenic nodules in the liver. These nodules were confirmed as hemangiomas. (*B*) Oblique ultrasound image in a 58-year-old man who had chronic hepatitis B shows a small homogeneous echogenic nodule in the liver. This nodule turned out to be an HCC at biopsy. (*From* Withers CE, Wilson SR. The liver. In: Rumack C, Wilson SR, Charboneau JW, et al, editors. Diagnostic Ultrasound. Philadelphia: Mosby; 2005. p. 77–147; with permission.)

estimated that approximately 67% to 79% of hemangiomas are hyperechoic (see Fig. 1A) [10,11], and of these, 58% to 73% are homogeneous [5,9]. Atypical features are also now familiar to most sonographers, and include: a nonhomogeneous central area containing hypoechoic portions that may appear uniformly granular (Fig. 2) or lacelike in character; an echogenic border, either a thin rim or a thick rind (Fig. 3); and scalloping of the margin [12]. Larger lesions tend to be heterogeneous with central hypoechoic foci corresponding to fibrous collagen scars, large vascular spaces, or both (see Fig. 2). A hemangioma may appear hypoechoic within the background of a fatty infiltrated liver [13]. Rapidly enhancing

hemangiomas seen on contrast-enhanced imaging also tend to be hypoechoic (Fig. 4).

Hemangiomas are characterized by slow blood flow that is not routinely detected by color or duplex Doppler. Occasionally lesions may demonstrate a low to midrange kHz shift from peripheral and central blood vessels. Cavernous hemangiomas are commonly observed on abdominal sonograms, and it is considered acceptable practice to manage some patients conservatively without confirmation of the diagnosis. When a hyperechoic lesion typical of a cavernous hemangioma is incidentally discovered, no further examination is usually necessary, or at most, a repeat ultrasound is performed in 3 to 6 months to document lack of change.

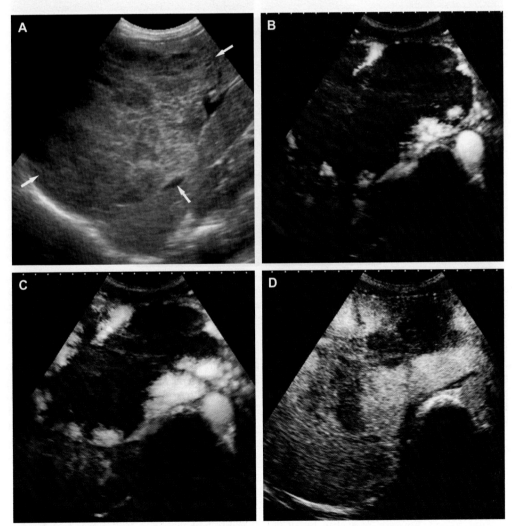

*Fig. 2.* Large atypical hemangioma in a 43-year-old man. (*A*) Oblique ultrasound image shows a large heterogeneous hyperechoic mass (*arrows*) in the right lobe of the liver. (*B*) CEUS image 22 seconds after injection demonstrates multifocal areas of nodular enhancement in the periphery of the mass. (*C*) At 39 seconds after injection, there is centripetal progression of peripheral nodular enhancement of the mass. (*D*) CEUS image at 133 seconds after injection shows further progression of centripetal enhancement without evidence of washout.

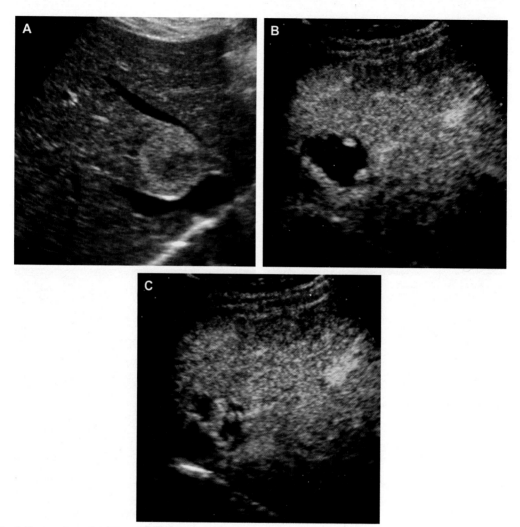

Fig. 3. Hemangioma in a 57-year-old woman. (A) Transverse ultrasound image shows a heterogeneous mass with central hypoechoic portion and peripheral thick echogenic rind in the right lobe of the liver. (B) CEUS image 58 seconds after injection demonstrating peripheral nodular enhancement of the mass. (C) At 115 seconds after injection there is central progression of nodular enhancement, producing a bridging of these enhancing nodules.

Conversely there are potentially significant lesions, such as metastases from a colon primary or a vascular primary, such as neuroendocrine tumor and small HCCs, that may mimic the morphology of a hemangioma on ultrasound and produce a single mass or multiple masses of uniform increased echogenicity (Fig. 1B). Caturelli and colleagues [14], in a prospective evaluation of 1982 patients who had newly diagnosed cirrhosis, found that 50% of echogenic liver lesions with a morphology suggestive of hemangioma had that ultimate diagnosis. Fifty percent, however, proved to be HCC. Furthermore, they also showed that in 1648 patients who had known cirrhosis and new appearance of an echogenic hemangioma-like mass, all were HCC. These results emphasize the extreme

necessity of establishing (or proving) the diagnosis of all echogenic masses in high-risk patients. In a patient who has a known malignancy, an increased risk for HCC, abnormal liver function tests, clinical symptoms referable to the liver, or an atypical sonographic pattern, confirmation of diagnosis is therefore recommended. In the authors' department, CEUS is routinely used for this indication.

### Microbubble-enhanced sonography

Following the injection of IV ultrasound contrast agents, hemangiomas demonstrate peripheral puddles and pools in the arterial phase that are brighter than the adjacent enhanced liver parenchyma. There are no linear vessels. Over time there is centripetal progression of the enhancement, resulting

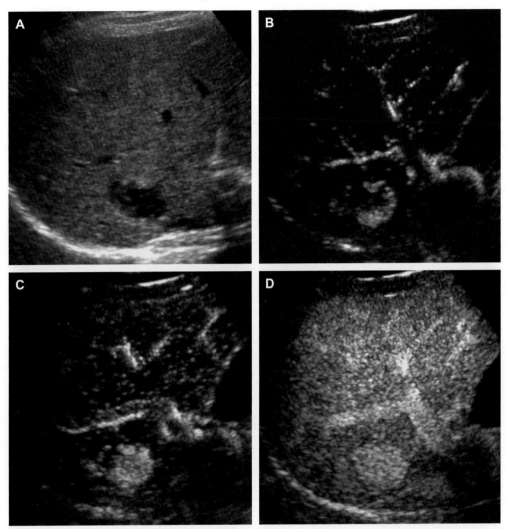

*Fig. 4.* Hypoechoic hemangioma with rapid enhancement in a 51-year-old woman. (*A*) Transverse ultrasound image shows a homogeneous hypoechoic mass in the right lobe of the liver. (*B*) CEUS image 9 seconds after injection shows peripheral nodular enhancement of the mass. (*C*) At 11 seconds after injection the mass shows homogeneous enhancement. (*D*) The mass shows persistent positive enhancement at 120 seconds after injection.

in complete globular fill-in, with sustained enhancement equal to or greater than the liver in the portal venous phase, which may last for several minutes (see Figs. 2–4) [2,3,15]. This enhancement may occur rapidly (see Fig. 4) or may be incomplete even in the delayed portal venous phase. In the authors' hands, we have accurately diagnosed close to 100% of hemangiomas, including those of very small size, obviating the necessity for CT, MR imaging, or labeled red blood cell scintigraphy for confirmation of diagnosis, particularly in incidentally detected lesions. The best approach to the diagnosis of hemangiomas depends on the clinical situation, the size and location of the lesion, the availability of alternative imaging modalities, such as MR imaging and single photon emission computed tomography (SPECT), and the experience of the imager. In general, the combination of two confirmatory studies is accepted as diagnostic of hemangioma [16]. The authors are hopeful that in the future, most hemangiomas initially depicted on ultrasound will be confirmed with CEUS.

## Focal nodular hyperplasia

FNH is the second most common benign liver mass after hemangioma. These masses are believed to be developmental hyperplastic lesions related to an area of vascular malformation, possibly a spider-like malformation or venous thrombosis [17]. Hormonal influence may be a factor, because FNH is more common in women than in men, particularly in the childbearing years [18–20]. Like hemangioma, FNH is invariably an incidentally detected liver mass in an asymptomatic patient (or is discovered as an incidental finding in an asymptomatic patient) [18]. Differentiation from hepatic adenoma is important. In contrast to hepatic adenoma, conservative management can be performed safely (recommended or just "is appropriate") in patients who have FNH irrespective of their size, because FNH neither undergoes malignant degeneration nor is likely to bleed or rupture [21].

FNH is typically a well-circumscribed and most often solitary mass that has a central scar [18]. Most lesions are less than 5 cm in diameter. Although usually single, patients have been reported to have multiple FNH. Microscopically, lesions include normal hepatocytes, Kupffer cells, biliary ducts, and the components of portal triads, although no normal portal venous structures are found. Because FNH is a hyperplastic lesion, proliferation of abnormally arranged but normal, non-neoplastic hepatocytes is observed. Bile ducts and thick-walled arterial vessels are prominent, particularly in the central fibrous scar. The excellent blood supply makes hemorrhage, necrosis, and calcification rare [18]. These lesions often produce a contour abnormality to the surface of the liver or may displace the normal blood vessels within the parenchyma.

On sonography, FNH is often a subtle liver mass that is difficult to differentiate in echogenicity (discriminate) from the adjacent liver parenchyma (Fig. 5). Considering the similarities in histology

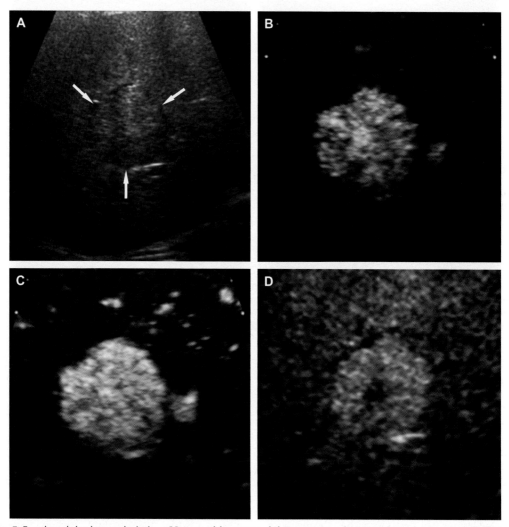

Fig. 5. Focal nodular hyperplasia in a 33-year-old woman. (A) Transverse ultrasound image shows a subtle isoechoic mass (arrows) in the right lobe of the liver. CEUS image at (B) 9 seconds and (C) 10 seconds after injection shows early filling of stellate arteries, followed by strong homogeneous enhancement of the mass. The enhancement direction is from the center to the periphery (centrifugal). (D) CEUS image at 253 seconds after injection shows persistent positive enhancement of the mass with a central nonenhancing area representing central scar.

of FNH to normal liver, this is not a surprising fact and has led to descriptions of FNH on all imaging modalities as a "stealth lesion" that may be extremely subtle or hide altogether (even invisible) [22]. Subtle contour abnormalities and displacement of vascular structures should immediately raise the possibility of FNH. The central scar may be seen on grayscale sonograms as a hypoechoic linear or stellate area within the central portion of the mass [23]. On occasion, the scar may appear hyperechoic. FNH may also display a range of grayscale appearances, ranging from hypoechoic to hyperechoic on rare occasion.

Doppler features are highly suggestive of FNH in that well-developed peripheral and central blood vessels are seen. Pathologic studies describe an anomalous arterial blood vessel in FNH larger than expected for the locale in the liver [17]. The authors' experience suggests that this feeding vessel is usually obvious on color Doppler imaging, although other vascular masses may seem to have unusually large feeding vessels also [24]. The blood vessels can be seen to course within the central scar with either a linear or stellate configuration. Spectral interrogation usually shows predominantly arterial signals centrally with a midrange (2–4 kHz) shift.

### Microbubble-enhanced sonography

Similar to hemangioma, FNH is consistently accurately diagnosed with the use of microbubble contrast agents. In the arterial phase, lesions are hypervascular, and two highly suggestive morphologic patterns include the presence of stellate vessels within the lesion and a tortuous feeding artery [15]. Arterial phase enhancement is homogeneous and in excess of the adjacent liver. Portal venous enhancement is sustained such that the lesion is enhanced equal to or greater than the adjacent liver with a nonenhancing scar (see Fig. 5). An unenhanced scar may be seen in arterial and portal phases. Ultrasound alone should be able to suggest the diagnosis of FNH without the necessity of referral for further imaging.

Biopsy may be required in a minority of patients who have FNH. The role of percutaneous needle biopsy for differentiation of FNH and adenoma is, however, often debated. A confident diagnosis of FNH can be made with a core biopsy if the sample is obtained under imaging control and the lesion contains benign-appearing hepatocytes and prominent arteries, lacks portal veins, and shows ductules at the interface between hepatocytes and fibrous regions [25]. It is not always possible, however, to obtain a sufficient sample from the center of the lesion by percutaneous needle biopsy. Because FNH rarely leads to clinical problems and does not undergo malignant transformation, noninvasive and conservative management is recommended [21].

### Hepatic adenoma

Hepatic adenomas are less common than FNH. Their incidence parallels the use of oral contraceptive agents. As would be expected, therefore, hepatic adenomas, similar to FNH, are more common in women. Hepatic adenomas have also been reported in association with glycogen storage disease [26]. The tumor may be asymptomatic, but often the patient or the physician feels a mass in the right upper quadrant. Pain may occur as a result of bleeding or infarction within the lesion. The patient may present acutely with shock caused by tumor rupture and hemoperitoneum. Because of its propensity to hemorrhage and risk for malignant degeneration, surgical resection is recommended [21].

Pathologically the hepatic adenoma is usually solitary and well encapsulated, and ranges in size from 8 to 15 cm. Microscopically the tumor consists of normal or slightly atypical hepatocytes. Bile ducts and Kupffer cells are either few in number or absent [27]. Hepatic adenomas may show calcification and fat (Fig. 6), both of which appear echogenic on sonography, making their grayscale appearance suggestive in some instances.

The sonographic appearance of hepatic adenoma is nonspecific. The echogenicity may be hyperechoic (see Fig. 6; Fig. 7), hypoechoic, isoechoic,

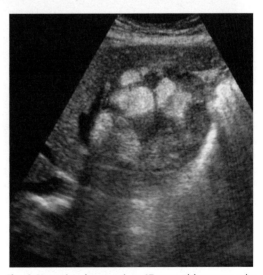

*Fig. 6.* Hepatic adenoma in a 47-year-old woman who had glycogen storage disease. Oblique ultrasound image shows a markedly heterogeneous mass with multifocal bright echogenic areas representing intratumoral fat.

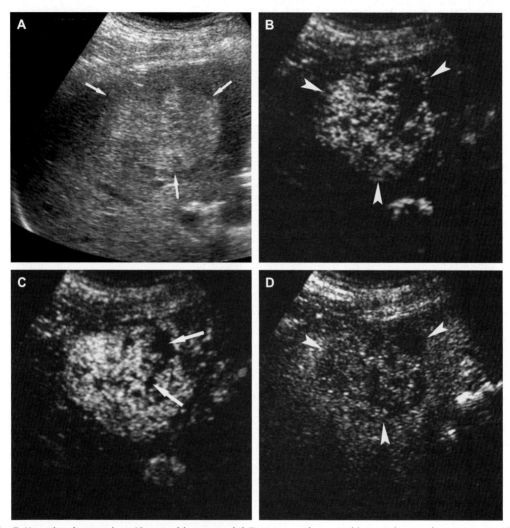

**Fig. 7.** Hepatic adenoma in a 48-year-old woman. (*A*) Transverse ultrasound image shows a heterogeneous hyperechoic mass (*arrows*) in the left lobe of the liver. CEUS image at (*B*) 8 seconds and (*C*) 10 seconds after injection shows diffuse hypervascularity of the mass (*arrowheads*) with small, irregular, nonenhancing areas (*arrows in C*) representing necrosis or hemorrhage. (*D*) CEUS image at 115 seconds after injection shows washout of the mass (*arrowheads*).

or mixed [28]. If hemorrhage occurs, a fluid component may be evident within or around the mass, and free intraperitoneal blood may be seen. The sonographic changes with bleeding are variable, depending on the duration and amount of hemorrhage. It is often not possible to distinguish hepatic adenomas from FNH by their grayscale or Doppler characteristics. Both demonstrate perilesional and intralesional well-defined blood vessels with kHz shifts in the midrange (2–4 kHz). In a patient who has right upper quadrant pain and possible hemorrhage, it is important to perform an unenhanced CT scan of the liver before contrast injection. Hemorrhage appears as high-density regions within the mass. The lesion often demonstrates rapid transient enhancement during the arterial phase [29]. Hepatic adenomas have a variable appearance on MR imaging, and it is not always possible to distinguish between hepatic adenoma, FNH, and HCC.

*Microbubble-enhanced sonography*

Most adenomas show strong enhancement in the arterial phase that can be somewhat heterogeneous in large lesions [15]. Adenomas are frequently isoechoic or slightly hyperechoic compared with the surrounding liver in the portal venous phase, but occasionally show mild washout in the portal venous phase. Intratumoral hypoechoic areas are occasionally seen and may represent necrosis or hemorrhage. Early arterial phase imaging of CEUS may demonstrate typical peritumoral arteries with

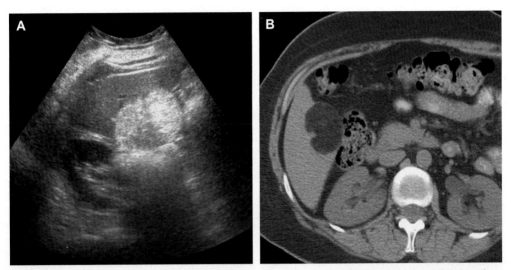

*Fig. 8.* Angiomyolipoma in a 47-year-old woman. (*A*) A transverse ultrasound image shows a bright echogenic mass in the right lobe of the liver. (*B*) On unenhanced CT scan the mass demonstrates marked hypoattenuation similar to subcutaneous fat. (*From* Withers CE, Wilson SR. The liver. In: Rumack C, Wilson SR, Charboneau JW, et al, editors. Diagnostic Ultrasound. Philadelphia: Mosby; 2005. p. 77–147; with permission.)

centripetal or diffuse intratumoral enhancement, which is different from the centrifugal enhancement of FNH (see Fig. 7) [15].

### Fatty lesions of the liver

Hepatic lipomas are extremely rare, and only isolated cases have been reported in the radiologic literature [30–32]. There is an association between hepatic lipomas and renal angiomyolipomas and tuberous sclerosis. The lesions are asymptomatic. Ultrasound demonstrates a well-defined and highly echogenic mass that may show differential sound transmission through the fatty mass with, for example, a discontinuous or broken diaphragm echo

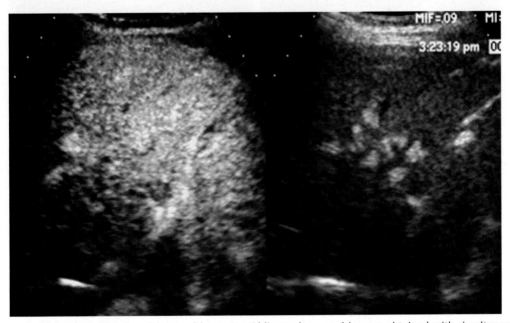

*Fig. 9.* Focal fat deposition in a 24-year-old woman. Oblique ultrasound images obtained with simultaneous dual-imaging display technique demonstrate an irregular echogenic focal lesion in the right lobe of the liver on grayscale image (*right side*), which demonstrates complete isovascularity relative to normal liver on CEUS image (*left side*). The lesion demonstrated isoechogenicity during all phases of contrast enhancement (not shown).

[31]. The diagnosis is confirmed using CT scanning, which demonstrates negative Hounsfield units (−30 HU) in the mass, indicating the presence of fat [30]. Angiomyolipomas, by comparison, may also appear echogenic on sonography (Fig. 8), although they may have insufficient fat to consistently demonstrate fatty attenuation on CT, making confirmation of their diagnosis more difficult without biopsy. MR imaging can be helpful for noninvasive characterization of angiomyolipoma with minimal fat content as in phase and out of phase imaging can detect even small amounts of fat.

Focal fat deposition in the liver is often easily recognized on the basis of the typical periligamentous or periportal location and homogeneous echogenicity without mass effect or distortion of traversing blood vessels. Patchy focal fat deposition may be mistaken for a neoplasm, however. CEUS is useful to characterize these lesions by demonstrating isovascularity of the lesions after injection of the contrast material (Fig. 9).

## Malignant hepatic neoplasms

### *Hepatocellular carcinoma*

HCC is one of the most common malignant tumors of the liver, most of which occur in a background of cirrhosis. Its major etiologic factors include viral infection with both hepatitis C and hepatitis B, although alcoholic cirrhosis remains a common

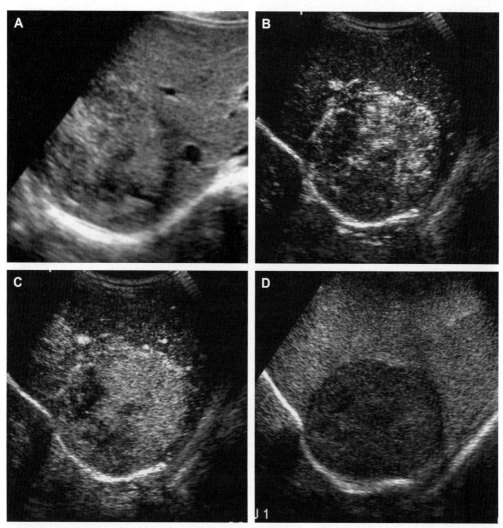

*Fig. 10.* Typical encapsulated HCC in a 53-year-old man. (*A*) Oblique ultrasound image shows a heterogeneous mass with hypoechoic halo in the right lobe of the liver. (*B*) CEUS image 11 seconds after injection demonstrates heterogeneous hypervascularity of the mass. (*C*) At 18 seconds after injection the mass shows diffuse enhancement with nonenhancing areas representing necrosis. (*D*) The mass shows washout (negative enhancement) relative to normal liver 148 seconds after injection.

predisposing cause for HCC in the Western population. The clinical presentation is typically delayed until the tumor reaches an advanced and often untreatable stage. Symptoms include right upper quadrant pain, weight loss, and abdominal swelling when ascites is present. Today, however, in most countries of the world, many high-risk patients have regular surveillance with 6-month interval ultrasound and serum alpha-fetoprotein levels, so many tumors are detected while small and before clinical presentation.

HCC may grow as a solitary or as multiple discrete nodules or as an ill-defined infiltrative mass. It is usually easy to make an imaging diagnosis of HCC when the tumor is large with expansive or infiltrative margins. Expansive HCCs are well demarcated, nodular, and frequently encapsulated (Fig. 10). Infiltrative HCCs, however, have irregular and indistinct margins with frequent invasion of the portal or hepatic veins (Fig. 11) [33]. A mixed expansive and infiltrative growth pattern is not uncommon. The portal vein is involved more commonly than the hepatic venous system in 30% to 60% of cases (Fig. 12) [34,35]. Expansive HCCs have a better prognosis and better response to the treatment.

Tumors have variable echogenicity on grayscale ultrasound. Small tumors without fatty metamorphosis are usually hypoechoic, but the echo pattern changes as the size increases. Most small (<5 cm) HCCs are hypoechoic (Fig. 13), corresponding histologically to a solid tumor without necrosis [36,37]. With time and increasing size, the masses tend to become more complex and inhomogeneous as a result of necrosis and fibrosis (see Fig. 10). HCCs with expansive growth patterns are usually seen as discrete heterogeneous nodules. A hypoechoic peripheral halo that corresponds to a fibrous capsule is a frequent finding (see Fig. 10) [38]. In contrast, infiltrative HCCs appear as heterogeneous areas that can be easily overlooked on ultrasound. It is important to evaluate the portal veins within any suspicious heterogeneous area on ultrasound, because portal vein thrombosis is frequently associated with infiltrative HCC (see Fig. 12). Calcification is uncommon but has been reported [39]. Small tumors may appear diffusely hyperechoic secondary to fatty metamorphosis or sinusoidal dilation, making them indistinguishable from focal fatty infiltration, cavernous hemangiomas, and lipomas (see Fig. 1B) [14,40]. Intratumoral fat also occurs in larger masses. Because it tends to be focal, however, it is unlikely to cause confusion in diagnosis. Rarely, lesions on the surface of the liver may present with spontaneous rupture and hemoperitoneum.

Studies evaluating focal liver lesions with duplex and color flow Doppler ultrasound suggest that HCC has characteristic high-velocity signals [41–43]. Doppler is also an excellent tool for detecting neovascularity within tumor thrombi in the portal veins, diagnostic of HCC even without demonstration of the parenchymal lesion (see Fig. 12).

*Microbubble-enhanced sonography*
The stepwise differentiation of a regenerative nodule to a dysplastic nodule to an HCC in the cirrhotic

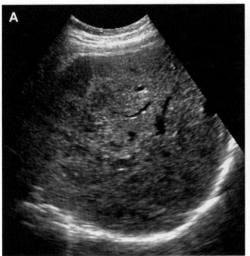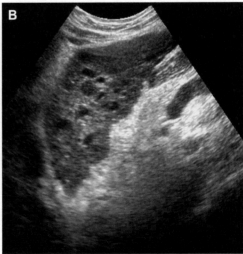

*Fig. 11.* Infiltrative HCC in a 49-year-old man. (*A*) Transverse ultrasound image of the right lobe and (*B*) sagittal ultrasound image of the left lobe show multiple ill-defined hypoechoic lesions throughout the liver. (*From* Withers CE, Wilson SR. The liver. In: Rumack C, Wilson SR, Charboneau JW, et al, editors. Diagnostic Ultrasound. Philadelphia: Mosby; 2005. p. 77–147; with permission.)

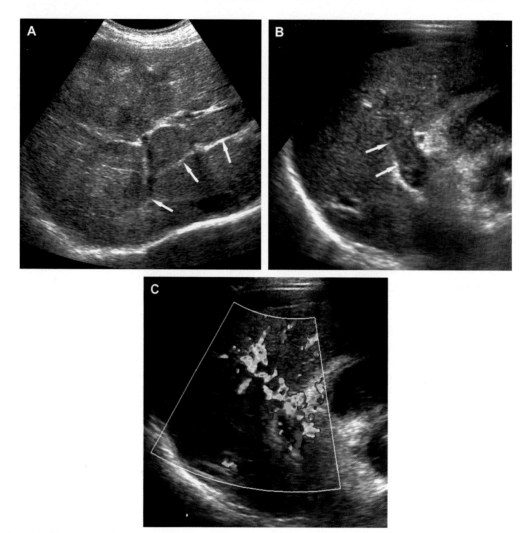

*Fig. 12.* HCC with portal vein thrombosis. (*A*) Transverse ultrasound image in a 44-year-old man shows a large infiltrative mass with invasion into the right and main portal veins, forming a tumor thrombi expanding the venous lumen (*arrows*). (*B*) Oblique ultrasound image and (*C*) color Doppler image of a 66-year-old man show hypoechoic thrombi in the right portal vein (*arrows*) with internal vascularity characteristic of tumor thrombosis.

liver is now well recognized. The evaluation of blood supply in a hepatic nodule is thus extremely important to characterize the lesion, because sequential changes in the supplying vessels and hemodynamic state occur during hepatocarcinogenesis [44]. Clinical use of microbubble contrast agents enables ultrasound to characterize HCCs based on enhancement features. Current real-time low-mechanical index (MI) techniques with second-generation contrast agents have remarkably improved the capability of CEUS in the characterization of HCCs and in their differentiation from various other types of hepatic nodules related to cirrhosis [45,46]. It is feasible to focus on a small indeterminate nodules on CT and MR scan from wash-in to wash-out of contrast, and CEUS can provide better understanding of the complex

hemodynamic changes within a nodule and the cirrhotic liver also.

Classic HCCs are typically supplied by abnormal arteries alone and show positive enhancement during the hepatic arterial phase and negative enhancement (washout) during the portal venous phase or delayed phase on contrast-enhanced imaging (see **Figs. 10 and 13**) [2,33,47–49]. Detection of arterial hypervascularity is important to make a diagnosis of HCC, because it is one of the most reliable characteristics of nodular HCC. There is a small subset of HCCs, however, that do not demonstrate arterial hypervascularity, particularly those that are well differentiated histologically [50].

Negative enhancement or washout during the venous phase is also an important characteristic of HCC, because typical tumors lack portal venous

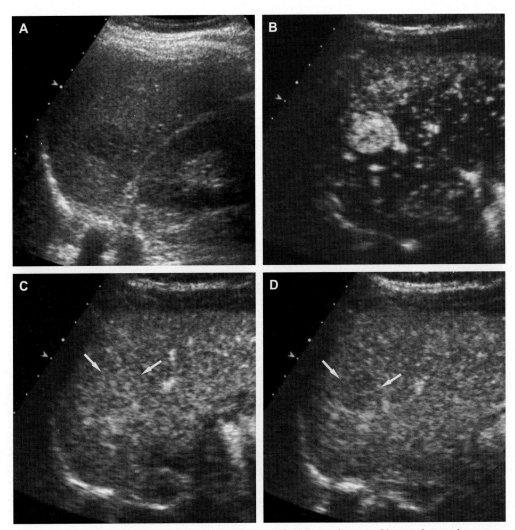

*Fig. 13.* Small HCC with late washout in a 56-year-old man. (*A*) Oblique ultrasound image shows a homogeneous hypoechoic mass in the right lobe of the liver. (*B*) CEUS image 8 seconds after injection shows homogeneous hypervascularity of the mass. (*C*) At 130 seconds after injection the mass (*arrows*) is not clearly seen because of isovascularity relative to adjacent liver. (*D*) The mass (*arrows*) shows slight washout at 221 seconds after injection.

supply. The intensity of enhancement of HCC in the portal venous phase, however, generally decreases more slowly than that in metastasis. In the authors' study with 115 hypervascular HCCs [50], only 50% showed the expected portal phase washout by 90 seconds. Extended evaluation over 3 minutes is important to characterize HCC by demonstrating "eventual" washout (see Fig. 13). Furthermore, sustained positive enhancement in the extended portal phase should not be considered diagnostic of a benign lesion, especially in patients at risk for HCC, because it may occur in well-differentiated HCCs in particular.

Any new nodular lesions in a cirrhotic liver are important because of the potential risk for HCC, and differential diagnosis between HCC and benign cirrhosis-related nodules is important clinically. Regenerative nodules (RN) generally do not stand out on any imaging modality. Most RNs in a mildly cirrhotic liver are isoechoic to the liver parenchyma during all phases on CEUS, although they may show transient hypovascularity in the arterial phase. As dysplastic nodules (DN) have more histologic atypia, the number of abnormal arteries increases, whereas normal arterial and portal supply decreases. The arterial and portal supply to DN are variable and inconsistent (Fig. 14) [51], and moreover there are significant overlaps of vascular supply patterns between DN and well-differentiated HCC. CEUS, CT, and MR imaging all suffer from similar problems in the imaging of these nodules. CEUS may have advantages from

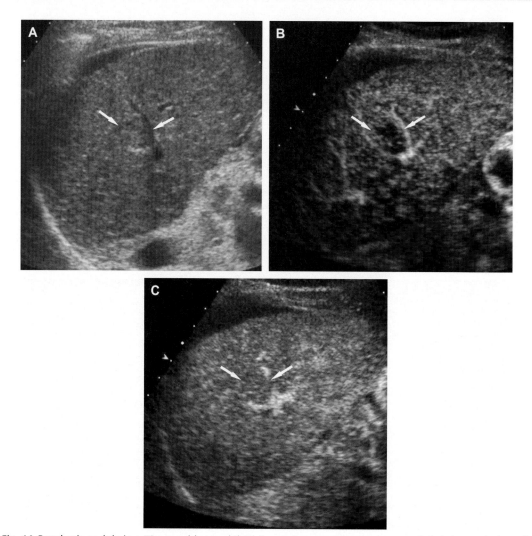

*Fig. 14.* Dysplastic nodule in a 59-year-old man. (*A*) Oblique ultrasound image shows a slightly hypoechoic nodule (*arrows*) in the right lobe of the liver. The liver is cirrhotic and there is a small amount of ascites. (*B*) CEUS image at 12 seconds after injection shows slight hypovascularity of the nodule (*arrows*) relative to adjacent liver. (*C*) The nodule (*arrows*) is not clearly seen at 90 seconds after injection because of isovascularity.

continuous observation in detecting subtle vascular differences of HCC from DN.

The authors' experience shows that CEUS is helpful for the diagnosis of newly detected small liver lesions on screening ultrasound or indeterminate lesions seen on CT or MR imaging scans. Immediate diagnosis of typical benign lesions decreases unnecessary visits for further investigation; diagnosis of malignant lesion prompts proper management. As a real-time procedure, ultrasound is better able to detect hypervascularity and washout in HCC regardless of the perfusion rate, whereas CT or MR imaging only allows imaging at fixed intervals in time, although hemodynamic changes are continuous. With excellent temporal and spatial resolution, CEUS can frequently depict characteristic intratumoral vascular patterns during the arterial phase, establishing the diagnosis of HCC.

CEUS may show additional small HCCs detected as nonenhancing nodules during multiple sweeps of the liver in the extended portal venous phase. These lesions are less conspicuous compared with metastases, however, and their detection is still challenging. In a cirrhotic liver with arterialization, there may be dysmorphology of all liver vessels in general, and the appreciation of focal areas of increased vascularity during arterial phase sweep in a small nodule is even more difficult. Further, there is a recognized tendency for washout of HCCs to be late. This may be partially related to the poor portal venous enhancement of a liver with cirrhosis making the

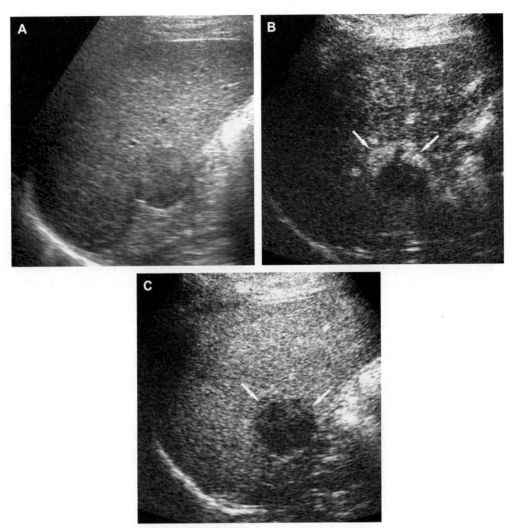

*Fig. 15.* Residual viable HCC after radiofrequency ablation in a 72-year-old man. (*A*) Oblique ultrasound image shows an exophytic mass in the right lobe of the liver representing an HCC treated with radiofrequency abla-tion. (*B*) Arterial-phase CEUS image obtained at 22 seconds after injection shows evidence of residual viable HCC that is seen as an eccentric area of enhancement in the anterior aspect of the mass (*arrows*). The remaining area of the mass is avascular because of necrosis. (*C*) At 55 seconds after injection the area of arterial enhance-ment shows washout relative to normal liver (*arrows*).

washout less conspicuous. CEUS is also useful to assess the therapeutic response to local treatment of HCCs, such as radiofrequency ablation or alcohol ablation (Fig. 15).

Fibrolamellar carcinoma is a histologic subtype of HCC that is found in younger patients (adoles-cents and young adults) without coexistent liver disease [52]. The serum alpha-fetoprotein levels are usually normal. The tumors are usually solitary, well differentiated, and often encapsulated by fibrous tissue. The prognosis is generally better for fibrolamellar carcinoma compared with HCC. Most patients, however, demonstrate advanced dis-ease at the time of diagnosis. The echogenicity of

fibrolamellar carcinomas is variable. Punctuate calcification and a central echogenic scar—features that are distinctly unusual in HCC—are more common in the fibrolamellar subtype.

### Hepatic epithelioid hemangioendothelioma

Epithelioid hemangioendothelioma (EHE) is a rare malignant tumor of vascular origin that occurs in adults. Soft tissues, lung, and liver are affected. The prognosis is variable. Many patients survive longer than 5 years with or without treatment [53]. Initially, multiple hypoechoic nodules are visualized in patients who have hepatic EHE. Over time the nodules grow and coalesce, forming larger confluent hypoechoic masses that tend to involve the periphery of the liver. Foci of calcification may be present [53,54]. The hepatic capsule overlying the lesions of EHE may be retracted inward secondary to fibrosis (desmoplastic reaction?) incited by the tumor. This is an unusual feature that is highly suggestive of this diagnosis. One should keep in mind that peripheral metastases postchemotherapy and tumors causing biliary obstruction may result in segmental atrophy and have a similar appearance [55]. The diagnosis is made by percutaneous liver biopsy, providing that immunohistochemical staining is performed.

## Metastatic disease

Metastasis is the most common malignancy in the liver. Its detection greatly alters the patient's prognosis and often the management. Most metastases to the liver are blood-borne by way of the hepatic artery or portal vein, but lymphatic spread of tumors from stomach, pancreas, ovary, or uterus may also occur. The portal vein provides direct access to the liver for tumor cells originating from the gastrointestinal tract and probably accounts for the high frequency of liver metastasis from organs that drain into the portal circulation.

Advantages of ultrasound as a screening test for metastatic liver disease include its relative accuracy, speed, lack of ionizing radiation, and availability. Sonography, however, is not uniformly used as a first-line imaging modality worldwide to search for metastatic disease, whereas CT has filled that role. Although many metastases can be easily seen on sonography, there are also many with such a similar backscatter that the lesions are virtually invisible on conventional unenhanced scans. This is now solved by the addition of contrast agents for ultrasound described subsequently.

On conventional grayscale sonography, metastatic liver disease may present as a single liver lesion, although more commonly multiple focal liver masses are seen (Fig. 16). Furthermore, metastatic involvement of the liver may take different forms, showing diffuse liver involvement and rarely also geographic infiltration. Knowledge of a prior or concomitant malignancy and features of disseminated malignancy at the time of a sonogram are helpful in correct interpretation of a sonographically detected liver mass or masses. Although there are no absolutely confirmatory features of metastatic disease on sonography, several are suggestive, including the presence of multiple solid lesions of varying size and the presence of a hypoechoic halo surrounding a liver mass. A halo around the periphery of a liver mass on sonography has been regarded as an ominous sign with a high association with malignancy (Figs. 17 and 18),

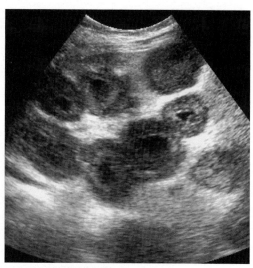

*Fig. 16.* Hepatic metastases with target pattern in a 56-year-old woman. Transverse ultrasound image shows numerous liver masses with alternating hypoechoic and hyperechoic rings around an internal hypoechoic center, a target-like appearance.

particularly metastatic disease but also HCC. In 1992, Wernecke and colleagues [56] described the importance of the hypoechoic halo in the differentiation of malignant from benign focal hepatic lesions. Its identification has a positive and negative predictive value of 86% and 88%, respectively. The authors therefore conclude that although

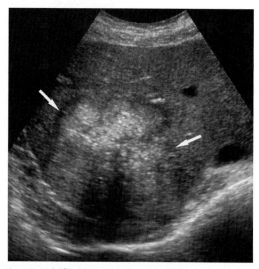

*Fig. 17.* Calcified hepatic metastasis from colon cancer in a 62-year-old man. Transverse ultrasound image shows a large echogenic mass containing central areas with posterior shadowing representing calcifications. There is a hypoechoic halo (*arrows*) surrounding the mass.

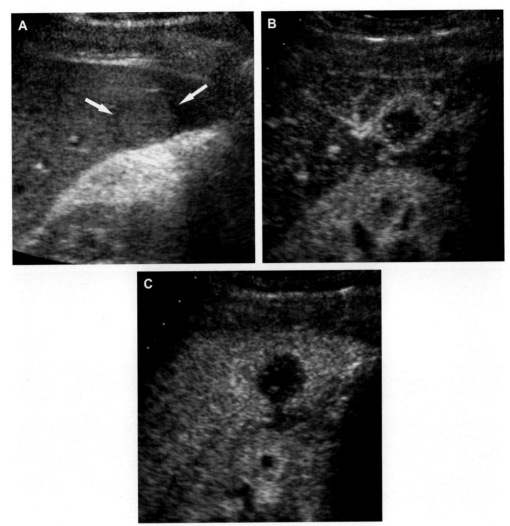

*Fig. 18.* Metastatic colon cancer in a 66-year-old man. (*A*) Sagittal ultrasound image shows a hyperechoic mass with surrounding hypoechoic halo (*arrows*) in the right lobe of the liver. (*B*) CEUS image obtained at 12 seconds after injection shows peripheral rim enhancement of the mass. (*C*) At 40 seconds after injection the mass shows complete washout.

a halo is not absolutely indicative of malignancy, it is seen with lesions that require further investigation and confirmation of their nature regardless of the patient's presentation or status. Radiologic–histologic correlation of a hypoechoic halo surrounding a liver mass has revealed that, in most cases, the hypoechoic rim corresponds to normal liver parenchyma that is compressed by the rapidly expanding tumor. Less commonly the hypoechoic rim represents proliferating malignant cells, tumor fibrosis, vascularization, or a fibrotic rim [57–59].

The following sonographic appearances of metastatic liver disease have been described: echogenic, hypoechoic, target, calcified, cystic, and diffuse. Although the ultrasound appearance is not specific for determining the origin of the metastasis, certain

generalities apply. Echogenic metastases tend to arise from gastrointestinal origin (see Fig. 17; Figs. 19 and 20) or from HCC. Also, the more vascular the tumor, the more likely the lesion is to be echogenic [60]. Metastases from renal cell carcinoma, carcinoid, choriocarcinoma, and islet cell carcinoma therefore tend to be hyperechoic. It is this particular group of tumors that may potentially mimic a hemangioma on sonography. Hypoechoic metastases are generally hypovascular and may be mono- and hypercellular without interstitial stroma. This is the typical pattern seen in untreated metastatic breast or lung cancer and gastric, pancreatic, and esophageal tumors. The bull's-eye or target pattern is characterized by a peripheral hypoechoic zone (see Fig. 16). The appearance is common but

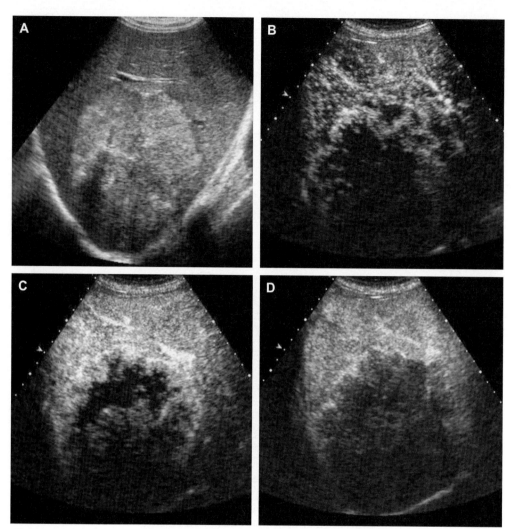

*Fig. 19.* Metastatic colon cancer in a 74-year-old man. (*A*) Oblique ultrasound image shows a large echogenic mass with a thin hypoechoic halo in the right lobe of the liver. CEUS images at (*B*) 14 seconds and (*C*) 21 seconds after injection show irregular rim-like enhancement of the mass. (*D*) CEUS at 87 seconds after injection shows complete washout of the mass.

nonspecific, although it is frequently identified in metastases from bronchogenic carcinoma [61]. Calcified metastases are distinctive by virtue of their marked echogenicity and distal acoustic shadowing (see Fig. 17). Calcified metastases are most commonly caused by mucinous adenocarcinoma of the colon. Calcium may appear as large echogenic, shadowing foci or more often innumerable tiny punctuate echogenicities without clear shadowing. Cystic metastases are fortunately uncommon and generally exhibit features that enable them to be distinguished from the ubiquitous benign hepatic cyst—for example, mural nodules, thick walls, fluid–fluid levels, and internal septations [62,63]. Metastatic neuroendocrine and carcinoid tumors are typically echogenic and often show secondary cystic change. Large colorectal metastases may also

rarely be necrotic, producing a predominantly cystic liver mass. Diffuse disorganization of the hepatic parenchyma reflects an infiltrative form of metastatic disease and is the most difficult to appreciate on sonography (Fig. 21), likely as a loss of the reference normal liver for comparison. In the authors' experience, breast and lung carcinoma and malignant melanoma are the most common primary tumors to give this pattern.

### Microbubble-enhanced sonography

On CEUS almost all hepatic metastases, including the ones known to be hypovascular, show obvious hypervascularity, often more pronounced in the periphery (see Figs. 18 and 19) but occasionally diffusely (see Fig. 20), particularly when the tumor is small. The time period for this hypervascularity is

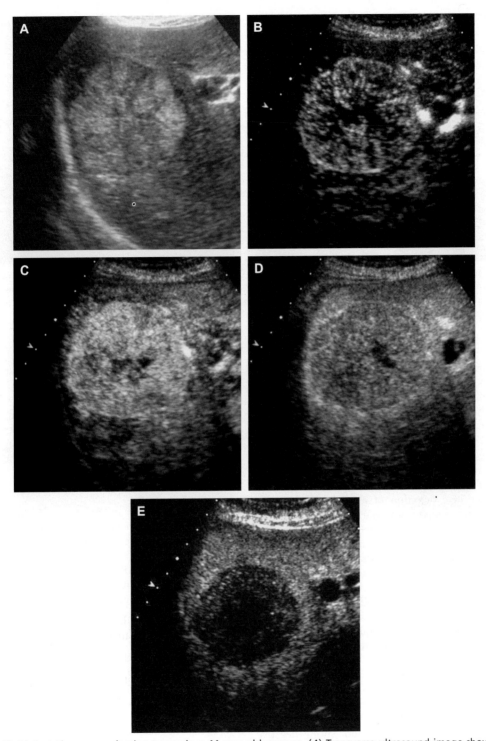

*Fig. 20.* Metastatic neuroendocrine tumor in a 44-year-old woman. (*A*) Transverse ultrasound image shows an echogenic mass surrounded by a thin hypoechoic halo in the right lobe of the liver. (*B*) CEUS image obtained at 6 seconds after injection shows heterogeneous enhancement of the mass with dysmorphic intratumoral arteries supplied by peripheral feeders. (*C*) At 9 seconds after injection there is diffuse staining of the tumor with small, central, nonenhancing areas representing necrosis. (*D*) CEUS image at 71 seconds after injection shows washout of the mass relative to normal liver. (*E*) Further washout of the mass is seen at 281 seconds after injection.

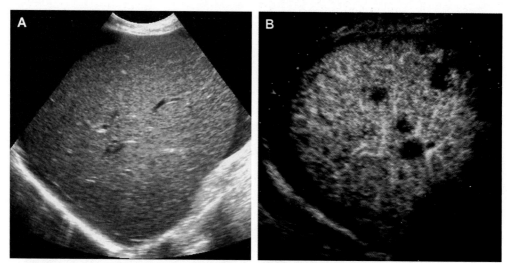

Fig. 21. Metastases from unknown primary tumor in a 72-year-old man. (*A*) Sagittal ultrasound image fails to demonstrate any evidence of focal liver lesions. There is a small amount of ascites. (*B*) CEUS image at 18 seconds after injection demonstrates multiple nodular perfusion defects in the liver representing metastases that are occult on grayscale ultrasound image.

short. The mass starts to washout within 20 seconds in most cases, and washout usually occurs from the center. Within 60 seconds, metastatic nodules usually show complete washout, appearing as punched-out perfusion defects with or without a thin, persistent rim enhancement (see Fig. 18) [64].

The capability of CEUS to depict such a rapid dynamic change is largely attributed to the real-time dynamic scan and high temporal resolution. The sensitive detection of arterial vascularity in metastases suggests potential usefulness of CEUS in the therapeutic assessment of metastasis after local ablation, because it is often difficult on contrast-enhanced CT or MR imaging because of the hypoattenuating or hypointense appearance of recurrent tumor similar to that of an ablated zone. CEUS is also useful in the differentiation of cystic metastasis from a non-neoplastic complex cyst by demonstrating vascular flow in the wall or mural nodules. It is especially helpful when the presence of contrast-enhancement on CT is obscured by hyperattenuating debris.

Regardless of arterial phase morphology, peripheral, diffuse, or centripetal, rapid and complete washout is a virtually invariable characteristic of metastasis on CEUS. This rapid, strong negative enhancement is helpful in differentiating metastasis from HCC, which shows washout generally later than metastasis, or in distinguishing metastasis from benign lesions that tend to show no washout or minimal washout [64].

Because virtually all metastases show complete washout during the portal venous phase on CEUS, liver survey during this phase can make metastases stand out as black holes contrasted to the well-perfused background liver (see Fig. 21). Early publications documented excellent results for first-generation air-based contrast agents and high MI imaging. More recent publications describe the use of second-generation perfluorocarbons and low MI imaging, both improving detection substantially over unenhanced scans [65].

## Summary

CEUS is useful in characterizing primary and secondary malignant hepatic lesions when found as an indeterminate lesion on baseline ultrasound or on previous CT or MR imaging scan. In the setting of surveillance for HCC or metastases in patients at high risk, the immediate diagnosis of benign disease on CEUS removes the necessity of referral for further imaging and unnecessary patient anxiety. Immediate characterization of malignant hepatic tumors detected incidentally or after a focused search can prompt appropriate further investigation and proper management. With careful analysis of characteristic enhancement patterns in the proper clinical context, CEUS can provide accurate diagnosis of hepatic malignancy.

## References

[1] Charboneau JW. There is a hyperechoic mass in the liver: what does that mean? In: Cooperberg PL, editor. Categorical course in diagnostic radiology: findings at US—what do they mean? Chicago: RSNA; 2002. p. 73–8.

[2] Brannigan M, Burns PN, Wilson SR. Blood flow patterns in focal liver lesions at microbubble-enhanced US. Radiographics 2004;24:921–35.

[3] Wilson SR, Burns PN. An algorithm for the diagnosis of focal liver masses using microbubble contrast-enhanced pulse-inversion sonography. AJR Am J Roentgenol 2006;186:1401–12.

[4] Gibney RG, Hendin AP, Cooperberg PL. Sonographically detected hemangiomas: absence of change over time. AJR Am J Roentgenol 1987; 149:953–7.

[5] Mungovan JA, Cranon JJ, Vacarro J. Hepatic cavernous hemangiomas: lack of enlargement over time. Radiology 1994;191:111–3.

[6] Nghiem HV, Bogost GA, Ryan JA, et al. Cavernous hemangiomas of the liver: enlargement over time. AJR Am J Roentgenol 1997;169: 137–40.

[7] Bree RL, Schwab RE, Neiman HL. Solitary echogenic spot in the liver: is it diagnostic of a hemangioma? AJR Am J Roentgenol 1983;140:41–5.

[8] McCardle CR. Ultrasonic appearances of a hepatic hemangioma. J Clin Ultrasound 1978;6: 122–3.

[9] Taboury J, Porcel A, Tubiana J-M, et al. Cavernous hemangiomas of the liver studied by ultrasound. Radiology 1983;149:781–5.

[10] Itai Y, Ohnishi S, Ohtomo K, et al. Hepatic cavernous hemangioma in patients at high risk for liver cancer. Acta Radiol 1987;28:697–701.

[11] Itai Y, Ohtomo K, Araki T, et al. Computed tomography and sonography of cavernous hemangioma of the liver. AJR Am J Roentgenol 1983;141:315–20.

[12] Moody AR, Wilson SR. Atypical hemangioma: a suggestive sonographic morphology. Radiology 1993;188:413–7.

[13] Marsh JI, Gibney RG, Li DKB. Hepatic hemangioma in the presence of fatty infiltration: an atypical sonographic appearance. Gastrointest Radiol 1989;14:262–4.

[14] Caturelli E, Pompili M, Bartolucci F, et al. Hemangioma-like lesions in chronic liver disease: diagnostic evaluation in patients. Radiology 2001;220:337–42.

[15] Kim TK, Jang HJ, Wilson SR. Benign liver masses: imaging with microbubble contrast agents. Ultrasound Q 2006;22:31–9.

[16] Nelson RC, Chezmar JL. Diagnostic approach to hepatic hemangiomas. Radiology 1990;176:11–3.

[17] Wanless IR, Mawdsley C, Adams R. On the pathogenesis of focal nodular hyperplasia of the liver. Hepatology 1985;5:1194–200.

[18] Saul SH. Masses of the liver. In: Sternberg SS, editor. Diagnostic surgical pathology. 2nd edition. New York: Raven; 1994. p. 1517–80.

[19] Knowles DM, Casarella WJ, Johnson PM, et al. The clinical, radiologic and pathologic characterization of benign hepatic neoplasms: alleged association with oral contraceptives. Medicine 1978;57:223–37.

[20] Ross D, Pina J, Mirza M, et al. Regression of focal nodular hyperplasia after discontinuation of oral contraceptives. Ann Intern Med 1976; 85:203–4.

[21] Herman P, Pugliese V, Machado MA, et al. Hepatic adenoma and focal nodular hyperplasia: differential diagnosis and treatment. World J Surg 2000;24:372–6.

[22] Buetow PC, Pantongrag-Brown L, Buck JL, et al. Focal nodular hyperplasia of the liver: radiologic–pathologic correlation. Radiographics 1996;16:369–88.

[23] Scatarige JC, Fishman EK, Sanders RC. The sonographic "scar sign" in focal nodular hyperplasia of the liver. J Ultrasound Med 1982;1:275–8.

[24] Golli M, Van Nhieu JT, Mathieu D, et al. Hepatocellular adenoma: color Doppler US and pathologic correlations. Radiology 1994;190:741–4.

[25] Bioulac-Sage P, Balabaud C, Wanless IR. Diagnosis of focal nodular hyperplasia: not so easy. Am J Surg Pathol 2001;25:1322–5.

[26] Brunelle R, Tammam S, Odievre M, et al. Liver adenomas in glycogen storage disease in children: ultrasound and angiographic study. Pediatr Radiol 1984;14:94–101.

[27] Kew MC. Tumors of the liver. In: Zakim D, Boyer TD, editors. Hepatology: a textbook of liver disease. Philadelphia: WB Saunders; 1982. p. 1048–84.

[28] Welch TJ, Sheedy PF, Johnson CM, et al. Focal nodular hyperplasia and hepatic adenoma: comparison of angiography, CT, US and scintigraphy. Radiology 1985;156:593–5.

[29] Grazioli L, Federle MP, Brancatelli G, et al. Hepatic adenomas: imaging and pathologic findings. Radiographics 2001;21:877–92.

[30] Roberts JL, Fishman E, Hartman DS, et al. Lipomatous tumors of the liver: evaluation with computed tomography and ultrasound. Radiology 1986;158:613–7.

[31] Marti-Bonmati L, Menor F, Vizcaino I, et al. Lipoma of the liver: ultrasound, computed tomography and magnetic resonance imaging appearance. Gastrointest Radiol 1989;14:155–7.

[32] Reinhold C, Garant M. Hepatic lipoma. Can Assoc Radiol J 1996;47:140–2.

[33] Kim TK, Jang HJ, Wilson SR. Imaging diagnosis of hepatocellular carcinoma with differentiation from other pathology. Clin Liver Dis 2005;9: 253–79.

[34] Subramanyam BR, Balthazar EJ, Hilton S, et al. Hepatocellular carcinoma with venous invasion: sonographic–angiographic correlation. Radiology 1984;150:793–6.

[35] LaBerge JM, Laing FC, Federle MP, et al. Hepatocellular carcinoma: assessment of resectability by computed tomography and ultrasound. Radiology 1984;152:485–90.

[36] Sheu J-C, Chen D-S, Sung J-L, et al. Hepatocellular carcinoma: ultrasound evaluation in the early stage. Radiology 1985;155:463–7.

[37] Tanaka S, Kitamura T, Imaoka S, et al. Hepatocellular carcinoma: sonographic and histologic correlation. AJR Am J Roentgenol 1983;140:701–7.

[38] Choi BI, Takayasu K, Han MC. Small hepatocellular carcinomas associated nodular lesions of the liver: pathology, pathogenesis and imaging findings. AJR Am J Roentgenol 1993;160: 1177–88.

[39] Teefey SA, Stephens DH, Weiland LH. Calcification in hepatocellular carcinoma: not always an indicator of fibrolamellar histology. AJR Am J Roentgenol 1987;149:1173–4.

[40] Yoshikawa J, Matsui O, Takashima T, et al. Fatty metamorphosis in hepatocellular carcinoma: radiologic features in 10 cases. AJR Am J Roentgenol 1988;151:717–20.

[41] Taylor KJW, Ramos I, Morse SS, et al. Focal liver masses: differential diagnosis with pulsed Doppler ultrasound. Radiology 1987;164:643–7.

[42] Tanaka S, Kitamura T, Fujita M, et al. Color Doppler flow imaging of liver tumors. AJR Am J Roentgenol 1990;154:509–14.

[43] Reinhold C, Hammers L, Taylor CR, et al. Characterization of focal hepatic lesions with Duplex sonography: findings in 198 patients. AJR Am J Roentgenol 1995;164:1131–5.

[44] Matsui O, Kadoya M, Kameyama T, et al. Benign and malignant nodules in cirrhotic livers: distinction based on blood supply. Radiology 1991;178:493–7.

[45] Giorgio A, Ferraioli G, Tarantino L, et al. Contrast-enhanced sonographic appearance of hepatocellular carcinoma in patients with cirrhosis: comparison with contrast-enhanced helical CT appearance. AJR Am J Roentgenol 2004;183: 1319–26.

[46] Nicolau C, Catala V, Vilana R, et al. Evaluation of hepatocellular carcinoma using SonoVue, a second generation ultrasound contrast agent: correlation with cellular differentiation. Eur Radiol 2004;14:1092–9.

[47] Lee KHY, O'Malley ME, Haider MA, et al. Triple-phase MDCT of hepatocellular carcinoma. AJR Am J Roentgenol 2004;182:643–9.

[48] Wilson SR, Burns PN, Muradali D, et al. Harmonic hepatic US with microbubble contrast agent: initial experience showing improved characterization of hemangioma, hepatocellular carcinoma, and metastasis. Radiology 2000;215: 153–61.

[49] Kim TK, Choi BI, Han JK, et al. Hepatic tumors: contrast agent-enhancement patterns with pulse-inversion harmonic US. Radiology 2000;216: 411–7.

[50] Jang HJ, Kim TK, Burns PN, et al. Enhancement patterns of hepatocellular carcinoma on contrast-enhanced ultrasound: correlation with pathologic differentiation. Radiology 2007;244: 898–906.

[51] Lim JH, Cho JM, Kim EY, et al. Dysplastic nodules in liver cirrhosis: evaluation of hemodynamics with CT during arterial portography and CT hepatic arteriography. Radiology 2000;214:869–74.

[52] Stevens WR, Johnson CD, Stephens DH, et al. Fibrolamellar hepatocellular carcinoma: stage at presentation and results of aggressive surgical management. AJR Am J Roentgenol 1995;164: 1153–8.

[53] Furui S, Itai Y, Ohtomo D, et al. Hepatic epithelioid hemangioendothelioma: report of five cases. Radiology 1989;171:63–8.

[54] Radin R, Craig JR, Colletti PM, et al. Hepatic epithelioid hemangioendothelioma. Radiology 1988;169:145–8.

[55] Oliver JH III. Malignant hepatic neoplasms, excluding hepatocellular carcinoma and cholangiocarcinoma. In: Freeny PC, editor. Radiology of the liver, biliary tract and pancreas. San Diego (CA): ARRS Categorical Course Syllabus; 1996. p. 27–32.

[56] Wernecke K, Vassallo P, Bick U, et al. The distinction between benign and malignant liver tumours on sonography: value of a hypoechoic halo. AJR Am J Roentgenol 1992;159:1005–9.

[57] Marchal GJ, Pylyser K, Tshibwabwa-Tumba EA. Anechoic halo in solid liver tumors: sonographic, microangiographic, and histologic correlation. Radiology 1985;156:479–83.

[58] Wernecke K, He ke L, Vassalo P, et al. Pathologic explanation for hypoechoic halo seen on sonograms of malignant liver tumours: an in vitro correlative study. AJR Am J Roentgenol 1992; 159:1011–6.

[59] Kruskal JB, Thomas P, Nasser I, et al. Hepatic colon cancer metastases in mice: dynamic in vivo correlation with hypoechoic rims visible at US. Radiology 2000;215:852–7.

[60] Rubaltelli L, Del Mashio A, Candiani F, et al. The role of vascularization in the formation of echographic patterns of hepatic metastases: microangiographic and echographic study. Br J Radiol 1980;53:1166–8.

[61] Yoshida T, Matsue H, Okazaki N, et al. Ultrasonographic differentiation of hepatocellular carcinoma from metastatic liver cancer. J Clin Ultrasound 1987;15:431–7.

[62] Wooten WB, Green B, Goldstein HM. Ultrasonography of necrotic hepatic metastases. Radiology 1978;128:447–50.

[63] Federle MP, Filly RA, Moss AA. Cystic hepatic neoplasms: complementary roles of computed tomography and sonography. AJR Am J Roentgenol 1981;136:345–8.

[64] Jang HJ, Kim TK, Wilson SR. Imaging of malignant liver masses: characterization and detection. Ultrasound Q 2006;22:19–29.

[65] Hohmann J, Albrecht T, Hoffmann CW, et al. Ultrasonographic detection of focal liver lesions: increased sensitivity and specificity with microbubble contrast agents. Eur J Radiol 2003;46: 147–59.

ELSEVIER
SAUNDERS

ULTRASOUND
CLINICS

Ultrasound Clin 2 (2007) 355–375

# Role of Vascular Ultrasound in the Evaluation of Liver Disease

Jennifer Swart, MD*, Sheila Sheth, MD

Imaging of the hepatic vasculature with color and duplex Doppler ultrasound (CDUS) provides invaluable structural and functional information in various hepatic diseases. Ultrasound is also routinely used for the monitoring of procedures used to treat liver disease, including liver transplantation and transjugular intrahepatic portosystemic shunts (TIPS).

In this article, the appearance of the normal hepatic vasculature is first described, followed by a review of the pathologic changes that can be observed with ultrasound in the setting of cirrhosis and portal hypertension, portal vein thrombosis, portal vein abnormalities and hepatic vein thrombosis, and Budd-Chiari syndrome. Finally, the

Department of Radiology, School of Medicine, Johns Hopkins Hospital, 600 North Wolfe Street, Baltimore, MD 21287, USA
* Corresponding author.
*E-mail address:* jswart2@jhmi.edu (J. Swart).

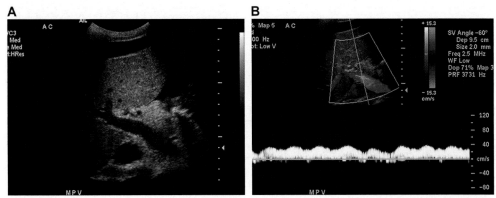

Fig. 1. Normal portal vein in a 48-year-old man who had a history of HIV and a lower gastrointestinal bleed. (*A*) Grayscale image demonstrates a normal portal vein coursing into the liver, with thin echogenic walls and anechoic lumen. The main portal vein divides into the right and left portal veins on entering the liver. (*B*) Color and duplex Doppler image demonstrates normal hepatopetal portal flow with venous waveform and a predominantly monophasic pattern with mild variation with respiration. Blood flow in the main and left portal vein is directed toward the transducer (*in red*). In the right portal vein, blood flows away from the transducer (*in blue*). The mean velocity is 35 cm/s.

contribution of CDUS in the evaluation of TIPS and liver transplantation is addressed.

## Normal hepatic vasculature

The liver has a dual blood supply from the portal vein and the hepatic artery. The portal vein carries 70% to 80% of partially oxygenated blood from the spleen and bowel to the liver, whereas the hepatic artery brings the remaining 20% to 30% [1,2]. Proper scanning technique requires 3.5-MHz or multifrequency curvilinear or sector transducers. Evaluation of the portal veins, common hepatic artery within the porta hepatis, and right hepatic vein is typically performed by way of a right intercostal approach [1]. The left portal vein and middle and left hepatic veins are usually imaged in the transverse plane at the level of the xiphoid process [1].

### Portal vein

The main portal vein is formed by the junction of the splenic vein and superior mesenteric vein and carries blood from the bowel, pancreas, and spleen to the liver. Its intrahepatic portion can be identified within the porta hepatis adjacent to the hepatic artery and the common hepatic duct. The portal vein and its intrahepatic branches have thin, mildly echogenic walls, and flow within the portal venous system should always be directed toward the liver (hepatopetal) [1]. With the usual intercostal or subcostal approach, blood flow in the main and left portal vein is thus directed toward the transducer, and flow in the right portal vein moves away.

Spectral Doppler demonstrates a monophasic pattern with little respiratory variation (Fig. 1). The fasting mean velocity within the main portal vein ranges from 13 to 23 cm/s [2].

### Hepatic artery

The extrahepatic portion of the hepatic artery, the proper hepatic artery, runs anterior to the main portal vein within the porta hepatis, and the intrahepatic branches of the hepatic arteries follow the portal veins. Although it provides only 20% to 30% of blood flow to the liver parenchyma, it is the main supplier of blood flow to the biliary tree. The normal hepatic artery has a low-resistance arterial waveform with continuous forward diastolic flow (Fig. 2). In the fasting state, the normal systolic

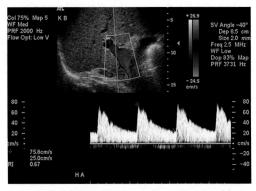

Fig. 2. Normal hepatic artery in a 48-year-old man who had a history of hepatitis C. Color and duplex Doppler image of the porta hepatis demonstrates the normal low-resistance spectral pattern of the hepatic artery.

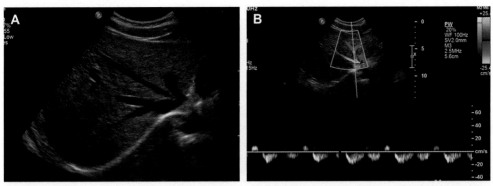

*Fig. 3.* Normal hepatic veins in a 28-year-old woman who had right upper quadrant pain. (*A*) Transverse gray-scale image shows the confluence of all three hepatic veins entering the hepatic IVC. (*B*) Color and duplex Doppler image demonstrates normal triphasic flow in the middle hepatic vein.

velocity measures approximately 30 to 40 cm/s with a diastolic velocity of 10 to 15 cm/s [2]. The Doppler measurement of resistive index (RI) in the hepatic artery varies in a normal fasting person from 0.55 to 0.81 (with a mean of 0.62 to 0.74) [2].

### Hepatic veins

The right, middle, and left hepatic veins and the hepatic venous confluence should be visible with ultrasound as tubular structures with no discernible walls and flow directed away from the

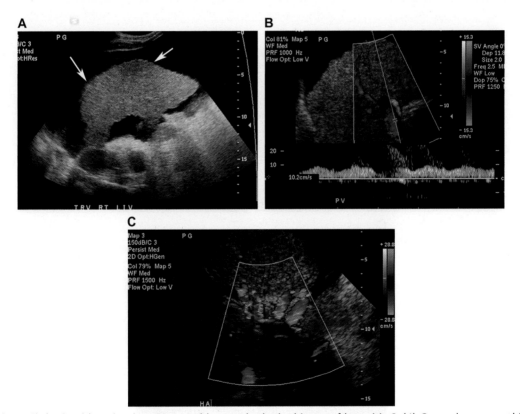

*Fig. 4.* Cirrhosis with ascites in a 50-year-old man who had a history of hepatitis C. (*A*) Grayscale sonographic image demonstrates a shrunken liver with a nodular contour and a large amount of surrounding ascites, compatible with cirrhosis. (*B*) Color and Doppler image of the portal vein demonstrates slow flow within the main portal vein, with a maximum velocity of 10 cm/s. (*C*) The hepatic artery is enlarged with a tortuous or "corkscrew" appearance. This occurs in the setting of cirrhosis when the blood flow increases within the hepatic artery to compensate for the decreased blood flow in the portal vein.

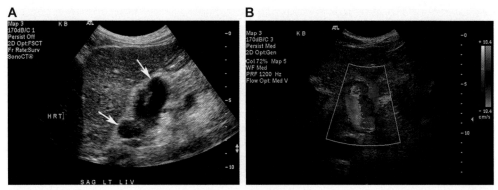

*Fig. 5.* Gastrohepatic varices in a 20-year-old woman who had a history of portal hypertension in the setting of sclerosing cholangitis associated with ulcerative colitis. (*A*) Grayscale image demonstrates multiple tubular anechoic structures posterior to the left lobe of the liver in the expected location of the esophageal–gastric junction (*arrows*). (*B*) Color image shows that these structures are tortuous blood vessels, compatible with gastrohepatic varices.

transducer in the direction of the inferior vena cava (IVC) [1]. The middle hepatic vein separates the right and left hepatic lobes, running between the anterior segment of the right hepatic lobe and the medial segment of the left hepatic lobe. The right hepatic vein is located between the anterior and posterior segments of the right hepatic lobe, and the left hepatic vein runs between the medial and lateral segments of the left hepatic lobe. The pulsations from the right

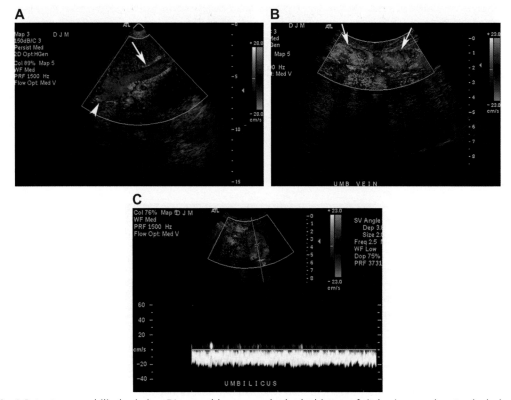

*Fig. 6.* Patent paraumbilical vein in a 51-year-old woman who had a history of cirrhosis secondary to alcohol use. (*A*) Sagittal color image through the left lobe of the liver depicts a large vessel coursing from the left portal vein (*arrowhead*) toward the anterior abdomen (*arrow*). (*B*) Sagittal color image using a curvilinear transducer demonstrates that this tortuous vessel courses underneath the abdominal wall toward the umbilicus. (*C*) Doppler image shows portal venous waveform within the vessel, confirming the diagnosis of patent paraumbilical vein.

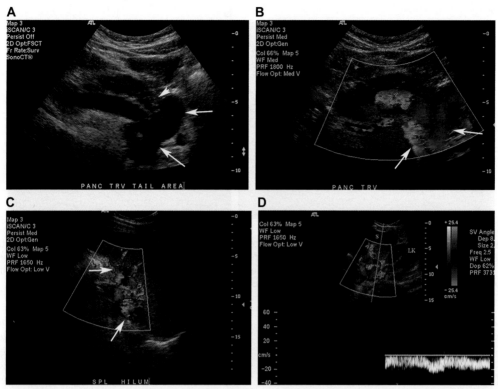

**Fig. 7.** Dilated upper abdominal varices with a spontaneous splenorenal shunt in a 23-year-old pregnant woman who had a history of appendiceal carcinoid tumor. The patient had a history of portal vein thrombosis after developing liver metastases. (*A*) Transverse grayscale image in the region of the pancreas demonstrates tortuous tubular vessels (*arrows*) near the pancreatic tail (*arrowhead*). (*B*) The color image confirms these are vascular structures (*arrows*). (*C*) Multiple dilated vessels are seen within the splenic hilum, consistent with varices (*arrows*). (*D*) A tortuous vessel with a portal venous Doppler waveform is seen coursing between the left kidney (*LK*) and the spleen (*S*) compatible with a large left splenorenal shunt.

heart are reflected in the waveform of the hepatic veins, with a triphasic flow pattern consisting of two periods of forward flow corresponding to the atrial diastole and ventricular systole [2]. The period of transient flow reversal corresponds to the right heart contraction of atrial systole (Fig. 3) [1].

## Cirrhosis and portal hypertension

Portal hypertension refers to an elevation of portal vein pressure to greater than the upper normal limit of 10 mm Hg [2,3]. Pathophysiologically, portal hypertension is subdivided into an extrahepatic form, most commonly caused by portal vein thrombosis, and an intrahepatic form. In the United States, portal hypertension most commonly results from hepatic fibrosis of the hepatic sinusoids, typically caused by alcoholic cirrhosis or chronic hepatitis [2]. Thrombosis of the hepatic veins of IVC or severe right heart failure can also result in centrilobular fibrosis and portal hypertension.

Patients who have cirrhosis often undergo repeated sonographic examinations to evaluate abnormalities in liver function tests, assess the hepatic vasculature, detect the manifestations of portal hypertension, and screen for hepatocellular carcinoma. Sonographic manifestations of advanced cirrhosis include a shrunken liver with nodular contour, slow flow in the portal vein, and a dilated corkscrew hepatic artery (Fig. 4) [2].

### *Portosystemic collaterals*

Sonographic manifestations of portal hypertension include splenomegaly, increased diameter of the portal vein, and visualization of portosystemic collateral vessels once the resistance to blood flow within the portal venous system exceeds that within the small veins connecting the portal and systemic circulations [1]. Spontaneous portosystemic shunts are reported to develop in approximately 38% of patients who have cirrhosis [4]. These varices divert splanchnic blood from the liver directly into the systemic circulation and are responsible for some

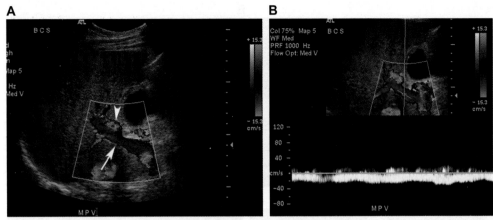

**Fig. 8.** Reversal of blood flow within the main portal vein in a 45-year-old man who had a history of portal hypertension secondary to cirrhosis stemming from alcohol abuse. (*A*) Color image demonstrates blood within the main portal vein flowing away from the transducer (blue away from the transducer) in a hepatofugal direction (*arrow*). Note the flow toward the transducer in the hepatic artery (*arrowhead*). (*B*) Doppler image confirms the reversal of flow with the waveform visualized below the baseline of the Doppler scale.

of the major complications of parenchymal liver diseases, such as gastrointestinal bleeding and hepatic encephalopathy. Although portosystemic varices are best demonstrated by contrast enhanced multidetector CT or MR imaging, ultrasound can identify many sites of portosystemic venous collaterals, including collateral vessels at the gastroesophageal junction, the paraumbilical collateral vein, splenorenal and gastrorenal shunts, pericholecystic or gallbladder varices within the wall of the gallbladder, and rectal varices [1].

### Gastroesophageal varices

Gastroesophageal junction collateral vessels develop from connections between the coronary and short gastric veins that drain into the systemic esophageal and paraesophageal veins, which then drain into the azygos and hemiazygos system [1]. These collateral vessels are important to identify, because they are the source of the potentially life-threatening hemorrhage resulting from the rupture of gastroesophageal varices. These tortuous dilated vessels are best visualized in the submucosal region of the gastric fundus and gastroesophageal junction on a sagittal image through the left lobe of the liver or between the greater curvature of the stomach and spleen (Fig. 5) [2]. Color and spectral Doppler demonstration of portal venous flow within these vessels confirms the diagnosis.

### Patent paraumbilical vein

The patent paraumbilical collateral vein is another common portosystemic collateral vessel easily visualized on ultrasound in the setting of portal hypertension, particularly in cases of alcohol-induced

liver cirrhosis [5]. This vessel traverses the ligamentum teres within the falciform ligament as it diverts blood away from the left portal vein to the superficial and deep epigastric veins of the abdominal wall [1]. It is believed that a patent paraumbilical vein may protect patients from severe hemorrhage from esophageal varices.

The patent paraumbilical vein can be recognized sonographically as a tubular anechoic structure measuring at least 3 mm in diameter coursing anteriorly and inferiorly from the left portal vein toward the anterior abdominal wall, demonstrating a monophasic venous blood flow spectral pattern [1]. Serpiginous dilated anterior abdominal veins,

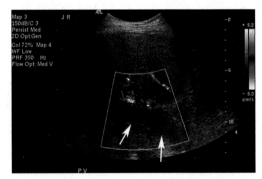

**Fig. 9.** Portal vein thrombosis in a 59-year-old woman who had a history of polycythemia vera who developed chest and abdominal pain. Color image at the porta hepatis demonstrates echogenic material filling the lumen of the main portal vein with absence of flow within the vessel, compatible with thrombosis of the main portal vein (*arrows*). Note that the image has been optimized for slow flow: low wall filter (*WF*), color priority at 72%, and color scale at 5.3 cm/s.

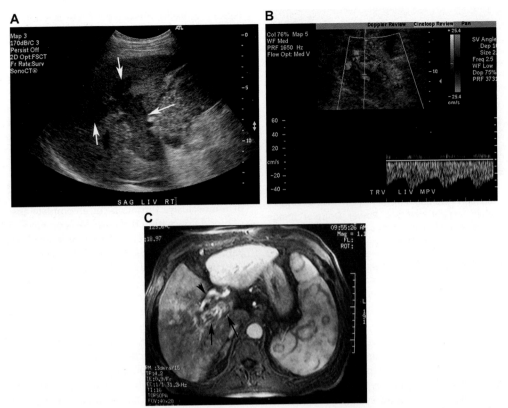

*Fig. 10.* Malignant portal vein thrombus in a 72-year-old man who had a history of hepatocellular carcinoma. Fine-needle aspiration of the portal vein thrombus confirmed hepatocellular carcinoma thrombus. (*A*) Grayscale image at the porta hepatic demonstrates echogenic material filling and expanding the lumen of the portal vein and its branches (*arrows*). (*B*) Color and Doppler images show vascularity within the thrombus filling the portal vein. The low-resistance arterial waveform suggests tumor thrombus. (*C*) Contrast-enhanced axial MR imaging in the arterial phase shows serpiginous enhancement within the thrombosed portal vein (*arrows*), confirming the diagnosis of malignant thrombus. The hepatic artery (*arrowhead*) is prominent.

the "caput medusa," may also be visualized within the subcutaneous tissues surrounding the umbilicus, particularly with the use of a linear or curvilinear transducer (Fig. 6). These vessels should be avoided when performing a paracentesis.

### Splenorenal varices

Splenorenal and gastrorenal shunts may be observed with ultrasound as tortuous veins lying within the splenic hilum and left renal fossa, best visualized through the left flank using the enlarged spleen as an acoustic window [2]. These represent a shunt from gastric or splenic veins to a frequently enlarged left renal vein into the IVC (Fig. 7) [1].

### Other portosystemic collaterals

Intestinal portosystemic collateral vessels, shunting blood from the superior and inferior mesenteric veins to the IVC, are rarely demonstrated by sonography because of their retroperitoneal location [1]. Rectal and perirectal varices, draining blood from

the superior hemorrhoidal vein to the hemorrhoidal plexus, can occasionally be visualized with transrectal ultrasound.

### Reversal of portal venous blood flow

Reversal of blood flow within the main portal vein or its branches, from the normal hepatopetal to a hepatofugal direction away from the liver parenchyma, can be a specific sign of portal hypertension and is more often present in patients who have advanced hepatic disease. An easy clue to diagnose this flow reversal is to notice that at the porta hepatic, the hepatic artery and the portal vein have blood flowing in opposite directions (Fig. 8) (Child-Pugh grade C cirrhosis) [4].

## Portal vein thrombosis

### Etiology of portal vein thrombosis

Various intra-abdominal or systemic disease processes are associated with portal vein thrombosis.

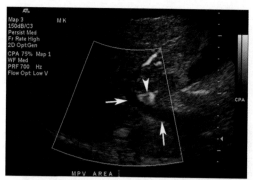

**Fig. 11.** False-positive portal vein thrombosis in a 55-year-old man who had a history of cirrhosis secondary to primary biliary cirrhosis. Power Doppler image shows absence of blood flow within the portal vein (*arrows*). Note flow in the hepatic artery (*arrowhead*). The liver is shrunken and there is ascites seen. Subsequent MR angiogram demonstrated a patent portal vein. The absence of blood flow on ultrasound may have been caused by extremely slow flow within the portal venous system.

Portal vein thrombosis can develop in various benign and malignant disease processes. Causes of bland thrombosis include hypercoagulable states (related to use of oral contraceptives, protein C deficiency, polycythemia rubra vera, and antiphospholipid syndrome), slow flow caused by portal hypertension and cirrhosis, intra-abdominal sepsis (pylephlebitis) caused by severe appendicitis, diverticulitis, pancreatitis, or inflammatory bowel disease, splenectomy, and trauma [1,6]. Dehydration, omphalitis, and umbilical vein catheterization are risk factors in small children. Direct invasion of the portal vein by hepatocellular carcinoma is the most common etiology of malignant thrombus in the portal vein. Cholangiocarcinoma of the hilar

region (Klatskin tumor) often encases the portal vein, but malignant thrombus is less common.

### Ultrasound appearance

Thrombus within the portal vein may be identified as echogenic material expanding the lumen of the involved vessel on grayscale sonography. Occasionally the clot may be anechoic or hypoechoic and the vessel lumen may appear normal in caliber, particularly in the case of a bland acute thrombus [6]. Color or power Doppler is therefore invaluable, because it demonstrates the thrombus by depicting either flow around the clot, in the setting of a partial or nonocclusive thrombus, or a complete absence of blood flow within the vessel in a complete occlusion [6]. Care should be taken to optimize Doppler parameters to detect slow blood flow (Fig. 9).

In patients who have cirrhosis or suspected hepatocellular carcinoma, it is imperative to distinguish between bland and tumor thrombus. The demonstration of arterial pulsatile hepatofugal flow within the portal vein thrombus itself has been found to be moderately sensitive (62% sensitivity) yet highly specific (95% specificity) in the diagnosis of malignant portal vein thrombus (Fig. 10) [7,8]. The distinction of benign from malignant thrombus is critical to accurately define the patient's prognosis and candidacy for surgical management. If needed, fine-needle aspiration of the portal vein thrombus for establishing the diagnosis of malignant invasion may be performed safely with ultrasound guidance [9].

### Potential pitfalls

Several potential pitfalls in the diagnosis of portal vein thrombosis should be avoided.

An important cause of false-positive diagnosis more commonly seen in patients who have

**A**

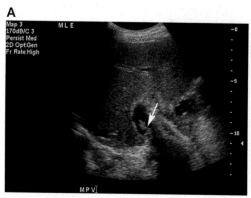

**B**

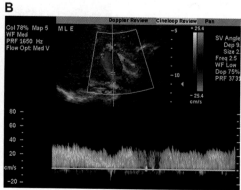

**Fig. 12.** Nonocclusive thrombus of the portal vein masked on color imaging in a 69-year-old woman who had a history of cholangitis status post biliary stent. (*A*) Grayscale image of the main portal vein demonstrates an echogenic thrombus partially filling the lumen (*arrow*). (*B*) Color image demonstrates complete filling of the main portal vein and obscures the clot.

cirrhosis is very slow flow within the portal vein: the velocity of portal blood flow may be below the detection threshold for color or even power Doppler. In these patients, further imaging with contrast-enhanced CT or MR imaging is useful to confirm or exclude the diagnosis of portal vein thrombosis (Fig. 11).

The following two technical or interpretative pitfalls should be avoided to prevent missing a portal venous clot. The portal vein should be imaged with grayscale and color to detect small thrombi, because color or power Doppler may "bleed" over and potentially obscure partial clots (Fig. 12).

A second cause of false negative diagnosis is to mistake a small collateral vessel in the porta hepatis for a patent main portal vein in patients who have cavernous transformation.

## Cavernous transformation of the portal vein

Cavernous transformation, or portal cavernoma, results from long-standing portal vein occlusion. Portal cavernoma is an important cause of extrahepatic portal hypertension in children in developing countries who have developed portal vein thrombosis as a result of umbilical cord infection with resultant dehydration and sepsis.

On ultrasound, multiple serpiginous or "worm like" collateral channels are seen within the porta hepatis, which demonstrate a portal venous waveform (Fig. 13). The flow within these vessels is hepatopetal, forming a bypass route from the splanchnic veins to the intrahepatic portal veins around the obstructed portal vein [10].

## Interpretation of abnormal flow patterns in the portal vein

Several hepatic or systemic conditions may alter the normal Doppler spectral pattern in the portal vein.

### Increased phasicity

Marked pulsatility in the portal venous flow is frequently an indication of right-sided heart failure (Fig. 14) [11,12]. A right upper quadrant

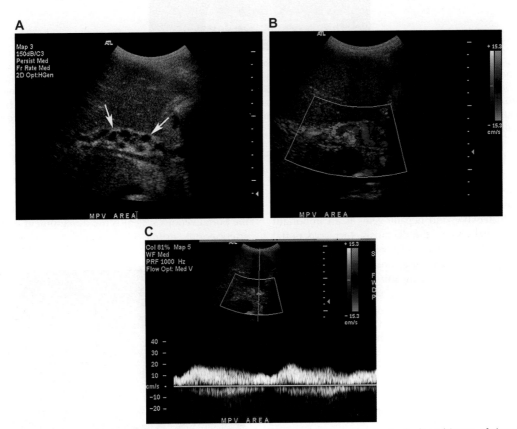

*Fig. 13.* Cavernous transformation of the portal vein in a 56-year-old woman who had a long history of chronic pancreatitis and multiple small bowel obstructions. (*A*) Grayscale image demonstrates multiple small tubular anechoic structures within the expected location of the main portal vein (*arrows*). (*B*) Color image shows that these tubular structures are small vessels, compatible with cavernous transformation of the portal vein. (*C*) Doppler interrogation demonstrates a portal venous waveform within these vessels.

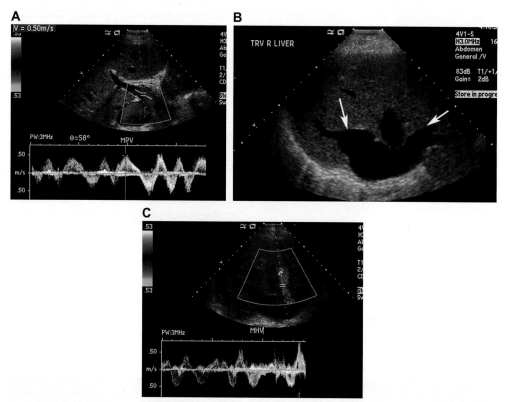

Fig. 14. Biphasic flow in the main portal vein in a 59-year-old woman who had a history of right heart failure and hepatitis C. (A) Color and Doppler image demonstrates biphasic blood flow within the main portal vein, with the waveform extending above and below the baseline. (B) Grayscale image shows enlarged hepatic veins draining into an enlarged IVC at the hepatic vein confluence (*arrows*) secondary to the right heart failure and resultant volume overload. (C) Increased pulsatility is also demonstrated within the middle hepatic vein on this color Doppler image.

ultrasound is often requested in these patients because of elevation of their liver function tests from passive congestion of the liver. The presence of dilated IVC and hepatic veins is an important additional clue to the diagnosis. Increased portal vein pulsatility has been observed to correlate with elevated right atrial pressure, particularly in cases of tricuspid regurgitation, severe pulmonary hypertension, large pericardial effusion, right atrial tumor, and constrictive pericarditis [13]. Increased pulsatility may also be observed in the setting of fistulas between the portal and hepatic veins and portocaval shunts [13]. Mild phasicity can be seen as a normal variant, particularly in young thin patients (Fig. 15).

## Reversal of flow in the portal vein and its branches

Reversal of the normal hepatopetal flow in the main portal vein is most frequently observed in patients who have advanced cirrhosis and portal hypertension. Flow reversal in the left or right portal venous

branch should, however, be expected in a normally functioning TIPS.

An uncommon cause of hepatofugal flow within the portal venous system is the development of an arterioportal fistula [14], a direct connection

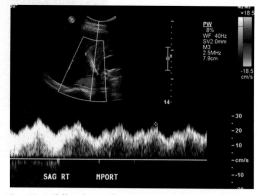

Fig. 15. Mildly phasic flow in the main portal vein in a 35-year-old woman who had right upper quadrant pain.

between the hepatic artery and portal vein. Congenital arterioportal malformations are rare and most of these fistulae are iatrogenic and form as a sequela from liver biopsy or trauma. Occasionally they are associated with a focal liver lesion [14]. The draining portal venous branch demonstrates hepatofugal flow, whereas the flow within the affected branch of the hepatic artery is turbulent with increased diastolic flow and a low RI (Fig. 16) [15]. Often the arterial RI within the affected lobe is decreased by at least 30% to 40% compared with the normal lobe [15].

Portal to hepatic venous fistulas are even less common and are iatrogenic or are associated with cirrhosis.

## Gas within the portal vein

The presence of gas within the portal venous system has traditionally been considered an alarming finding, associated with life-threatening conditions, such as mesenteric ischemia in the elderly patient or necrotizing enterocolitis in infants. It is now recognized that portal venous gas can be an incidental finding in an asymptomatic patient, particularly in cases of blunt abdominal trauma, liver transplantation, or postoperative ileus [16–19].

Ultrasound is the most sensitive imaging modality for detecting portal venous gas. On grayscale sonography, portal venous gas manifests as tiny, bright, echogenic foci that move rapidly within a portal vein branch (Fig. 17). High-amplitude,

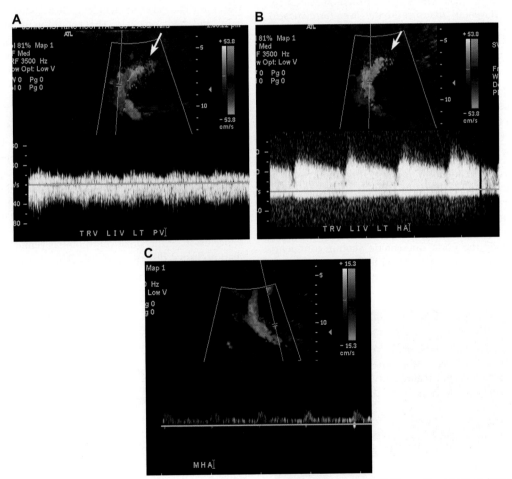

*Fig. 16.* Arterioportal fistula in a 26-year-old man who had a history of hepatitis C. The patient had undergone a percutaneous liver biopsy several months before this sonogram. (*A*) Color and duplex Doppler image of the left portal vein shows reversal of flow in the left portal vein. Note the flow is turbulent and there is a focal color bruit (*arrow*). (*B*) Color and duplex Doppler image of the left hepatic artery shows turbulent arterial flow with increased diastolic flow compared with the main hepatic artery. Note the focal color bruit (*arrow*). (*C*) Color and duplex Doppler image of the main portal vein and hepatic artery shows normal hepatopetal flow in the vein and normal flow in the artery. (*From* American College of Radiology (ACR). Ultrasound (Third Edition). American College of Radiology; 2005. Reproduced with permission of the American College of Radiology. No other representation of this material is authorized without expressed, written permission from the American College of Radiology.)

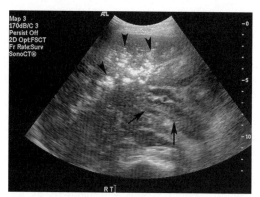

Fig. 17. Portal venous air found incidentally in a 49-year-old woman who had a history of renal failure and HIV. Grayscale image shows bright echogenic foci in the main portal vein (*arrows*) and air in the portal venous branches in the liver (*arrowheads*). The echoes in the portal vein were observed to be mobile on real-time ultrasound. Air within the portal vein was confirmed on CT (not shown).

spike-like artifacts superimposed on the Doppler portal vein waveform are specific for portal venous gas (Fig. 18) [16].

### Yin yang sign of portal venous aneurysm

Portal vein aneurysm is a rare abnormality seen as a segmental fusiform or saccular expansion of the portal vein greater than 2 cm in diameter that is usually extrahepatic in location [20,21]. It is often detected incidentally. The most common locations include the portal–mesenteric venous confluence and the main portal vein within the porta hepatis, with the less frequent intrahepatic portal vein

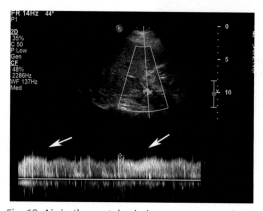

Fig. 18. Air in the portal vein in an asymptomatic 53-year-old woman after liver transplantation. Color Doppler image of the transplant liver demonstrates high amplitude spike artifacts (*arrows*) superimposed on the main portal vein waveform. Rapidly mobile echogenic foci were observed in the portal vein at real-time ultrasound (not shown).

aneurysm occurring at the bifurcation site [22]. It can be congenital in origin, or acquired in association with portal hypertension, trauma or liver transplantation.

The sonographic manifestations of portal vein aneurysm include focal dilatation of the vein or a cystic mass closely related to the portal vein. On color Doppler the aneurysm demonstrates turbulent or bidirectional flow (Fig. 19) [21].

## Hepatic vein thrombosis and Budd-Chiari syndrome

### Budd-Chiari syndrome

Budd-Chiari syndrome is a rare condition that is secondary to hepatic venous outflow obstruction. The classic clinical triad includes ascites, abdominal pain, and hepatomegaly. The condition is most common in young women, and presentation ranges from a fulminant acute syndrome manifested by jaundice and hepatic encephalopathy to a subacute or chronic form resulting in the gradual onset of cirrhosis [23].

Approximately 75% of the cases in the United States result from hypercoagulable states, including polycythemia vera or other myeloproliferative disorders and paroxysmal nocturnal hemoglobinuria [24]. Other causes include postpartum state or use of oral contraceptives, vasculitis, and malignancy. In IVC, webs and stenosis account for almost 50% of cases in Asian patients. The cause remains unknown in one third of patients [3,23].

Occlusion of the small centrilobular venules, or veno-occlusive disease, is considered by most to represent a separate entity. It is characterized by non-portal fibrosis causing obstruction of the small centrilobular venules and was first described following ingestion of pyrrolizidine alkaloids contained in "bush-tea" drinks. It is now most commonly caused by the toxicity of chemotherapy agents and radiation administered to bone marrow transplant patients [3].

### Ultrasound appearance of Budd-Chiari syndrome

On grayscale imaging the diagnosis should be suspected if the hepatic veins cannot be visualized. Additional findings include thickened hepatic vein walls, irregular caliber of the veins, and tortuous collateral veins. Hepatomegaly and ascites are common. Predominant hypertrophy of the caudate lobe is characteristic and occurs because of its separate venous drainage directly into the IVC.

Color and spectral Doppler ultrasound may demonstrate absent, decreased, reversed, or turbulent flow with elevated velocities within the hepatic veins [23]. When blood flow is present in the

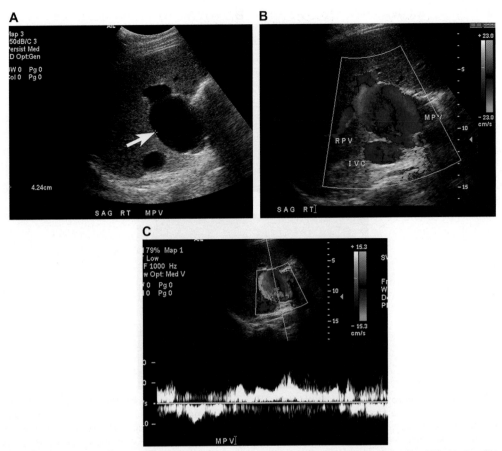

*Fig. 19.* Aneurysm of the portal vein in a 22-year-old man who underwent a liver transplant 11 years earlier. (*A*) Grayscale sonographic image of the main portal vein shows a focal dilatation of the main portal vein (*arrow*) measuring 4 cm in diameter. (*B*) The color Doppler image shows bidirectional flow within the aneurysm, representing the blood swirling around in the dilated portion of the portal vein. Note the blood in the right portal vein is flowing in the normal hepatopetal direction. (*C*) The duplex Doppler image shows portal venous type flow within the aneurysm. This aneurysm had been stable for at least 4 years and the patient was managed conservatively. (*From* American College of Radiology (ACR). Ultrasound (Third Edition). American College of Radiology; 2005. Reproduced with permission of the American College of Radiology. No other representation of this material is authorized without expressed, written permission from the American College of Radiology.)

hepatic veins and the IVC, the waveform morphology changes to reflect the downstream obstruction from the normal triphasic pattern to a flattened appearance resembling the portal vein—the "pseudoportal Doppler signal" [1,25]. This pattern is not specific, however, and can be observed with conditions resulting in increased pressure within the hepatic parenchyma, such as fatty infiltration, acute hepatitis, and cirrhosis [25].

Approximately 50% of Budd-Chiari patients also demonstrate an enlarged caudate vein greater than 3 mm in diameter, and this may be considered a specific sign when observed in the absence of heart failure (Fig. 20) [25]. This caudate vein dilatation occurs because the caudate lobe is the only segment of the liver that drains directly into the IVC, and the shunting of blood from the remainder of the hepatic

parenchyma through collateral vessels results in enlargement of the caudate lobe and vein [25].

Demonstration of intrahepatic venovenous collaterals is a specific sign of Budd-Chiari syndrome and can include subcapsular veins, vessels shunting between hepatic veins, large venovenous collaterals draining directing into the IVC, and the classic spiderweb collaterals (Fig. 21) [23,25]. The development of spontaneous portocaval collaterals may also occur and may in some cases obviate the need for a TIPS placement [25].

Besides the changes in the hepatic venous system and IVC, the venous obstruction may also manifest in thrombosis caused by the underlying hypercoagulable state or hepatofugal flow within the portal vein (10% to 20% of patients) in cases of severe portal hypertension [26].

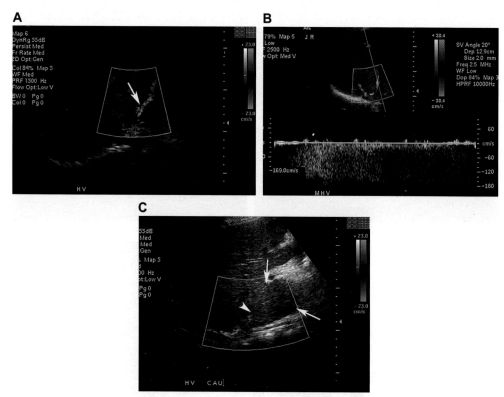

**Fig. 20.** Budd-Chiari syndrome in a 30-year-old man who had a history of paroxysmal nocturnal hemoglobinuria and who presented with abdominal swelling. (*A*) Color image demonstrates narrowing of the middle hepatic veins with color aliasing near its junction with the IVC (*arrow*). (*B*) Color and Doppler image shows that although the middle hepatic vein is patent, the flow velocity is markedly increased. (*C*) Color and grayscale image demonstrates an enlarged caudate lobe (*arrows*) with its vein draining directly in the IVC (*arrowhead*). MR imaging and liver biopsy confirmed the diagnosis of Budd-Chiari syndrome.

### Ultrasound appearance of veno-occlusive disease

In this entity the hepatic veins are usually normal, because the obstruction occurs at the level of the centrilobular hepatic venules. The usefulness of ultrasound in the evaluation of this complication is controversial. In some cases the venous outflow obstruction may manifest by alterations in the hepatic artery Doppler waveform with an elevated hepatic artery RI of greater than 0.75 to 0.8 caused by increased peripheral resistance in the liver parenchyma. In severe cases portal hypertension leads to reversal of portal venous flow.

## Evaluation of liver transplantation

### Normal appearance

Liver transplantation has become the treatment of choice in patients who have irreversible liver failure and is increasingly performed in children and adults. When vascular complications occur, it is frequently during the early postoperative period. Ultrasound plays a crucial role in assessing the post-transplantation liver and its vasculature. In whole liver transplantation, the most common vascular anastomoses typically consist of an end-to-end anastomosis of the donor and recipient hepatic arteries and the main portal veins. The piggyback technique of IVC anastomosis obviates the need for sectioning and cross clamping the recipient IVC by preserving the recipient IVC and performing and end-to-side anastomosis between the recipient and donor IVC (Fig. 22) [27]. Post-transplant, the normal hepatic artery Doppler waveform should depict the typical rapid systolic upstroke and continuous diastolic flow, with an RI between 0.5 and 0.7 and an acceleration time (time from end diastole to the first systolic peak) less than 80 ms [28].

### Hepatic artery thrombosis or occlusion

Hepatic artery thrombosis is the most serious vascular complication in liver transplantation. It occurs in approximately 8% of patients and is a particularly

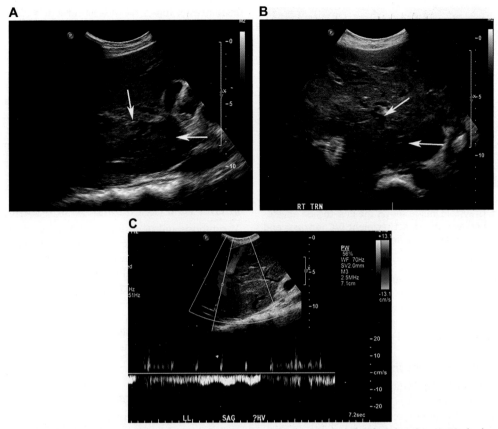

*Fig. 21.* Budd-Chiari syndrome in a 36-year-old woman who had a history of polycythemia vera and who presented with abdominal pain and swelling. The patient had received a TIPS previously, which was occluded at the time of this examination. (*A*) Grayscale image demonstrates an enlarged caudate lobe (*arrows*) with multiple serpiginous anechoic structures within the liver. (*B*) Grayscale image again demonstrates multiple serpiginous venous channels within the liver, compatible with hepatic vein collateral vessels. (*C*) Color and Doppler image confirms flow within the collateral vessels.

devastating complication, because the hepatic artery represents the sole arterial supply to the transplant liver and its biliary tree. Patients may present with sepsis and fulminant hepatic failure, recurrent abscesses or bacteremia, biliary leak or obstruction, and ischemic biliary strictures. Hepatic artery thrombosis results in necrosis of the biliary epithelium and eventual infarction and necrosis of the hepatic parenchyma [28]. Doppler depiction of the complete absence of hepatic arterial flow is diagnostic (Fig. 23); however, a "syndrome of impending thrombosis" has also been described in the acute post-transplantation period and is important to recognize [28,29]. This syndrome of impending thrombosis consists of a progression over 3 to 10 days from a normal hepatic artery waveform to the development of loss of diastolic flow to a dampening of the systolic peak to the eventual complete loss of the arterial waveform [28,29].

Hepatic artery stenosis develops in approximately 11% of recipients. It most frequently occurs at the anastomotic site and may be recognized by a focal narrowing of the lumen diameter or turbulence at the stenotic site as demonstrated by aliasing on color Doppler [28]. Spectral analysis at the site of narrowing demonstrates a focal area of accelerated systolic velocity greater than 200 cm/s (Fig. 24) [28].

In the setting of hepatic artery stenosis, or if arterial collateral vessels develop after hepatic artery thrombosis, the intrahepatic arteries demonstrate a tardus-parvus pattern with an RI less than 0.5 and an acceleration time greater than 80 ms [27,28]. This sign is often easier to detect sonographically and should trigger a more thorough evaluation of the more central hepatic artery. Care must be taken, however, because a tardus-parvus pattern within the hepatic parenchyma within the first 72 hours after transplant may be the result of normal postoperative edema at the anastomosis site and can be observed to resolve within 3 to 4 days after transplant [27]. A rare arterial

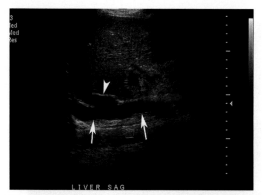

Fig. 22. Piggyback anastomosis in a normal liver transplant. Grayscale image shows the end-to-side anastomosis between the intact recipient IVC (*arrows*) and the donor vessel (*arrowhead*).

complication after transplant includes the development of hepatic artery pseudoaneurysms at the anastomotic site that may eventually result in the formation of a fistula between the aneurysm and the biliary tree or portal vein [28].

### Portal vein thrombosis or occlusion

Portal vein complications include portal vein thrombosis and stenosis, with an acute portal vein thrombus in children frequently manifesting as an anechoic thrombus that is not detectable on grayscale ultrasound [27]. Color and spectral Doppler reveal absence of flow within the portal vein. An echogenic intraluminal thrombus and vessel narrowing may also occasionally be observed [27]. Portal vein stenosis occurs at the anastomotic site and can be diagnosed when there is a reduction

in the vessel lumen by at least 50% or a diameter less than 2.5 mm at the site of narrowing [27,30]. Focal turbulence with color aliasing and a velocity within the stenotic segment that is 3 to 4 times greater than that in the prestenotic segment can be demonstrated with Doppler evaluation [27]. High-velocity jet flow may also be noted distal to the area of stenosis [30]. Portal vein aneurysms have also been described in the post-transplant setting as saccular dilatations of 2 to 3 cm with turbulent venous flow [30].

### Inferior vena cava thrombosis or occlusion

Thrombosis and stenosis of the IVC after transplantation are rare complications, more often seen in pediatric patients or in cases of retransplantation [28]. Findings of vessel narrowing or intraluminal echogenic material suggest the diagnosis, as does a focal increase in blood velocity at the site of the stenosis [28]. Suprahepatic IVC stenosis can cause a reversal of flow or absence of the normal phasicity within the hepatic veins [28].

### Nonvascular complications

These include biliary complications, such as leaks, strictures, stones, and sludge, and the development of perihepatic fluid collections, such as abscess, biloma, and ascites. Neoplastic disease may also develop in the form of recurrence of the neoplasm for which the liver transplant was initially performed or post-transplantation lymphoproliferative disorder.

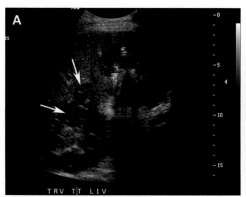
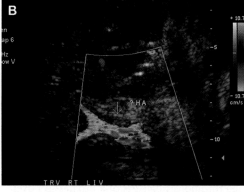

Fig. 23. Hepatic infarcts caused by thrombosis of the main hepatic artery in a 71-year-old man who was status post-orthotopic liver transplant the previous day for primary sclerosing cholangitis. This was the patient's second liver transplant, because the first had also failed because of hepatic artery thrombosis. (*A*) Grayscale image demonstrates multiple hypoechoic areas within the liver parenchyma caused by developing infarcts secondary to hepatic artery thrombosis. (*B*) Color image demonstrates echogenic material within the hepatic artery and absence of vascular flow. The adjacent main portal vein demonstrates normal blood flow. The diagnosis was confirmed by angiography (not shown).

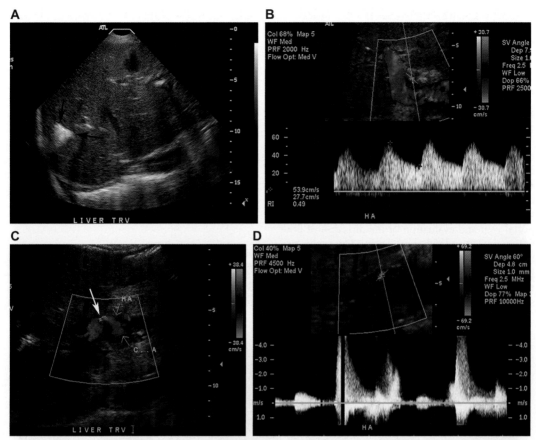

**Fig. 24.** Hepatic abscesses caused by stenosis of the main hepatic artery in a 52-year-old woman who was status post-orthotopic liver transplant and septic. (*A*) Grayscale image shows a collection of air within the right lobe of the liver, compatible with an abscess (*arrow*). Multiple abscesses were confirmed on CT (not shown). (*B*) Doppler image of the hepatic artery in the porta hepatic shows an abnormal waveform with increased diastolic flow and low RI and a parvus tardus appearance. (*C*) Color Doppler image shows a focal narrowing in the proximal hepatic artery (*arrow*). (*D*) Doppler spectrum confirms the presence of a significant hepatic artery stenosis with markedly elevated peak systolic velocity greater than 4 m/s. Hepatic angiogram confirmed the diagnosis (not shown) and the stenosis was dilated with balloon angioplasty.

## Evaluation of transjugular intrahepatic portosystemic shunts

TIPS are used primarily in the management of severe portal hypertension and its complications, specifically uncontrollable bleeding from gastroesophageal varices and intractable ascites [31]. Other indications include Budd-Chiari syndrome and veno-occlusive disease. A stent is deployed over a tract created within the liver parenchyma between the portal venous and hepatic venous system, typically between a branch of the right portal vein and right hepatic vein. The objective of TIPS placement is to decrease the portosystemic gradient to less than 12 mm Hg [31].

The incidence of TIPS malfunction is high, reported to be 23% to 78% after 1 year. Monitoring of shunt function by ultrasound within the months

after the procedure is often necessary. A postprocedure ultrasound within 24 hours after TIPS placement is frequently helpful to document patency and to obtain baseline flow velocity [8].

### Technique

Ultrasound examination of TIPS can be challenging: the cirrhotic liver is often shrunken with the stent placed deep within the organ. Scanning with a low-frequency transducer, a 2.5-MHz sector transducer, through a right intercostal approach is often the best technique. The lower frequency affords the best penetration and optimal Doppler evaluation. When measuring blood flow velocities within the TIPS, care should be taken to properly adjust the Doppler angle. The author typically records velocities in the main portal vein at the porta hepatis and velocities in the proximal (or portal venous end), mid, and distal (or hepatic venous end) of the TIPS. Flow direction within the left and if visualized right portal venous branches should also be documented.

### Normal ultrasound findings

Sonographically the TIPS stent appears as two parallel echogenic lines with an intraluminal diameter of 8 to 9 mm. Blood flow within the stent should be directed from portal vein to hepatic vein and extend from the near wall to the far wall [31]. Complete evaluation of TIPS function includes measurements of angle-corrected velocities within the proximal, mid, and distal shunt and the velocity in the main portal vein and evaluation of the direction of flow within the left and right portal veins. Flow velocities within the TIPS as measured by spectral Doppler may vary considerably and have some degree of pulsatility, with a mean velocity within patent shunts of 95 cm/s at the portal venous end and

120 cm/s in the shunt midportion [2]. The flow direction within the main portal vein should be hepatopetal, and the velocity within this vein is increased, with a portal vein velocity slightly greater than 40 cm/s [2,31]. This occurs because the shunt provides a low-pressure outflow for the high-pressure portal venous system, thereby redirecting portal venous flow from the pre-existing portosystemic collaterals, with a resultant increased flow volume through the main portal vein toward the shunt [31]. Flow in the right and left portal veins is typically directed away from the liver parenchyma and toward the TIPS, although this may vary depending on the degree of cirrhosis (Fig. 25) [32].

### Transjugular intrahepatic portosystemic shunts dysfunction

Complications of TIPS include thrombosis, diffuse stenosis secondary to pseudointimal hyperplasia,

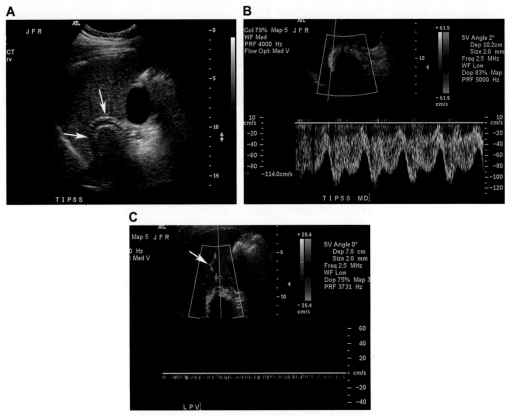

*Fig. 25.* Patent TIPS in a 42-year-old man who had a history of severe gastrointestinal bleeding secondary to varices from cirrhosis induced by hepatitis C and alcohol abuse. (*A*) Grayscale image demonstrates the TIPS, with the echogenic walls of the stent well depicted and no evidence of thrombus within the lumen (*arrows*). (*B*) Color and Doppler image depicts pulsatile blood flow within the patent TIPS, with a peak velocity of 114 cm/s. This velocity is within the normal expected range of 90 to 120 cm/s. (*C*) Doppler image of the left portal vein depicts blood flow reversal within the left portal vein, with blood directed away from the liver (hepatofugal) and into the stent. This confirms the TIPS is functioning properly. Note the large left hepatic artery (*arrow*).

and focal stenosis, usually at the hepatic venous end [2].

Stent thrombosis is easily diagnosed if there is complete absence of flow within the TIPS on color or power and spectral Doppler (Fig. 26). A potential pitfall to recognize is a paradoxic loss of sensitivity when the Doppler scale is set very low, leading to false-positive diagnosis of thrombosis [31]. In addition, the role of ultrasound surveillance for the new covered stents may be more limited, as suggested by a recent study [33].

Criteria described in the literature for the diagnosis of TIPS stenosis are not uniformly accepted. Different groups use various thresholds for stent velocity when assessing shunt malfunction. A TIPS velocity below the lower limit of normal for stent velocity ranges of 50 to 90 cm/s has been described to indicate a significant narrowing [31,32]. Flow velocity should be measured at the end of expiration, because a recent study has documented that intra-TIPS velocity decreases by approximately 22 cm/s during deep inspiration [32]. Alternatively if there is a focal stenosis, one may identify an area of increased velocity with focal turbulence resulting in color aliasing at the stenotic site (see Fig. 26) [31]. The upper limit of normal for shunt velocity has been reported as 185 to 220 cm/s, with Middleton and colleagues [31] suggesting using a cut-off of 190 cm/s as the maximum peak velocity measured on angle-corrected pulsed Doppler waveforms. Because the peak velocity increases and the minimum velocity decreases in a stenotic shunt, assessment of the velocity gradient may be the most sensitive means of detecting shunt malfunction [31].

Malfunction of the TIPS also results in a decrease in the velocity within the main portal vein, with Middleton and colleagues [31] setting 30 cm/s as their threshold for the lower limit of normal. Hepatopetal flow in the left or right portal vein, away from the TIPS, confirms the diagnosis [31].

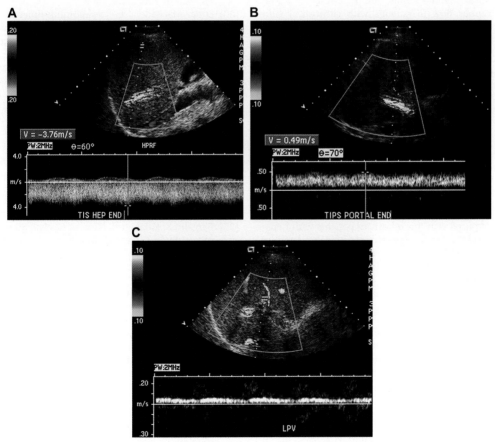

Fig. 26. Stenosis of the distal TIPS in a 56-year-old woman. (*A*) Color and Doppler image shows markedly elevated velocity at 376 cm/s in the distal TIPS. (*B*) In the portal (proximal) TIPS, the velocity is only 49cm/s; this indicates a significant gradient within the shunt. (*C*) Flow in the left portal vein is red, hepatopetal, and away from the TIPS, confirming shunt dysfunction.

## Summary

Sonography can provide a considerable amount of information concerning the structure and function of the hepatic vasculature, aiding in the detection of the sequelae of liver disease resulting from local hepatic or systemic processes. Evaluation of postprocedure hepatic vasculature may also provide a safe, noninvasive means of assessing and monitoring patients after liver transplantation or TIPS procedure.

## References

[1] Killi RM. Doppler sonography of the native liver. Eur J Radiol 1999;32(1):21–35.

[2] Martinez-Noguera A, Montserrat E, Torrubia S, et al. Doppler in hepatic cirrhosis and chronic hepatitis. Semin Ultrasound CT MR 2002; 23(1):19–36.

[3] Okuda K. Non-cirrhotic portal hypertension versus idiopathic portal hypertension. J Gastroenterol Hepatol 2002;17:S204–13.

[4] Von Herbay A, Frieling T, Haussinger D. Color Doppler sonographic evaluation of spontaneous portosystemic shunts and inversion of portal venous flow in patients with cirrhosis. J Clin Ultrasound 2000;28(7):332–9.

[5] Chen C-H, Wang J-H, Lu S-N, et al. Comparison of prevalence for paraumbilical vein patency in patients with viral and alcoholic liver cirrhosis. Am J Gastroenterol 2002;97(9):2415–8.

[6] Tchelepi H, Ralls P, Radin R, et al. Sonography of diffuse liver disease. J Ultrasound Med 2002;21: 1023–32.

[7] Dodd GD, Memel DS, Baron RL, et al. Portal vein thrombosis in patients with cirrhosis: does sonographic detection of intrathrombus flow allow differentiation of benign and malignant thrombus? AJR Am J Roentgenol 1995;165: 573–7.

[8] Tanaka K, Numata K, Okazaki H, et al. Diagnosis of portal vein thrombosis in patients with hepatocellular carcinoma: efficacy of color Doppler sonography compared with angiography. AJR Am J Roentgenol 1993;160:1279–83.

[9] Vilana R, Bru C, Bruix J, et al. Fine-needle aspiration biopsy of portal vein thrombosis: value in detecting malignant thrombosis. AJR Am J Roentgenol 1993;160:1285–7.

[10] De Gaetano AM, Lafortune M, Patriquin H, et al. Cavernous transformation of the portal vein: patterns of intrahepatic and splanchnic collateral circulation detected with Doppler sonography. AJR Am J Roentgenol 1995;165:1151–9.

[11] Catalano D, Caruso G, DiFazzio S, et al. Portal vein pulsatility ratio and heart failure. J Clin Ultrasound 1998;26(1):27–31.

[12] Gallix BP, Taourel P, Dauzat M, et al. Flow pulsatility in the portal venous system: a study of Doppler sonography in healthy adults. AJR Am J Roentgenol 1997;169(1):141–4.

[13] Gorg C, Riera-Knorrenschild J, Dietrich J. Colour Doppler ultrasound flow patterns in the portal venous system. Br J Radiol 2002;75(899): 919–29.

[14] Wachsberg RH, Bahramipour P, Sofocleous CT, et al. Hepatofugal flow in the portal venous system: pathophysiology, imaging findings, and diagnostic pitfalls. Radiographics 2002;22:123–40.

[15] Bolognesi M, Sacerdoti D, Bombonato G, et al. Arterioportal fistulas in patients with liver cirrhosis: usefulness of color Doppler US for screening. Radiology 2000;216:738–43.

[16] Lafortune M, Trinh BC, Burns PN, et al. Air in the portal vein: sonographic and Doppler manifestations. Radiology 1991;180(3):667–70.

[17] Brown MA, Hauschildt JP, Casola G, et al. Intravascular gas as an incidental finding at US after blunt abdominal trauma. Radiology 1999; 210(2):405–8.

[18] Chezmar JL, Nelson RC, Bernardino ME. Portal venous gas after hepatic transplantation: sonographic detection and clinical significance. AJR Am J Roentgenol 1989;153(6):1203–5.

[19] Chevallier P, Peten E, Souci J, et al. Detection of portal venous gas on sonography, but not on CT. Eur Radiol 2002;12:1175–8.

[20] Lopez-Machado E, Mallorquin-Jimenez F, Medina-Benitez A, et al. Aneurysms of the portal venous system: ultrasonography and CT findings. Eur J Radiol 1998;26:210–4.

[21] Ascenti G, Zimbaro G, Mazziotti S, et al. Intrahepatic portal vein aneurysm: three-dimensional power Doppler demonstration in four cases. Abdom Imaging 2001;26:520–3.

[22] Ohnami Y, Ishida H, Konno K, et al. Portal vein aneurysm: report of six cases and review of the literature. Abdom Imaging 1997;22:281–6.

[23] Chaubal N, Dighe M, Hanchate V, et al. Sonography in Budd-Chiari syndrome. J Ultrasound Med 2006;25:373–9.

[24] Menon NKV, Shah V, Kamath P. The Budd-Chiari syndrome. N Engl J Med 2004;350:578–85.

[25] Bargallo X, Gilabert R, Nicolau C, et al. Sonography in Budd-Chiari syndrome. AJR Am J Roentgenol 2006;187:W33–42.

[26] Valla DC. The diagnosis and management of the Budd-Chiari syndrome: consensus and controversies. Hepatology 2003;38:793–803.

[27] Berrocal T, Parron M, Alvarez-Luque A, et al. Pediatric liver transplantation: a pictorial essay of early and late complications. Radiographics 2006;26(4):1187–209.

[28] Crossin JD, Muradali D, Wilson SR. US of liver transplants: normal and abnormal. Radiographics 2003;23:1093–114.

[29] Nolten A, Sproat IA. Hepatic artery thrombosis after liver transplantation: temporal accuracy of diagnosis with duplex US and the syndrome of impending thrombosis. Radiology 1996;198: 553–9.

[30] Tamsel S, Demirpolat G, Killi R, et al. Vascular complications after liver transplantation:

evaluation with Doppler US. Abdom Imaging 2006;32(3):1–9.

[31] Middleton WD, Teefey SA, Darcy MD. Doppler evaluation of transjugular intrahepatic portosystemic shunts. Ultrasound Q 2003;19(2):56–70.

[32] Feldstein VA, Patel MD, LaBerge JM. TIPS shunts: accuracy of Doppler US in determination of patency and detection of stenoses. Radiology 1996;201:141–7.

[33] Carr CE, Tuite CM, Soulen MC, et al. Role of ultrasound surveillance of transjugular intrahepatic portosystemic shunts in the covered stent era. J Vasc Interv Radiol 2006;17(8): 1297–305.

# ULTRASOUND CLINICS

Ultrasound Clin 2 (2007) 377–390

# The Role of Sonography in Liver Transplantation

Susan J. Ackerman, MD*, Abid Irshad, MD

- Use of ultrasound for preoperative assessment
- Ultrasound in the immediate postoperative period
- Ultrasound of postoperative complications: vascular
  *Hepatic artery complications*
  *Hepatic artery thrombosis*
  *Hepatic artery stenosis*
  *Hepatic artery pseudoaneurysm*
  *Portal vein complications*
  *Inferior vena cava complications*
  *Hepatic vein complications*

- *Biliary complications*
- *Postoperative fluid collections*
- *Infection*
- Malignancy in liver transplantation
  *De novo nonlymphoid malignancies*
  *Posttransplant lymphoproliferative disorders*
  *Recurrent hepatocellular cancer*
- Rejection in transplantation
  *Acute rejection*
  *Chronic rejection*
- Summary
- References

Liver transplantation (LT) involves the surgical placement of a portion of or whole donor liver into a patient to restore hepatic function. There are two types of donor organs for LT. Cadaveric donor organs (OLTX) are taken from patients declared brain dead. The main requirement for this type of donation is that the donor liver is of appropriate size and the donor has a compatible ABO blood type. Alternatively a living donor liver transplant (LDLTX) can be performed when a healthy person donates a liver segment to a transplant patient. This is possible because the liver has the ability to regenerate. The donated segment and the remaining portion of the donor liver grow to a normal size in several weeks.

The first successful LT was performed in 1967. According to the database of the Organ Procurement and Transplantation Network (OPTN),

77,775 liver transplants were performed in the United States from January 1988 to May 2006. Of these, 74,682 were cadaveric and 3,093 were living donor liver transplants [1]. Most liver transplants are orthotopic, which means the damaged native liver is removed and replaced by the donor liver in the recipient's native hepatic bed. For patients who have end-stage chronic liver disease or acute liver failure, LT is the primary treatment option. The major indications for adult LT are alcoholic cirrhosis, cirrhosis associated with hepatitis B and hepatitis C, autoimmune hepatitis, acute liver failure, primary sclerosing cholangitis, primary biliary cirrhosis, and some neoplasms. The most common precipitating cause for LT is cirrhosis caused by hepatitis C [2]. Contraindications for LT include active infection (spontaneous bacterial peritonitis or positive human immunodeficiency virus), active

Department of Radiology, Medical University of South Carolina, 169 Ashley Avenue, Charleston, SC 29425, USA
* Corresponding author.
E-mail address: ackerman@musc.edu (S.J. Ackerman).

1556-858X/07/$ – see front matter © 2007 Elsevier Inc. All rights reserved.                    doi:10.1016/j.cult.2007.07.001
ultrasound.theclinics.com

substance or alcohol abuse, and extrahepatic malignancy. The 1-year survival rate for liver transplant patients is approximately 85% to 90%. The 5-year survival rate is 65% to 75% [3]. The survival rates for cadaveric donor transplants are within 1% of the survival rates for living related donor transplants [3]. The major complications following OLTX are identical to those of LDLTX and include hepatic artery stenosis and thrombosis, bile leaks, and biliary stenosis. The most common causes of liver transplant failure include acute or chronic rejection, technical problems, primary graft dysfunction, and infection. Ultrasound is an excellent screening modality for evaluating the post-transplant liver and for the detection and follow-up of LT complications.

## Use of ultrasound for preoperative assessment

A potential candidate for LT is first evaluated clinically to determine the severity of the liver disease. There are several scoring systems that can be used to grade the severity of liver disease, including the Child-Turcotte-Pugh (CTP) scoring system and the Model for End-Stage Liver Disease (MELD) scoring system. Although the CTP system is useful for grading the severity of liver disease, the OPTN uses the MELD system for allocation of livers to patients on the LT waiting list. Patients are screened with multiple imaging studies, including chest radiography, duplex ultrasonography, abdominal computed tomography (CT), and occasionally magnetic resonance angiography (MRA) or selective arteriogram. After the diagnosis of end-stage liver disease (ESLD) is established, any contraindications to the surgical procedure must be excluded.

Ultrasound is frequently used to exclude contraindications to transplantation and has multiple advantages compared with other imaging modalities, such as low cost, ready availability, and lack of ionizing radiation. Because cirrhosis is the most common reason for LT and cirrhosis is frequently associated with the development of hepatocellular carcinomas (HCC), ultrasound evaluation begins with initial gray-scale imaging of the liver parenchyma. Patients who have cirrhosis usually demonstrate a coarse, heterogenous echotexture on ultrasound examination. HCCs are variable in appearance depending on the size and extent of liver involvement. If a mass lesion is detected, further evaluation with cross-sectional imaging such as CT or MR imaging is warranted. Generally accepted absolute contraindications to LT include extrahepatic malignancy and secondary liver metastases with the exception of metastatic neuroendocrine tumors such as carcinoid tumors. Relative contraindications include advanced stage hepatocellular carcinomas greater than stage II. Given the new techniques in chemoembolization and radiofrequency ablation procedures, however, this may change in the near future.

In addition to evaluating the liver parenchyma, it is important to image the hepatic vasculature. Portal venous thrombosis is a common complication of chronic liver disease, with an incidence of 5% to 10% [4]. Ultrasound is sensitive and specific in the detection of portal vein thrombosis [4–7]. Although portal vein thrombosis is not an absolute contraindication to LT, the superior mesenteric vein must be patent for transplantation to be feasible if the portal vein is thrombosed or if there is cavernous transformation of the portal vein. If ultrasound cannot delineate the venous anatomy, then conventional angiography or MRA should be done. In patients who have cirrhosis and PHT, the portal vein waveform demonstrates reduced respiratory pulsatility and velocity. The patency of the recipient inferior vena cava (IVC) is also important in patients undergoing standard orthotopic LT. The hepatic veins should also be assessed for extension of thrombus, particularly in patients who have Budd-Chiari syndrome. In patients who have cirrhosis, the hepatic vein Doppler waveform may also demonstrate a loss of pulsatility. The hepatic artery is important in the donor liver but not in the recipient. Cirrhosis may cause blunting of the hepatic artery systolic component [8] with an increase in the resistive index (RI) [9]. If the portal vein is thrombosed, however, the RI in the hepatic artery usually decreases [10].

Ultrasound of the abdomen is also routinely performed as part of the imaging workup of a living donor. In addition to evaluating the solid organs to exclude mass lesions, it is important to establish that all of the donor hepatic vessels are patent. The precise anatomy and configuration of the hepatic veins is important to document, because this may dictate the surgical technique. The presence of anomalous hepatic veins should be documented. The size of the liver graft is also important. A graft should be no more than 20% larger than the explant, because larger grafts may cause compression of adjacent vessels, resulting in poor perfusion [4]. A graft should be no less than 50% of the size of the native liver, however, because the incidence of hepatic failure is increased when smaller grafts are placed [4]. At the authors' institution, CT, including computed tomography angiography (CTA) is routinely used in the assessment of living related donors.

## Ultrasound in the immediate postoperative period

Ultrasound is usually the initial imaging modality performed in the evaluation of the post-transplant liver. It is used routinely as a screening tool for early detection of occult complications and as a diagnostic tool in situations in which there is clinical evidence of graft dysfunction or systemic symptoms. There are many variations of liver transplants ranging from a segment or lobe to a whole liver transplant and numerous potential variations in vascular anastomoses, dependent on donor and recipient anatomy. It is thus important for the sonographer to understand the exact surgical procedure performed and the anatomy. The structures requiring anastomosis between the recipient and the graft are as follows: the suprahepatic IVC, the infrahepatic IVC, the portal vein, the hepatic artery, and the common bile duct. The type of anastomosis depends on the anatomy of the donor and recipient vessels and the patient's underlying disease process.

In the immediate postoperative period, ultrasound is used to evaluate the hepatic parenchyma, the hepatic vasculature, and the biliary system. At many institutions including the authors', all LT recipients have a routine ultrasound examination 24 hours after surgery. Occasionally if the liver is not perfusing well after the anastomosis, an intraoperative Doppler ultrasound of the graft vessels is required. The timing and frequency of postoperative ultrasound is variable, but there is evidence to suggest that routine color doppler ultrasound of all hepatic vessels within 24 hours following transplantation is beneficial [7]. This is because abnormalities in the initial postoperative period may be clinically occult but sonographically evident. The authors' imaging protocol includes gray-scale ultrasound of the hepatic parenchyma, biliary system, and perihepatic spaces, and color and pulse Doppler ultrasound of the hepatic artery, portal vein, IVC, and hepatic veins. Postoperative complications can be mechanical or nonmechanical. Mechanical complications involve the anastomotic sites, such as the hepatic artery, main portal vein, IVC, and common bile duct. Nonmechanical complications include rejection, allograft dysfunction, infection, and hematoma. Ultrasound plays an important role in the detection of mechanical complications [11].

## Ultrasound of postoperative complications: vascular

### Hepatic artery complications

The biliary tree of the allograft is totally dependent on hepatic artery perfusion. Poor perfusion of the hepatic artery results in biliary ischemia or necrosis, bile leaks or bilomas, biliary strictures, and infection or abscess formation. Sepsis, hepatic infarction, and hepatic failure can then occur. Complications of the hepatic artery include hepatic artery thrombosis (HAT), hepatic artery stenosis (HAS), pseudoaneurysms, and arteriovenous fistulas.

### Hepatic artery thrombosis

HAT is one of the most serious early complications post-LT, usually occurring within the first 6 weeks. The incidence of HAT is approximately 5% in adults and 9% to 18% in pediatric transplant patients [12]. The mortality rate is high, 20% to 50%, and retransplantation is often required [13]. Predisposing factors include technical or surgical problems at the anastomosis, underlying HAS, vascular redundancy, and allograft rejection. HAT should be considered in a patient who has recently undergone transplantation, has a sudden onset of high fever and an elevation in AST, or who has evidence of a bile leak. Doppler ultrasound is estimated to be 60% to 80% sensitive in detecting HAT [14]. A study by Ryan and Sidhu [15] reports increased visualization of the hepatic artery with the use of microbubble contrast medium, up to 98%. Another more recent study by Horn and colleagues [16] showed 100% sensitivity, specificity, and accuracy of contrast enhanced ultrasound in visualizing the hepatic artery. Doppler findings of HAT include absent flow in the donor hepatic artery with abnormal or absent intrahepatic flow (Fig. 1A,B). Especially in pediatric patients, however, collaterals to the liver may form from branches of the superior mesenteric artery resulting in intrahepatic parenchymal arterial flow even when the hepatic artery is thrombosed. Collateralized intrahepatic flow may be distinguished from normal intrahepatic flow on Doppler ultrasound, however, by the demonstration of a tardus parvus Doppler waveform [17], although this waveform pattern may also be seen in patients who have HAS. The normal Doppler waveform of the hepatic artery has a sharp systolic upstroke with high diastolic velocity and, thus, a low RI. In the early postoperative period, however, the Doppler waveform can be variable, particularly the diastolic component. The RI is usually increased secondary to reperfusion edema that increases peripheral vascular resistance and decreases compliance. This abnormal Doppler waveform usually resolves after 72 hours. Any cause of edema or inflammation in the transplanted liver, however, can dampen the hepatic arterial waveform. Additionally, an abnormal ultrasound in the presence of a patent artery may be seen in patients who have rejection, hepatic necrosis, or massive hypotension [12]. Although the hepatic artery waveform can be variable in the early postoperative period, the progression of a previously normal Doppler waveform to that of one characterized by absent diastolic flow or a dampened waveform is worrisome for impending HAT. Although thrombolysis and angioplasty

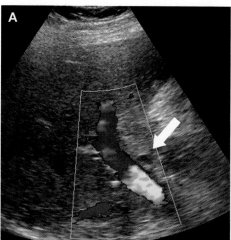 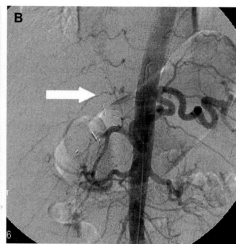

**Fig. 1.** Hepatic artery thrombosis. (A) Color Doppler image demonstrates flow in the main portal vein but no flow in the main hepatic artery (*arrow*). (B) Arteriogram confirming absence of flow in the hepatic artery (*arrow*) consistent with thrombosis.

have been used to successfully treat HAT, a large number of patients require emergent retransplantation for graft or patient survival.

### Hepatic artery stenosis

The incidence of HAS is approximately 5% to 10% [13]. It usually occurs in the early postoperative period, but may be seen several years after transplantation. HAS usually occurs at the anastomotic site and can be caused by anastomotic ischemia, intimal injury caused by catheters, clamp injury, or rejection [18]. Clinically, HAS may lead to biliary ischemia, thus causing hepatic dysfunction and possibly liver failure. Significant HAS (>50% stenosis) thus has a similar outcome to HAT. Doppler ultrasound of HAS demonstrates an intrahepatic arterial tardus parvus waveform defined as an RI of less than 0.5 and a delayed systolic acceleration time of equal to or greater than 0.08 s. Additionally, if the arterial anastomosis can be visualized, a peak systolic velocity greater than 200 cm/s is diagnostic of a stenosis. Proximal to the stenosis, a high-resistance, low-velocity pattern can be detected in the common hepatic artery. Direct Doppler visualization of the hepatic artery anastomosis, however, may be difficult secondary to tortuosity of the vessel or artifact from bowel gas. If a low RI is detected in the hepatic artery in an immediate postoperative patient who has normal hepatic function, an interval follow-up Doppler ultrasound is recommended (Fig. 2A–C), because this waveform pattern may be common transiently in the first 24 hours post-transplantation because of reperfusion edema. If there is high clinical suspicion of HAS, angiography may be done for confirmation. Treatment options

include balloon angioplasty, vascular reconstruction, or retransplantation [18].

### Hepatic artery pseudoaneurysm

The incidence of hepatic artery pseudoaneurysm following OLTX is 1% [17]. Hepatic artery pseudoaneurysms can be extrahepatic/periportal or intrahepatic. Intrahepatic artery pseudoaneurysms are usually secondary to percutaneous needle biopsy. Fistulae can also form between the aneurysm and biliary tree or portal vein. Extrahepatic pseudoaneurysms usually occur at the donor–recipient arterial anastomosis and may be caused by infection or technical failure. Regardless of their location, pseudoaneurysms are visualized as round anechoic fluid collections adjacent to the hepatic artery on gray scale ultrasound (Fig. 3A,B). Spectral and color Doppler ultrasound demonstrate flow within the lumen (if it is not thrombosed) and a "to and fro" or disorganized waveform pattern in the neck. The potential for rupture and life-threatening hemorrhage makes early diagnosis and treatment critical. Intrahepatic lesions can be treated by embolization or stent placement. Extrahepatic pseudoaneurysms are usually treated surgically, because the mortality is approximately 70% [19].

### Portal vein complications

Portal vein occlusion occurs in up to 2% of OLTX [20]. The transplanted portal vein often has abnormal flow characteristics secondary to tortuosity at the anastomosis. Predisposing factors to portal vein thrombosis include technical difficulties, misalignment or redundant length, previous portal

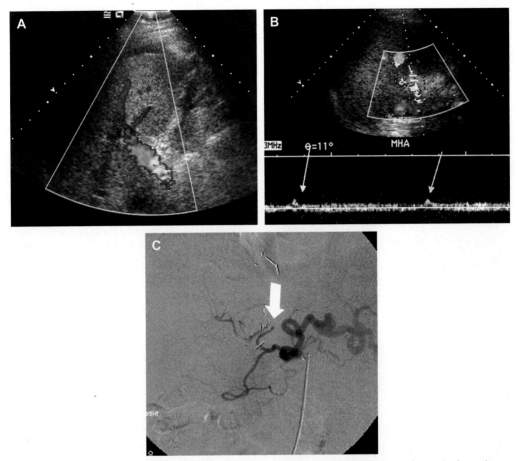

*Fig. 2.* Hepatic artery stenosis. (*A*) Color Doppler image demonstrates no flow in the main hepatic artery. (*B*) Doppler waveform in the distal hepatic artery demonstrates a low RI and abnormally decreased PSV. (*C*) Selective hepatic arteriogram confirming HAS (*arrow*).

vein thrombosis, prior shunt surgery, and hypercoagulable states [15]. Ultrasound of acute portal vein thrombosis demonstrates distention of the vessel or intraluminal echogenic thrombus and no flow. A secondary sign of portal vein thrombosis is decreased RI in the hepatic artery. Portal vein stenosis (Fig. 4) usually occurs at the donor–recipient anastomosis and can lead to portal vein thrombosis. A peak velocity of greater than 1 m/s or a three- to fourfold increase in velocity across the narrowed segment relative to velocity in the prestenotic segment is suggestive of clinically significant stenosis, at least in the setting of abnormal liver function [21]. Portal vein thrombosis and significant portal vein stenosis can cause graft dysfunction and portal hypertension (Fig. 5). Interval enlargement of the spleen and ascites may be secondary signs of portal hypertension. The treatment options for portal vein complications include angioplasty, stent placement, portosystemic shunt, and surgical revision of the venous anastomosis.

### Inferior vena cava complications

Stenosis or thrombosis of the IVC post-transplantation is rare, occurring in less than 1% of cases [22]. IVC stenosis and thrombosis may occur at either the superior or inferior IVC anastomosis. Predisposing factors for IVC stenosis include size discrepancy between donor and recipient IVC or technical problems. IVC thrombosis may occur secondary to extrinsic from an enlarged, edematous liver or fluid collection, such as a biloma or hematoma. Patients who have suprahepatic IVC stenosis/thrombosis may present with hepatomegaly, ascites, and pleural effusions. Lower extremity edema may be a complication of infrahepatic stenosis. Ultrasound of patients who have IVC thrombosis may demonstrate intraluminal echoes consistent with thrombus (Fig. 6). A stenosis of the IVC is diagnosed on ultrasound when narrowing is noted on gray-scale or color/power Doppler images associated with a three- to fourfold increase in velocity compared with the velocity in the prestenotic segment.

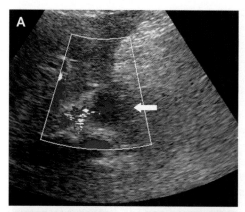

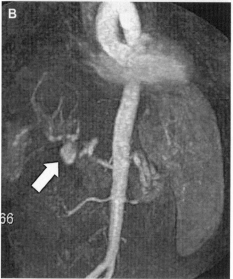

Fig. 3. Hepatic artery pseudoaneurysm. (A) Color Doppler image demonstrates flow within fluid collection adjacent to the main hepatic artery (*arrow*). (B) Coronal T1 post-gadolinium MR image of the pseudoaneurysm (*arrow*).

Indirect findings of suprahepatic IVC stenosis or thrombosis include distension, reversal of flow, and loss of phasicity in the hepatic veins [23]. Treatment options for IVC stenosis include balloon angioplasty and stent placement.

## Hepatic vein complications

Hepatic vein thrombosis is a rare complication, occurring in less than 1% of LT recipients, because the hepatic veins are not directly involved in a surgical anastomosis [24]. Any process that alters liver compliance may change hepatic vein pulsatility. Ischemia, rejection, and cholangitis may cause dampening of the spectral Doppler waveform. In recipients whose transplant was performed because of liver failure secondary to Budd-Chiari syndrome, hepatic vein and IVC thrombosis may recur (Fig. 7A,B).

## Biliary complications

Biliary complications are an important cause of morbidity and mortality following postoperative LT, occurring in 20% of patients [25]. The major complications are bile leakage, strictures of the bile ducts, and biliary obstruction. Eighty percent of biliary complications occur within the first 6 months after transplantation, although bile duct strictures can occur years later [26]. Factors that influence the frequency and severity of complications include surgical anastomosis, prolonged cold ischemic time, and vascular insufficiency. Most bile leaks or bilomas are secondary to anastomotic complications and occur early, within the first 30 days of LT [15]. Bile may extravasate freely or form a perihepatic fluid collection. Ultrasound is sensitive in detecting perihepatic fluid but may not be able to differentiate bland ascites from hematoma or infected fluid (Fig. 8A). Ultrasound-

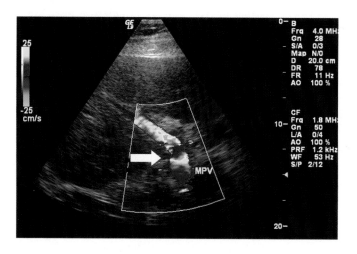

Fig. 4. Portal vein stenosis. Color Doppler image of stenosis of the main portal vein. Note narrowing and focal color aliasing at the stenosis (*arrow*).

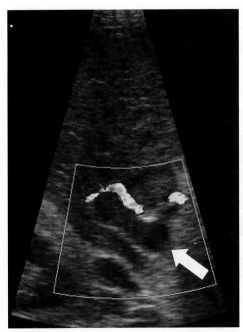

*Fig. 5.* Portal vein thrombosis. Sagittal color Doppler image showing no flow within the main portal vein (*arrow*).

guided aspiration can be performed for diagnosis. Additionally, bilomas can mimic periportal edema. The presence of a biloma usually indicates severe or extensive bile duct necrosis and is associated with graft dysfunction and failure [27]. Clinically, patients may present with abdominal pain or signs and symptoms of sepsis. A bile leak or biloma can be confirmed by nuclear medicine hepatobiliary scans or by endoscopic retrograde cholangiopancreatography (ERCP) (Fig. 8B). Small bile leaks can seal spontaneously. Large bile leaks, however, typically require intervention or surgical correction. Bile duct strictures can be anastomotic or

nonanastomotic. Nonasastomotic strictures have a worse prognosis and usually reflect diffuse biliary injury, such as with rejection or HAT and HAS. Compromise of the hepatic artery can result in ischemia or necrosis of the biliary system. This is suspected if ultrasound reveals dilated bile ducts with intraluminal debris. Patients may present with abnormal liver function tests or progressive obstructive jaundice. Anastomotic strictures may result from technical difficulties or scarring. Ultrasound usually shows dilatation of the proximal bile duct to the level of the anastomosis with dilated intrahepatic ducts (Fig. 9A,B).

Intrahepatic ductal dilatation has a higher predictive value for biliary obstruction than the dilatation of the common bile duct [28]. Ultrasound may not be able to identify a bile duct stricture in the absence of dilatation of the biliary tree. Stricture or dilatation can occur without obstruction or leakage and may be associated with acute rejection, ischemia, or cholangitis. Ultrasound may demonstrate irregular intrahepatic ducts that do not taper normally and demonstrate increased periductal echogenicity [29]. Bile duct strictures may be treated by percutaneous transhepatic cholangiography (PTC), ERCP, or surgical revision. Recurrence of primary sclerosing cholangitis occurs in approximately 20% of cases, usually within 1 year of transplantation [11]. Ultrasound demonstrates dilated, irregular bile ducts with a normal hepatic artery Doppler waveform.

### Postoperative fluid collections

Fluid collections and ascites occur commonly post-transplantation, usually in the gallbladder fossa and subhepatic space. Hematomas are one of the most common postoperative fluid collections. On ultrasound these appear as complex, avascular fluid collections. Occasionally acute hemorrhage can be uniformly echogenic and may resemble a solid

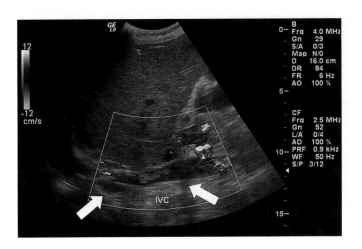

*Fig. 6.* IVC thrombus. Color Doppler image of thrombus (*arrow*) in the IVC at the level of the hepatic veins.

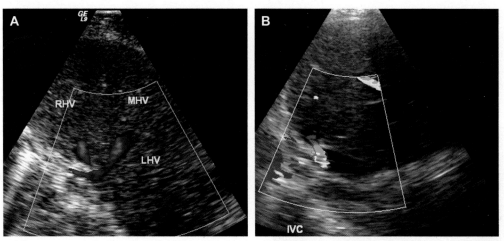

**Fig. 7.** Hepatic vein and IVC thrombus in a patient whose transplant was performed because of liver failure secondary to Budd-Chiari syndrome. (*A*) Color Doppler image of thrombosis of the left hepatic vein. Note color flow in the right and middle hepatic veins. (*B*) Color Doppler image of nonocclusive thrombosis of the IVC.

mass (Fig. 10). Hematomas usually resolve spontaneously without the need for aspiration or drainage unless they become infected. Interval increase in the size of a fluid collection or the development of a new collection may indicate a bile leak or may be a consequence of portal vein or IVC abnormalities [30]. If the patient has tense ascites, ultrasound-guided drainage can be performed to prevent hepatic dysfunction caused by compression. Abdominal bleeding after the immediate postoperative period may be caused by hepatic artery pseudoaneurysm, leakage of a vascular anastomosis, or hemobilia, and is seen in less than 10% of patients [31]. Occasionally intraparenchymal fluid collections are noted within the transplanted liver. These may represent hematomas, bilomas, fluid within the ligamentum teres, or contusions (Fig. 11A,B).

## Infection

In the early post-transplantation period, infections usually result from surgical complications, such as biliary leaks (Fig. 12A,B), hemorrhage, hepatic artery thrombosis, acute graft failure, or pre-existing latent infections [25,30–34]. Postoperative fluid collections are common and usually occur near the vascular anastomoses. The risk for superinfection of these fluid collections is high, given the immunocompromised state of liver transplant patients. The most common site for early postoperative infection in the liver transplant recipient is the abdomen. Intrahepatic and extrahepatic abscesses, peritonitis, wound infections, and cholangitis may complicate LT. The incidence of hepatic abscesses is 2.6% to 3.9% in adult liver transplant recipients [30,33,34]. Abscesses are solitary in approximately two thirds of cases and most are caused by bacterial

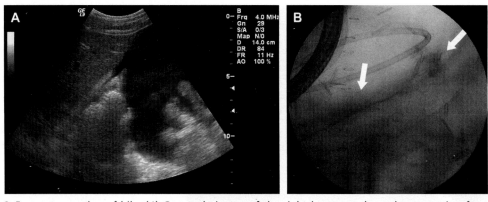

**Fig. 8.** Free extravasation of bile. (*A*) Gray-scale image of the right lower quadrant demonstrating free fluid with multiple low-level internal echoes. (*B*) ERCP confirms a bile leak (*arrow*).

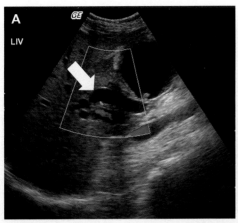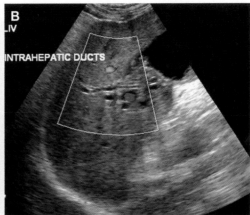

Fig. 9. Patient who had progressive obstructive jaundice and an anastomotic stricture of the central bile duct. (A) Dilatation of the bile duct (*arrow*). (B) Note dilated intrahepatic ducts.

pathogens with Gram positive species recovered more frequently than Gram negative species [33,34]. Polymicrobial abscesses are not uncommon. HAT is the most common predisposing condition, although the presentation of abscess secondary to HAT may be delayed by several months [33,34]. Abscesses may also occur in patients who have cholangitis caused by biliary obstruction [32,34]. The classic sonographic findings of hepatic abscess include single or multiple parenchymal hypoechoic or hyperechoic lesions. Doppler interrogation does not reveal flow centrally, but increased flow may be noted peripherally and the outer margin may be irregular [15,34]. The lesion may contain echogenic areas with "dirty" shadowing consistent with gas (Fig. 13). The major risk factor for development of infection in the time frame of 2 to 6 months after LT is the immunosuppressive therapy necessary to treat or prevent transplant rejection. Depression of cell-mediated immunity makes the liver transplant recipient particularly vulnerable to viral infections, including cytomegalovirus, varicella, and recurrent hepatitis B and C [34]. The imaging findings of hepatic viral infections are nonspecific; therefore, the diagnosis relies on liver function tests, serology, high clinical suspicion, and liver biopsy.

## Malignancy in liver transplantation

Malignancy is the second leading cause of death in liver transplant patients, following age-related cardiovascular disease [35]. Similar to other solid organ transplant recipients, the incidence of malignancy is increased following LT. There have been several studies that have documented increased risk for various malignancies [35–38]. The post-transplant malignancies may be divided into the following categories:

1. De novo nonlymphoid malignancies
2. Post-transplant lymphoproliferative disorder (PTLD)
3. Recurrent hepatocellular cancer (in patients transplanted for primary HCC or cirrhosis)

### De novo nonlymphoid malignancies

The most common de novo malignancies seen after LT are skin cancers [39]. These include squamous cell cancer, basal cell cancer, Kaposi sarcoma, and melanoma. Other common de novo nonlymphoid malignancies include oropharyngeal, lung, gastrointestinal, and genitourinary tumors. Immunosuppression plays a key role in the development of these tumors. Viral infections, especially Epstein-Barr virus (EBV), play an important role in the development of post-transplant proliferative disorder (PTLD), skin cancers, and Kaposi sarcoma [35]. The incidence of skin cancer varies with the

Fig. 10. Hematoma in the hepatorenal space simulating a solid mass.

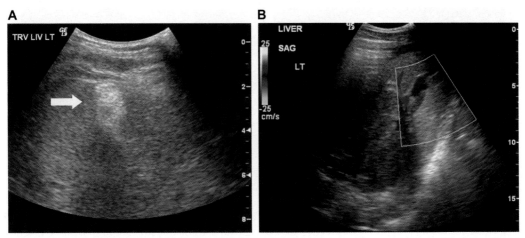

*Fig. 11.* Intraparenchymal hematoma (*A*) gray-scale image of an echogenic mass (*arrow*). (*B*) Color Doppler image of fluid within the ligamentum teres in a different patient.

time interval after transplantation and ranges from 13% at 5 years to 26% at 8 years [38]. Increasing age is a risk factor for developing these cancers. Most of these cancers have a high mortality rate, except skin cancers, which have shown better survival rates. Most cancers occur 2 to 6 years post-transplantation. Among the primary causes of explanted liver failure, alcoholic cirrhosis was found to have a significantly higher association with subsequent development of these nonlymphoid malignancies [37]. The type of immunosuppression may not play a key role in determining the incidence of nonlymphoid tumors; however, the degree of immunosuppression is probably related to the amount of increased risk. Careful long-term screening protocols are required for surveillance of these patients

for tumors. Ultrasound may show relevant findings in the involved internal organs and ultrasound-guided biopsy is useful to establish a definitive diagnosis.

### Posttransplant lymphoproliferative disorders

PTLD may present clinically as an increase in total gamma globulin level and the appearance of mono or oligoclonal immunoglobulins. It thus has a broad clinical spectrum ranging from mononucleosis-like illness to frank lymphoma [40]. PTLD including lymphoma may involve the liver or extrahepatic structures. The overall incidence of PTLD in -LT patients is approximately 4% to 5% [41]. The incidence is much higher in children (approximately 10%) compared with adults

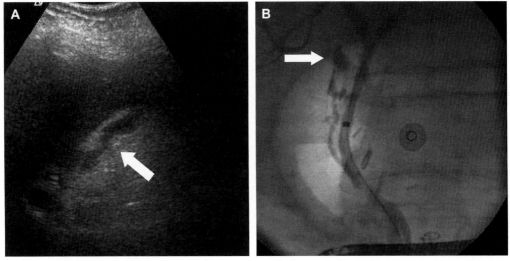

*Fig. 12.* Bile leak resulting in peritonitis. (*A*) Gray-scale image depicting a fluid collection in the gallbladder fossa (*arrow*). (*B*) ERCP image confirming a bile leak (*arrow*).

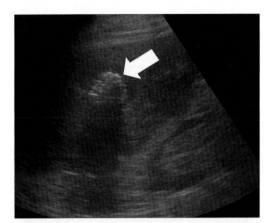

Fig. 13. Hepatic abscess. Gray-scale image showing echogenic area with "dirty" shadowing in the right hepatic lobe classic for gas.

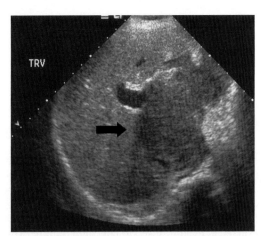

Fig. 14. Hypoechoic mass in the porta hepatic (*arrow*), biopsy proven to be PTLD.

(approximately 3%). PTLD is associated with decreased survival rates. In adults, the type of immunosuppression may not make a significant difference in the incidence of developing PTLD. In children, however, a higher incidence was noted with tacrolimus than with cyclosporine [41]. The average time to development of PTLD is approximately 10 months. This time frame is much shorter in children than in adults. PTLD may involve a single or multiple sites. Lymph nodes are the most common site of involvement (35%). Other common sites involved are the gastrointestinal tract, liver, spleen, and central nervous system (CNS). EBV plays an important role in the development of PTLD [41,42], because 60% to 80% of patients test positive. Depending on the site of involvement, ultrasound may show nodal masses in the abdomen or may show hypoechoic focal masses within the liver or at the porta hepatis (Fig. 14). Treatment involves reducing the immunosuppressive drugs together with antiviral therapy and immunotherapy.

## Recurrent hepatocellular cancer

In patients in whom liver transplant was originally performed for treatment of HCC, recurrent tumor may be noted in approximately 10% to 25% of cases [43–45]. Recurrence usually occurs within 2 years of transplantation and is associated with decreased survival rates. Although recurrent HCC usually occurs in the early post-transplant period, some tumors may occur later, when it may be difficult to differentiate a recurrence from a de novo HCC. Biopsy of the tumor with DNA testing may establish whether the cancer is recurrent, is derived from the patient's explant liver HCC, or is a de novo occurrence of a new cell line of HCC. Recurrence

most commonly occurs in the lungs, liver, and lymph nodes [46].

Routine ultrasound or CT surveillance helps detect focal mass lesions within the liver or extrahepatic nodes. Recurrent and de novo HCC may present as a focal mass lesion or as multifocal involvement of the liver. Metastatic disease to the transplanted liver may have a similar ultrasound appearance.

## Rejection in transplantation

### Acute rejection

Clinically, acute rejection is associated with jaundice and abnormal liver function tests. It may be associated with fever, liver tenderness, and eosinophilia. It is usually treated with high-dose steroids. The incidence of rejection has decreased during the past 20 years, as has the time period to first acute rejection episode [47]. The incidence of acute rejection varies from 20% to 70% [47]. The average time to acute rejection is 7 to 20 days. Multiple episodes of rejection may occur. Approximately 7% of episodes of rejections may be steroid-resistant. It has been suggested that large volume blood loss during surgery is associated with a decreased occurrence of acute rejection [47]. This most likely is secondary to a temporary immunosuppressive effect from bleeding.

The diagnostic role of ultrasound in acute rejection is limited, and usually a liver biopsy is required to establish the diagnosis. It has been suggested that decreased portal blood velocity and slightly increased splenic pulsatility index on Duplex sonography is associated with acute rejection, showing a good accuracy of approximately 88% [48]. The authors, however, have not noted this at our institution. More studies are required to confirm these findings. In cases of living donor LT, the attenuation indices of the liver on noncontrast CT scans in the early post-transplant period have been correlated with early graft dysfunction and hence decreased 1-year survival rate [49]. Conversely, findings on duplex Doppler ultrasound of the hepatic artery have not been shown to be predictive of acute or chronic rejection [50].

## Chronic rejection

Chronic hepatic allograft rejection occurs infrequently, in less than 10% of cases, and is characterized pathologically by obliterative vasculopathy, foam cell changes, and bile duct loss. Chronic rejection is a major cause of late graft failure. The incidence of graft loss caused by chronic rejection, however, has decreased over time. Clinically chronic rejection manifests as a cholestatic pattern of liver injury often accompanied by jaundice or pruritus. No gray-scale or duplex ultrasound features specific to chronic rejection have been described, and the diagnosis is usually established at liver biopsy.

## Summary

The role of ultrasound in LT is well established, and ultrasound is routinely used for pre- and post-liver transplant evaluation. The role of ultrasound in pretransplant evaluation is primarily to identify any contraindication to transplantation, because vascular and biliary tract abnormalities are now primarily evaluated by MR imaging, MRA, magnetic resonance venogram and magnetic resonance choliangopancreatography. The major role of ultrasound in evaluating patients in the immediate to early post-transplant period is to search for vascular or biliary complications that may require surgical intervention to save the graft. CT is helpful in detecting or confirming postoperative complications. Over the long term, routine ultrasound surveillance helps to identify potential delayed complications of LT, such as bile duct strictures, hepatic artery or portal vein stenoses, and malignancy. The value of ultrasound in acute or chronic graft rejection or dysfunction is limited, and more studies may be required to establish the role of duplex ultrasound in these clinical situations.

## References

[1] U.S. Department of Health and Human Services. 2005 Annual Report of the U.S. Organ Procurement and Transplantation Network and the Scientific Registry of Transplant Recipients. Transplant Data 1995–2004. Rockville, MD: Health Resources and Services Administration, Healthcare Systems Bureau, Division of Transplantation.

[2] Keefee EB. Selection of patients for liver transplantation. In: Maddrey WC, Schiff ER, Sorrell MR, editors. Transplantation of the liver. 3rd edition. Philadelphia: Lippincott Williams & Wilkins; 2001. p. 5–34.

[3] Manzarbeitia C. Liver transplantation, e Medicine. Available at: www.emedicine.com. Accessed January 26, 2006.

[4] Shaw A, Siddhu PS. Ultrasound assessment of the liver transplant candidate. In: Siddhu PS, Baxter GM, editors. Ultrasound of abdominal transplantation. 1st edition. Stuttgart: Thieme; 2002. p. P76–87.

[5] Tessler FN, Gehring BJ, Gomes AS, et al. Diagnosis of portal vein thrombosis: value of color Doppler imaging. AJR Am J Roentgenol 1991; 157:293–6.

[6] Kolmannskog F, Jakobsen JA, Schrumpf E, et al. Duplex Doppler sonography and angiography in the evaluation for liver transplantation. Acta Radiol 1994;35:1–5.

[7] Alpern MB, Rubin JM, Williams DM, et al. Porta hepatic: duplex Doppler US with angiographic correlation. Radiology 1987;162:53–6.

[8] Iwao T, Toyonaga A, Shigermori H, et al. Hepatic artery hemodynamic responsiveness to altered portal blood flow in normal and cirrhotic livers. Radiology 1996;200:793–8.

[9] Schneider AW, Kalk JF, Klein CP. Hepatic arterial pulsatility index in cirrhosis: correlation with portal pressure. J Hepatol 1999;30:876–81.

[10] Platt JF, Rubin JM, Ellis JH. Hepatic artery resistance changes in portal vein thrombosis. Radiology 1995;196:95–8.

[11] Russ P, Elliott D, Durham J, et al. Liver transplantation complications, e Medicine. Available at: www.emedicine.com. Accessed September 9, 2005.

[12] Karani JB, Heaton ND. Imaging in liver transplantation. Clin Radiol 1998;53:317–22.

[13] Nolten A, Sproat IA. Hepatic artery thrombosis after transplantation; temporal accuracy of diagnosis with duplex ultrasound and the syndrome of impending thrombosis. Radiology 1996;198: 553–9.

[14] Kok T, Slooff MJH, Thijn CJ, et al. Routine Doppler ultrasound for the detection of clinically unsuspected vascular complications in the early post operative phase after orthotopic liver transplantation. Transpl Int 1998;11:272–6.

[15] Ryan SM, Siddhu PS. Early postoperative liver transplant ultrasound. In: Siddhu PS, Baxter GM, editors. Ultrasound of abdominal transplantation. 1st edition. Stuttgart: Thieme; 2002. p. 90–103.

[16] Horn BK, Shrestha R, Palmer S, et al. Prospective evaluation of vascular complications after liver transplantation: comparison of conventional and microbubble contrast-enhanced US. Radiology 2006;241:267–74.

[17] Dodd GD, Mernel DS, Zaijko AB, et al. Hepatic artery stenosis and thrombosis in transplant recipients: Doppler diagnosis with resistive index and systolic acceleration time. Radiology 1994; 192:657–61.

[18] Wozney P, Zajko AB, Bron KM, et al. Vascular complications after liver transplantation: a 5-year experience. AJR Am J Roentgenol 1986; 147:657–63.

[19] Rollins NK, Timmons C, Superina RA, et al. Hepatic artery thrombosis in children with liver transplants: false positive findings at Doppler sonography and arteriography in four patients. AJR Am J Roentgenol 1993;160:291.

[20] Abbasoglu O, Levy MR, Vodapally MS, et al. Hepatic artery stenosis after liver transplantation—incidence, presentation, treatment, and long term outcome. Transplantation 1997;27: 250–5.

[21] Marshall MM, Muiesan P, Kane PA, et al. Hepatic pseudoaneurysms following liver transplantation: incidence, presenting figures and management. Clin Radiol 2001;56:579–87.

[22] Glockner JF, Forauer AR. Vascular or ischemic complications after liver transplantation. AJR Am J Roentgenol 1999;173:1055–9.

[23] Lerut J, RTzakis A, Bron KM, et al. Complications of venous reconstruction in human orthotopic liver transplantation. Ann Surg 1987;205: 404–14.

[24] Meire H. Transplant liver assessment. In: Meire H, Cosgrove DO, Dewbury K, et al, editors. Abdominal and general ultrasound. 2nd edition. London: Churchill Livingstone; 2000. p. 280–94.

[25] Ngheim H, Tran K, Winter TC, et al. Imaging of complications in liver transplantation. Radiographics 1996;16:825–40.

[26] Crossin J, Muradali D, Wilson S. US of liver transplants: normal and abnormal. Radiographics 2003;23:1093–114.

[27] Everson GT, Kam I. Immediate postoperative care. In: Maddrey WC, Schiff ER, Sorrell MF, editors. Transplantation of the liver. 3rd edition. Philadelphia: Lippincott Williams and Wilkins; 2001. p. 31–162.

[28] Gow PJ, Chapman RW. Liver transplantation for primary sclerosing cholangitis. Liver 2000;20: 97–103.

[29] Woods RP, Shaw BW, Starzl TE. Extrahepatic complications of liver transplantation. Semin Liver Dis 1985;5:377–84.

[30] Winston D, Emmanoulides C, Busuttil R. Infections in liver transplant recipients. Clin Infect Dis 1995;21:1077–91.

[31] Bowen A, Hungate R, Kaye R, et al. Imaging in liver transplantation. Radiol Clin North Am 1996;34:757–78.

[32] Boraschi P, Donati F. Complications of orthotopic liver transplantation: imaging findings. Abdom Imaging 2004;2:189–202.

[33] Tachopoulou Oa, Vogt DP, Henderson JM, et al. Hepatic abscess after liver transplantation. Transplantation 2003;75:79–83.

[34] Poghosyan T, Ackerman S, Ravenel J. Infectious complications of solid organ transplantation. Semin Roentgenol 2006;42(1):11–2.

[35] Fung JJ, Jain A, Kwak EJ, et al. De novo malignancies after liver transplantation: a major cause of late death. Liver Transpl 2003;7(11B):s109–18.

[36] Yao FY, Gautam M, Palese C, et al. De novo malignancies following liver transplantation: a case-control study with long-term follow-up. Clin Transplant 2006;20(5):617.

[37] Saigal S, Norris S, Muiesan P, et al. Evidence of differential risk for posttransplantation malignancy based on pretransplantation cause in patients undergoing liver transplantation. Liver Transpl 2002;8(5):482–7.

[38] Xiol X, Guardiola J, Menendez S, et al. Risk factors for development of de novo neoplasia after liver transplantation. Liver Transpl 2001;7(11): 971–5.

[39] Morrison VA, Dunn DL, Manivel JC, et al. Clinical characteristics of post-transplant lymphoproliferative disorders. Am J Med 1994;97:14–24.

[40] Otley CC, Pittelkow MR. Skin cancer in liver transplant recipients. Liver Transpl 2000;6(3): 253–62.

[41] Jain A, Nalesnik M, Reyes J, et al. Posttransplant lymphoproliferative disorders in liver transplantation: a 20-year experience. Ann Surg 2002; 236(4):429–37.

[42] Sokal EM, Antunes H, Beguin C, et al. Early signs and risk factors for the increased incidence of Epstein-Barr virus-related posttransplant lymphoproliferative diseases in pediatric liver transplant recipients treated with tacrolimus. Transplantation 1997;64(10):1438–42.

[43] Roayaie S, Schwartz JD, Sung MW, et al. Recurrence of hepatocellular carcinoma after liver transplant: patterns and prognosis. Liver Transpl 2004;10(4):534–40.

[44] Klinmalm GB. Liver transplantation for hepatocellular carcinoma. A registry report of the impact of tumor characteristics on outcome. Ann Surg 1998;228:479–90.

[45] Yao FY, Ferrel L, Bass NM, et al. Liver transplantation for hepatocellular carcinoma: expansion of the tumor size limits does not adversely impact survival. Hepatology 2001;331:1394–403.

[46] Ferris JV, Baron RL, Marsh JW Jr, et al. Recurrent hepatocellular carcinoma after liver transplantation: spectrum of CT findings and recurrence patterns. Radiology 1996;198(1):233–8.

[47] Matinlauri LH, Nurminen MN, Hockerstedt KA, et al. Changes in liver graft rejections over time. Transplant Proc 2006;38(8):2663–6.

[48] Bolognesi M, Sacerdoti D, Mescoli C, et al. Acute liver rejection: accuracy and predictive values of Doppler US measurements—initial experience. Radiology 2005;235(2):651–8.

[49] Cho JY, Suh KS, Lee HW, et al. Hypoattenuation in unenhanced CT reflects histological graft dysfunction and predicts 1-year mortality after living donor liver transplantation. Liver Transpl 2006;12(9):1403–11.

[50] Longley DG, Skolnick ML, Sheahan DG. Acute allograft rejection in liver transplant recipients: lack of correlation with loss of hepatic artery diastolic flow. Radiology 1988; 169(2):417–20.

# ULTRASOUND CLINICS

Ultrasound Clin 2 (2007) 391–413

# Ultrasound Imaging of the Biliary Tract

Deborah J. Rubens, MD

Patients who have disease of the biliary tract commonly present with acute right upper quadrant pain, nausea or vomiting, mid-epigastric pain, and/ or jaundice. Etiologies include inflammation with or without infection, noninflammatory disorders, and benign or malignant neoplasms of the gallbladder or bile ducts. Ultrasound (US) is now accepted as the initial imaging modality of choice for the work-up of suspected biliary tract disease.

This article reviews the most common diseases of the gallbladder and bile ducts, strategies for evaluating the biliary tract with ultrasound, and specific imaging patterns that aid in diagnosis.

## Inflammatory disorders: cholecystitis

Acute cholecystitis most often occurs secondary to obstruction of the gallbladder with resultant inflammation of the gallbladder wall. There may or may not be associated infection and necrosis. Ninety to ninety-five percent of all cases of acute cholecystitis are caused by obstruction of either the cystic duct or the neck of the gallbladder by gallstones [1]. Acute cholecystitis, however, occurs in only approximately 20% of patients who have gallstones [2]. This means that most gallstones are asymptomatic. Thus, right upper quadrant pain in a patient who has gallstones often is caused by something other than acute cholecystitis [3]. Furthermore, studies have shown that only 20%–35% of patients presenting with right upper quadrant pain are subsequently shown to have acute cholecystitis [1,2]. Therefore, it is important to understand the sensitivity and specificity of common US findings in patients who have acute cholecystitis, because the presence of gallstones alone is not adequate to

University of Rochester Medical Center, Department of Imaging Sciences, 601 Elmwood Avenue, Rochester, NY 14642-8648, USA
E-mail address: deborah_rubens@urmc.rochester.edu

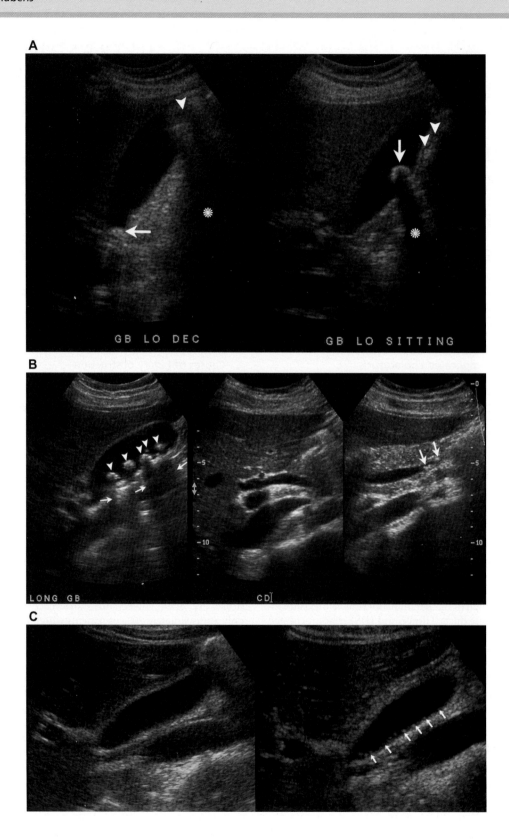

A

GB LO DEC          GB LO SITTING

B

LONG GB          CD

C

make the diagnosis of acute cholecystitis. The combination of US findings that is most predictive of acute cholecystitis is the presence of a positive sonographic Murphy' sign plus the presence of gallstones. Secondary signs on US examination of acute cholecystitis include gallbladder wall thickening (>3 mm), a distended or hydropic gallbladder (loss of the normal tapered neck and development of an elliptic or rounded shape), and pericholecystic fluid.

## The sonographic Murphy's sign

The sonographic Murphy sign is defined as reproducible point tenderness specifically over the gallbladder upon application of pressure by the transducer. Ralls and colleagues [4] wrote a classic article that reported a sonographic Murphy sign was 87% specific for the diagnosis of acute cholecystitis, in a patient population which only included patients who had right upper quadrant pain, fever and an elevated white blood cell count. Laing and colleagues [5] reported that the presence of a positive sonographic Murphy's sign in combination with the presence of gallstones has a positive predictive value of 92% for the diagnosis of acute cholecystitis. In order to avoid false positive examinations, one must be careful to elicit pain directly over the gallbladder, not diffusely in epigastrium, or over the liver edge. False negative examinations may occur in patients who have received pain medicine, patients who are taking steroids, para or quadriplegics, or any patient who is not able to give a reliable history or pain response. In addition, the sonographic Murphy's sign may be absent in denervated gallbladders, for example, in patients who have diabetes or gangrenous cholecystitis. A sonographic Murphy's sign also may be significantly diminished if the gallbaldder ruptures because this will relieve the obstruction. Therefore, careful attention to the patient's clinical status is important when assessing for a sonographic Murphy's sign.

## Gallstones

Gallstones are diagnosed on US by the presence of gravity-dependent, mobile, echogenic foci within the gallbladder lumen that cast a posterior shadow (Fig. 1). Although ultrasound has been demonstrated to have an accuracy (>95%) for the identification of gallstones, stones that are too small, (usually <1 mm to cast a posterior shadow soft stones lacking strong internal echoes [1], or gallstones impacted in the gallbladder neck or in the cystic duct that may not be as readily detectable on US examination as they silhouette with the surrounding echogenic bowel gas or intraperitoneal fat (see Fig. 1) [5]. If the gallbladder is focally tender but no gallstones are appreciated, the patient should be examined from multiple positions and scanning planes, including prone, upright and decubitus positions and intercostal scanning, to facilitate complete visualization of the neck of the gallbladder [3,6].

Harmonic imaging significantly improves visualization of small gallstones. This type of ultrasound transmits the insonating US beam at a fundamental frequency, such as 2.5 or 3 MHz, and receives the returning echoes not only at the fundamental frequency but also at the second harmonic frequency that is twice the fundamental frequency creating the image with the higher harmonic frequency [7–9]. By eliminating the fundamental frequency, this technique significantly reduces degradation of the image by noise, since lower frequencies easily can be filtered out. In addition, scattering of the US beam from fat in the anterior abdominal wall is diminished because the harmonic frequencies are generated after the beam enters the body. The narrower harmonic beam also has fewer side lobes, and therefore, improved lateral resolution and signal to noise ratio. Harmonic imaging increases the echogenicity of gallstones and strengthens their posterior shadows, permitting visualization of stones not seen with conventional grayscale ultrasound (see Fig. 1). Another technique that improves visualization of stones is spatial compounding. Multiple images are acquired slightly off axis from one another, which increases the signal from the persistent echoes that comprise the image and blurs out some of the random noise. The disadvantage of compounding is that posterior shadowing is diminished, which may be a better visual cue to detect typical gallstones than the actual echoes

*Fig. 1.* Gallstones. (A) (*Left*) Gallstone in the gallbladder neck (*arrow*) casts no significant shadow and is nearly invisible. Gas in the duodenum (*arrowhead*) obscures the fundus of the gallbladder and casts a strong sharp shadow (*asterisk*). (*Right*) With patient in sitting position, stone (*arrow*) moves out of the neck and casts a clear shadow (*asterisk*). Adjacent duodenum (*arrowheads*) is now separate from the gallbladder but still casts a strong shadow, equivalent to the gallbladder. (B) (*Left*) Multiple gallstones (*arrowheads*), some of which cast shadows (*arrows*), whereas others do not. (*Right*) Normal caliber common duct (6 mm at the porta) with stones (*arrows*) in the same patient. Choledocholithiasis may be difficult to detect, especially in the distal duct, if the stones do not shadow or are not outlined by fluid. (C) (*Left*) Longitudinal ultrasound shows a normal gallbladder. (*Right*) Harmonic imaging reveals multiple small stones (*arrows*). (*From* Rubens D. Hepatobiliary imaging and its pitfalls. Radiol Clin North Am 2004;42:257–78; with permission.)

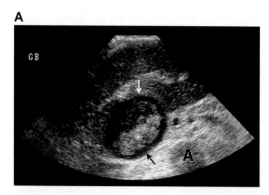

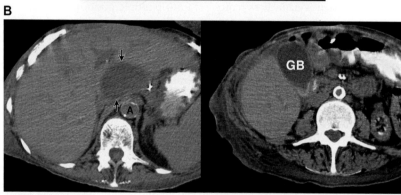

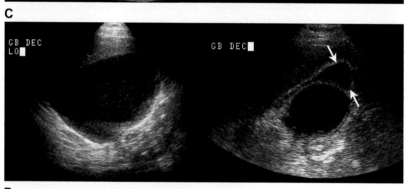

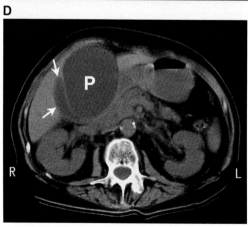

from the stones themselves. So, while harmonic imaging definitely improves detection, spatial compounding remains optional on an individual case basis.

Other stones such as soft pigment stones may not shadow with any technique. Soft pigment stones are less echogenic than the more common cholesterol gallstones and may simulate soft tissue masses. Pigmented stones are commonly associated with recurrent pyogenic cholangiohepatitis and are more often seen in the bile ducts than in the gallbladder. Because of their lack of shadowing, they may be misinterpreted as sludge or debris and result in a false negative examination.

False positive US diagnosis of gallstones may occur secondary to side lobe artifacts that can generate echoes appearing to arise within the gallbladder lumen but actually originate from the wall or outside the wall [1]. Similarly, gas in adjacent bowel can create a brightly echogenic mass-like area with posterior shadowing, which appears to be within the gallbladder lumen because of a partial volume artifact and thereby mimics gallstones (Fig. 1A). A calcium bile salt precipitate may form in patients taking the antibiotic ceftriaxone and may mimic gallstones on sonographic examination. These precipitates resolve after the patient ends therapy.

Other fluid-containing structures such as the duodenum, gastric antrum, colon, hematomas, pancreatic pseudocysts (Fig. 2), or even dilated vascular collaterals may be mistaken for the gallbladder on US examination, especially if the gallbladder is out of its normal position or is small and contracted. Mistaking these structures for the gallbladder may result in missing pathology in the true gallbladder or a false-positive diagnosis of gallbladder disease (ie, obstructed gallbladder or acalculous cholecystitis).

## Gallbladder wall thickening and pericholecystic fluid

Gallbladder wall thickening is defined as a wall diameter greater than 3 mm and is present in 50% of patients who have acute cholecystitis (Fig. 3) [1]. However, this is a very non-specific

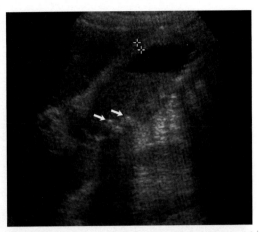

Fig. 3. Acute cholecystitis. This patient presented with RUQ pain and had a positive sonographic Murphy sign. Longitudinal ultrasound shows stones (*arrows*) and diffuse gallbladder wall thickening (*cursors*) measuring 5 mm. (*From* Harrow A. The gallbladder and biliary tree. In: Dogra V, Rubens D, editors. Ultrasound secrets. Philadelphia: Hanley and Belfus; 2004. p. 113–29; with permission.)

finding, because numerous other etiologies such as hepatic congestion or edema, congestive heart failure, or hypoproteinemia (often associated with renal disease or hepatic dysfunction) can cause thickening of the gallbladder wall. Adenomyomatosis and cancer of the gall bladder also may result in thickening of the gallbladder wall [3]. A thickened gallbladder wall also can occur in association with viral infections and adjacent inflammatory conditions, including hepatitis, peptic ulcer disease (Fig. 4), pancreatitis, perihepatitis (Fitz-Hugh-Curtis syndrome), and pyelonephritis (Fig. 5). In patients who have thickening of the gallbladder wall caused by etiologies other than acute cholecystitis, the gallbladder often is nondistended, implying a nonobstructive (non-biliary) cause of wall thickening (Fig. 6).

A thickened gallbladder wall demonstrating a striated appearance with alternating hyper- and hypoechoic layers in the setting of acute cholecystitis is strongly associated gangrenous cholecystitis [10]. However, striations in the gallbladder wall without

Fig. 2. Pseudo gallbladders. (A) Transverse image in the right upper quadrant (RUQ) with structure identified as the gallbladder (*arrows*) containing debris (*asterisk*). Note that the "gallbladder" does not extend anteriorly and that the aorta (A) is immediately adjacent. (B) (*Left*) CT image of the same area as in (A) showed a fluid-containing structure with similar attenuation to blood in the aorta (A). This was a retroperitoneal hematoma in an anticoagulated patient. (B) (*Right*) The true gallbladder (GB) is lateral to the aorta and extends anteriorly. (C) (*Left*) Fluid and debris-containing structure believed to represent an abnormal gallbladder (GB) in this patient who had RUQ pain. (*Right*) The true gallbladder (*arrows*) is compressed and displaced by the adjacent mass, a pancreatic pseudocyst. (D) CT of the pancreatic pseudocyst (P) displacing the gallbladder (*arrows*). (*From* Rubens D. Hepatobiliary imaging and its pitfalls. Radiol Clin North Am 2004;42:257–78; with permission.)

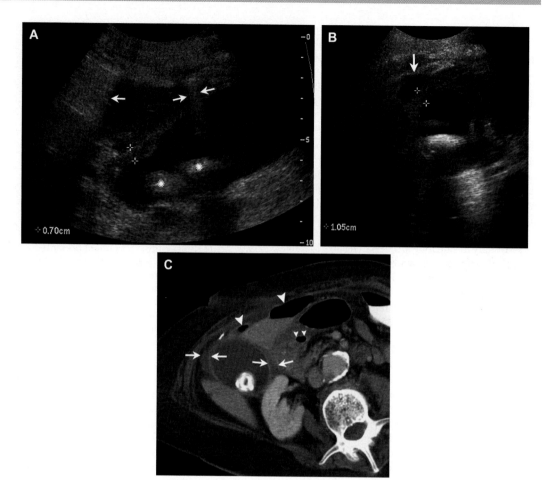

Fig. 4. Peptic ulcer perforation and thick gallbladder wall. (A) Patient who had RUQ pain, fever, and elevated white blood cell count (WBC). Ultrasound shows focal gallbladder wall thickening (7 mm; *cursors*) and gallstones (*asterisks*) and could be interpreted as cholecystitis. The free air with reverberation shadows (*arrows*) that leads to the correct diagnosis could be easily overlooked. (B) Transverse ultrasound shows wall thickening (*cursors*) and simple pericholecystic fluid (*arrow*). (C) CT image shows pericholecystic fluid (*arrows*), free air (*arrowheads*), and extraluminal accumulated air (*paired arrowheads*) in perforated duodenal ulcer. (*From* Rubens D. Hepato-biliary imaging and its pitfalls. Radiol Clin North Am 2004;42:257–78; with permission.)

evidence of acute cholecystitis is a nonspecific find-ing and is often noted in patients who have hepati-tis [11] (see Fig. 6).

Pericholecystic fluid is also a nonspecific finding, often occurring secondary to localized inflamma-tion from other causes, such as peptic ulcer disease [3] (see Fig. 4) or identified in patients who have ascites. Teefey and colleagues [10] have described two specific patterns of pericholecystic fluid. Type I, a thin anechoic crescent-shaped collection adja-cent to the gallbladder wall, is a nonspecific find-ing (see Fig. 4B). Type II, a round or irregularly shaped collection with thick walls, septations, or internal debris, is more likely to be associated with gallbladder perforation and abscess formation (Fig. 7).

## Acute acalculous cholecystitis

Acute acalculous cholecystitis account for up to 5%–14% of cases of acute cholecystitis [11]. It is seen most commonly in critically ill patients often following trauma, surgery, or major burns. The ex-act etiology is unknown, but ischemia, hypotension or sepsis are likely cotributing factors [12]. These critically ill patients are often medicated with narcotics, placed on ventilators, and receive hyper-alimentation that contribute to biliary stasis and functional obstruction of the cystic duct obstruc-tion. Gangrene of the gallbladder develops in ap-proximately 40% to 60% of patients who have an associated increased risk for perforation [2]. Mortal-ity ranges from 6% to 44% but can be reduced by

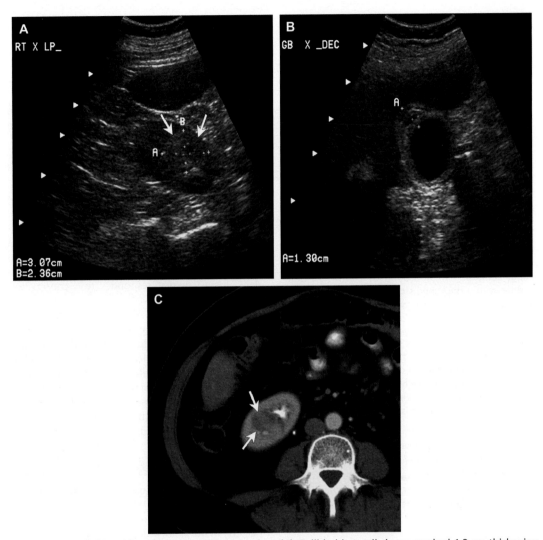

*Fig. 5.* Pyelonephritis with gallbladder wall thickening. (*A*) Gallbladder wall shows marked 1.3-cm thickening (*cursors*) and hypoechoic fluid within the wall. (*B*) Transverse ultrasound of the lower pole of the right kidney shows a 3-cm echogenic mass (*arrows*). (*C*) CT through the right lower pole shows a characteristic round, heterogeneous, decreased attenuation area of focal pyelonephritis (*arrows*). (*From* Rubens D. Hepatobiliary imaging and its pitfalls. Radiol Clin North Am 2004;42:257–78; with permission.)

early diagnosis and therapy [12]. However, the diagnosis of acalculous cholecystitis is difficult to make clinically and by US, because gallstones are absent and the sonographic Murphy sign may not be detected because of diminished mental status, medication and co-morbid illness. In the series reported by Cornwall and colleagues [12], only 50% of patients who had acalculous cholecystitis had a positive Murphy's sign. The diagnosis is, therefore, made by distension of the gall bladder in a suspicious clinical setting, the presence of intraluminal debris, gallbladder tenderness when present (~50%) and gallbladder wall thickening when other etiologies, such as hypoalbuminemia,

congestive heart failure (CHF), or liver disease are considered unlikely to be the cause (Fig. 8). CT can be used to assess for pericholecystic inflammation to improve diagnostic specificity in patients who have a thick gallbladder wall and multiple potential etiologies [2,13].

## Complicated cholecystitis

Gangrenous cholecystitis, emphysematous cholecystitis, and perforation of the gallbladder occur in up to 20% of patients who have acute cholecystitis [5]. These complications are important to recognize, because they are associated with increased

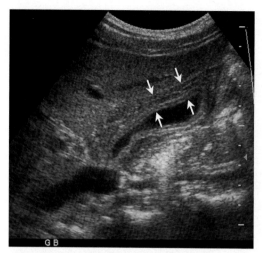

**Fig. 6.** Hepatitis with striated gallbladder wall thickening. Longitudinal ultrasound of contracted gallbladder with a thickened striated wall (*arrows*) with alternating echogenic and hypoechoic layers. This patient had RUQ pain, fever, abnormal liver function tests, and a negative sonographic Murphy sign. She tested positive for hepatitis B and also had clinically acute alcoholic hepatitis. The striated wall is not specific for gallbladder disease. (*From* Ghazle H, Rubens D. The liver. In: Dogra V, Rubens D, editors. **Ultrasound secrets**. Philadelpha: Hanley and Belfus; 2004. p. 130–49; with permission.)

morbidity (10%) and mortality (15%) [14] and require emergency surgery [2]. There is also approximately a 30% conversion rate for laparoscopic cholecystectomy to an open procedure in the setting of complicated cholecystitis [14].

## Gangrenous cholecystitis

Gangrenous cholecystitis is defined histologically as coagulative necrosis of the mucosa or the entire gallbladder wall associated with acute or chronic inflammation [10]. It occurs in up to 20% of patients who have acute cholecystitis and has an increased risk for perforation [3]. Unfortunately ultrasound is nonspecific for the diagnosis of gangrenous cholecystitis. This is because the sonographic Murphy sign is absent in up to two thirds of patients [15]. A specific finding is the presence of intraluminal membranes or stranding caused by sloughing of the gallbladder mucosa, necrosis of the gallbladder wall or fibrous exudate (Fig. 9). This finding is present on US examination, however, in only 5% of patients [10].

## Gallbladder perforation

Perforation of the gallbladder occurs in 5% to 10% of patients who have acute cholecystitis, most often

in association with gangrenous cholecystitis [3]. The fundus is the most common site for perforation, because it has the least blood supply. Acute gallbladder perforation with an intraperitoneal bile leak will result in peritonitis but is much less common than subacute perforation, which typically leads to pericholecystic abscess formation [2]. These abscesses may occur within or adjacent to the gallbladder wall in the gallbladder fossa, within the liver, parrenchyma, or along the free margin of the gallbladder within the peritoneal cavity [10]. These are complex fluid collections. Inflammatory changes in the adjacent fat can be detected on ultrasound or CT (Fig. 7C) [2]. Patients who have intraperitoneal abscesses require immediate surgery, although liver abscesses can be treated effectively with percutaneous drainage. Abscesses in the gallbladder wall or gallbladder fossa may respond to conservative management [16].

Pericholecystic fluid adjacent to the gallbladder wall may mimic perforation. However, with careful inspection, the gallbladder wall will be intact, and the fluid is typically anechoic (see Fig. 4B). Fluid collecting within the gallbladder wall has been reported in one case to precede perforation [17]. However, no other specific ultrasound features have been identified that will accurately predict which inflamed gallbladders will perforate.

## Emphysematous cholecystitis

This is a rare complication of acute cholecystitis, accounting for less than 1% of all complicated cases of acute cholecystitis, and is caused by gas-forming bacteria in the gallbladder lumen or in the gallbladder wall. As many as 40% of patients who have emphysematous cholecystitis have diabetes [2]. Emphysematous cholecystitis is more common in men and patients often do not have gallstones. The clinical course is rapidly progressive, with a 75% incidence of gallbladder gangrene and a 20% incidence of gallbladder perforation [18]. Emphysematous cholecystitis can be recognized on US examination by the extremely echogenic gas which casts a distal shadow and layers nondependently within the gallbladder lumen (Fig. 10). Intramural gas is more difficult to identify, because it may mimic the mural calcification seen in a porcelain gallbladder. The type of shadowing (ie, "clean" versus "dirty") does not differentiate between calcium and air. The nondependent location of the mobile echoes within the lumen or mobile bubbles within the wall can document gas. If the US findings are equivocal, either CT or plain film radiography can be used to differentiate between gas and calcification [19].

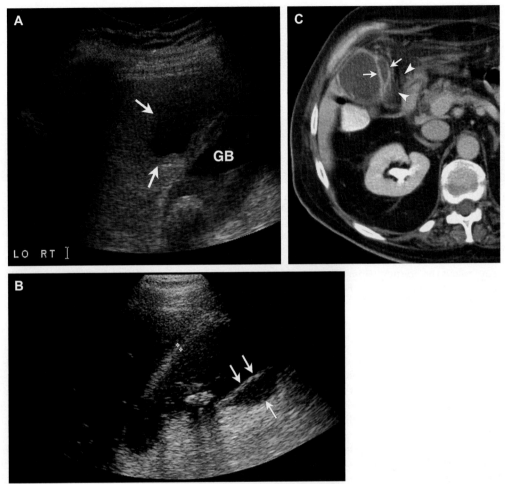

*Fig. 7.* Complicated cholecystitis with gallbladder perforation. (*A*) Longitudinal ultrasound of the gallbladder with adjacent irregularly marginated pericholecystic intrahepatic fluid (*arrows*). This patient presented with sepsis 2 weeks after prostate surgery and was found to have acute cholecystitis with an adjacent liver abscess. (*B*) Longitudinal ultrasound of gallbladder containing stones shows a pericholecystic collection (*arrows*) containing debris. The collection abuts the free wall of the gallbladder and is not contained within the gallbladder wall (*double arrow*). (*C*) CT shows an enhancing rim around the fluid (*arrows*) and inflammatory edema in the adjacent fat consistent with abscess (*arrowheads*). (*From* Rubens D. Hepatobiliary imaging and its pitfalls. Radiol Clin North Am 2004;42:257–78; with permission.)

## Chronic cholecystitis

Chronic cholecystitis is defined histologically as chronic inflammation of the gallbladder wall and is routinely associated with gallstones. It can generally be differentiated from acute cholecystitis by the absence of acute clinical symptoms, although it can be exacerbated by episodes of superimposed acute cholecystitis. The chronic inflammation causes thickening and fibrosis of the gallbladder wall and, ultimately, contraction of the gallbladder which when severe can result in almost complete obliteration of the gallbladder lumen. This produces an US image with two brightly colored arcs and a posterior shadow, the so-called "double arc"

sign or wall-echo-shadow (WES) complex [20] (Fig. 11). The first echogenic arc of the WES complex is created by the near wall of the gallbladder and the second by the gallstone. The two echoes are discernible because they are separated by a thin crescent of anechoic bile in the residual gallbladder lumen. The WES complex can be mimicked by a collapsed duodenum (Fig. 12) or, rarely, by a porcelain gallbladder. Porcelain gallbladder is more common in males, is seen in conjunction with chronic cholecystitis, and is the result of mural calcification of the gallbladder wall. It is a rare disorder, seen in 0.06% to 0.8% of cholecystectomy specimens [2]. The calcification pattern on ultrasound may involve the entire wall or only a portion

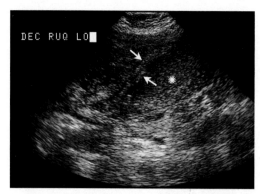

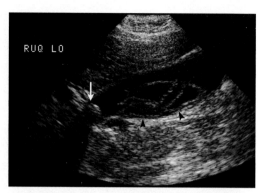

*Fig. 8.* Acalculous cholecystitis. A 50 year old woman presents with fever and right upper quadrant pain and a positive sonographic Murphy's sign on US examination. Longitudinal ultrasound shows a debris-filled (*asterisk*) gallbladder with a thick, striated wall (*arrows*). No stones are visualized. At surgery, this was acute acalculous cholecystitis. (*From* Rubens D. Hepatobiliary imaging and its pitfalls. Radiol Clin North Am 2004;42:257–78; with permission.)

*Fig. 9.* Gallbladder gangrene/mucosal sloughing. Longitudinal ultrasound of a patient who had acute cholecystitis secondary to stone (*arrow*) impacted in the gallbladder neck. Note the intraluminal membranes (*arrowheads*) that are associated with gangrene of the gallbladder. (*From* Rubens D. Hepatobiliary imaging and its pitfalls. Radiol Clin North Am 2004;42: 257–78; with permission.)

of it. In either case, the calcified wall causes only a single echogenic arc, not the double arc seen in the WES complex. If calcification in the wall is heavy, there is a single echo with a strong posterior shadow obscuring the gallbladder. With lesser degrees of calcification, the gallbladder lumen may be discerned posteriorly (Fig. 13). Another manifestation of chronic cholecystitis is xanthogranulomatous cholecystitis (XGP), in which the gallbladder wall is infiltrated by foamy histiocytes, lymphocytes, polymorphonuclear leukocytes, fibroblasts, and giant cells [19]. It presents sonographically as diffuse or focal thickening of the gallbladder wall, with mural nodularity (Fig. 14). Although this is rare, occurring in only 2% of cholecystectomy specimens [21], the imaging appearance is often difficult to distinguish from noninflammatory lesions, such as adenomyomatosis and gallbladder carcinoma. Because the hepatic surface of the gallbladder lacks a serosal layer, the inflammatory process more easily extends to the adjacent liver, and the liver–gallbladder margin is frequently indistinct [2,19].

## Noninflammatory non-neoplastic gallbladder disorders: the hyperplastic cholecystoses—cholesterolosis and adenomyomatosis

Hyperplastic cholecystoses are common, often asymptomatic processes that involve various layers of the gallbladder wall. Cholesterolosis, which may be diffuse or polypoid, has been reported in up to 25% of surgical specimens [2], whereas

adenomyomatosis (diffuse, focal, or polypoid) has been reported in 8.7% [22]. Cholesterolosis is caused by deposition of lipid-laden macrophages in the lamina propria, beneath the normal epithelium in the mucosa of the gallbladder wall. The diffuse form, which is more common, is difficult to appreciate on imaging [2]. Cholesterol polyps represent 20% of cholesterolosis but comprise approximately one half of all gallbladder polyps [2,19]. They are usually less than 1 cm in size, often multiple, and have no malignant potential. On ultrasound they appear brightly echogenic, round or lobulated, immobile, non-shadowing masses abutting the gallbladder wall (Fig. 15). Adenomyomatosis, also known as adenomyomatous hyperplasia, involves the mucosa and the muscular and connective tissue layers of the gallbladder wall. The epithelium and muscular layers proliferate, and invagination of the epithelial-lined spaces into the gallbladder wall produce intramural diverticula, termed Rokitansky-Aschoff sinuses. These may accumulate bile, cholesterol crystals, or even stones. On US examinations they may be anechoic if large enough and bile containing but more frequently are small and contain cholesterol, biliary sludge, or gallstones that create echogenic foci (Fig. 16), often with ring-down or comet tail reverberation artifacts [23]. The most common form of adenomyomatosis is a focal polypoid lesion, also known as an adenomyoma, typically located at the tip of the gallbladder fundus. The segmental form consists of localized gallbladder wall thickening that typically narrows the gallbladder body in an hourglass configuration. Diffuse adenomyomatosis involving

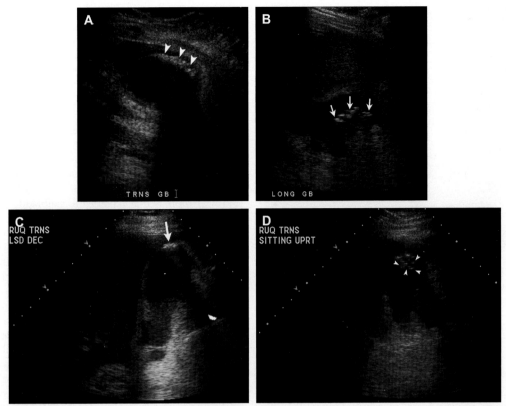

**Fig. 10.** Emphysematous cholecystitis. (*A*) Transverse supine view of the gallbladder reveals nondependent echoes anteriorly (*arrowheads*), which cast a dense posterior shadow. (*B*) When viewed longitudinally from the flank, the dependent echogenic gallstones (*arrows*) can be seen. Note that the shadow cast by the gas in (*A*) is denser and sharper than that from the stones (*B*). Bowel gas does not necessarily cast a "dirty" or reverberant echo-filled shadow. The shadow thus cannot be used to distinguish gas from the stones. (*C*) Emphysematous cholecystitis in another patient. Sagittal image of the gallbladder shows echoes anteriorly (*arrow*) that could be in either the lumen or the wall. (*D*) When the patient is turned into the upright position, the gas moves and breaks into bubbles (*arrowhead*), distinguishing it from mural air or calcium. 10A and B (*From* Rubens D. Hepatobiliary imaging and its pitfalls. Radiol Clin North Am 2004;42:257–78; with permission.)

the entire gallbladder wall is less common than focal or segmental diseases.

### Benign neoplasms of the gallbladder

Adenomas are well-demarcated, polypoid gallbladder lesions, usually less than 2 cm in size, and are rare compared with cholesterol polyps or polyps of adenomyomatous hyperplasia. They are found in 0.3% to 0.5% of cholecystectomy specimens and are usually solitary. They are classified as tubular, papillary, or tubulopapillary, depending on their growth pattern. On US they are typically echogenic when small, but become more heterogeneous as they enlarge [19]. Their premalignant potential is believed to be low, although this is somewhat controversial. There is a much stronger relationship between chronic cholecystitis and gallbladder carcinoma than between

adenoma and carcinoma. On imaging alone, however, it is impossible to identify coexistent dysplasia or carcinoma in situ within an adenoma, or to determine whether a polypoid mass is benign or malignant (Fig. 17). The current surgical literature therefore recommends excision of polyps greater than 1 cm in size in patients older than age 50 years or any polyp that is clearly growing, even if less than 1 cm [24,25].

### Malignant neoplasms of the gallbladder

Gallbladder carcinoma represents 98% or more of all gallbladder malignancies; the rest are comprised of nonepithelial tumors arising from the muscular or neurologic components of the wall, metastases or lymphoma (lymphoma) [26]. The median age at presentation is 72 years, with a 2:1 female-to-male ratio [26]. The major risk factor is

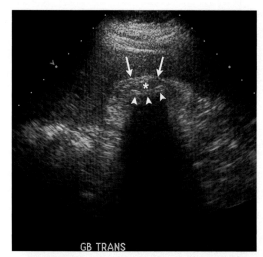

*Fig. 11.* Wall-echo-shadow complex. Transverse image of the gallbladder demonstrates the anterior echo of the gallbladder wall (*arrow*), the small space of the residual lumen containing bile (*asterisk*) and the second, posterior parallel echo of the stone (*arrowheads*).

chronic cholecystitis, which is associated with dysplasia and carcinoma in situ, and which subsequently progresses to invasive carcinoma [27]. Other risk factors include primary sclerosing cholangitis, anomalous junction of the pancreaticobiliary ducts, and choledochal cysts [27]. Gallbladder carcinoma is found incidentally in 1% of cholecystectomy specimens and in up to 6% of cholecystectomies performed for polypoid lesions [25]. It is usually not suspected clinically nor detected on preoperative imaging. When gallbladder carcinoma is

diagnosed by imaging, it is usually advanced [27,28]. The lack of serosa in the portion of the gallbladder wall adjacent to the liver means that the connective tissue of the gallbladder wall in this region is in direct continuity with the hepatic interlobar fissure. This permits early tumor invasion into the bloodstream, lymphatics, adjacent liver parenchyma, and hepatoduodenal ligament [27]. The most common imaging presentation of the gallbladder is that of a mass completely replacing the gallbladder (40%–65%), Less commonly focal or diffuse wall thickening (20%–30%) or an intraluminal polypoid mass (15%–25%) may be seen [27]. Carcinomas that replace the gallbladder are often heterogeneous, obliteration of the normally distinct plane which separates the gallbladder from the adjacent liver, caused by direct invasion of the adjacent hepatic parenchyma. Immobility of gallstones displaced by the mass may be a clue to diagnosis. Hepatic arterial Doppler waveforms within an intraluminal mass are also suspicious for malignancy (Fig. 18). Any solitary mass greater than 1 cm with internal vascularity should raise suspicion for carcinoma [28] (Fig. 17). Wall thickening alone may be difficult to distinguish from more common benign disorders, such as chronic cholecystitis or adenomyomatosis. Pronounced wall thickening greater than 1 cm or loss of the normal mural layers of the wall [27,28] should raise concern for malignancy (Fig. 18). If adenomyomatosis is suspected, the characteristic echoes from the Rokitansky-Aschoff sinuses should be sought, or MR imaging can be used to improve specificity [27]. Similarly, if a focal polypoid mass is present, the characteristics of adenomyomatosis should be absent.

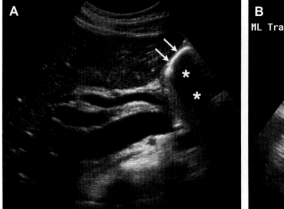
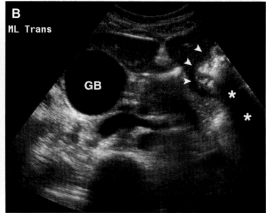

*Fig. 12.* WES mimic. (*A*) Longitudinal ultrasound image shows a sharp shadow (*asterisk*) behind a strong echo (*arrow*) that could be mistaken for a WES complex. (*B*) Transverse image confirms a normal gallbladder (*GB*) laterally. Unlike the gallbladder wall, which is echogenic, the duodenal wall (*arrowhead*) anterior to the echo of the luminal gas is actually hypoechoic.

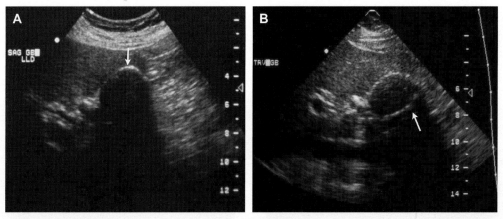

*Fig. 13.* Porcelain gallbladder. (*A*) Sagittal image of the gallbladder shows a densely echogenic anterior wall (*arrow*) with a sharp shadow that obliterates the gallbladder lumen and posterior wall. (*B*) Transverse ultrasound of the gallbladder in the same patient. The anterior wall is bright, but, without enough reflection or attenuation to eliminate visualization of the lumen and posterior wall (*arrow*), which is also echogenic and casts a posterior acoustic shadow. (*From* the Armed Forces Institute of Pathology/American Registry of Pathology; with permission.)

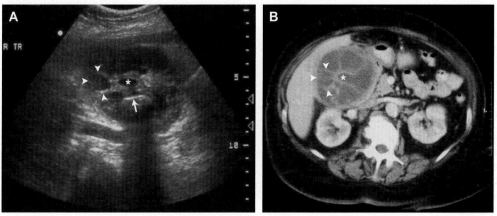

*Fig. 14.* Xanthogranulomatous cholecystitis. (*A*) Transverse image of the gallbladder with a compressed lumen (*asterisk*). The walls are markedly thickened with multiple hypoechoic mural inflammatory nodules (*arrowheads*) that envelop the adjacent stone (*arrow*). (*B*) CT axial image of the gallbladder shows the compressed lumen (*asterisk*) and the multiple large mural nodules (*arrowheads*) separated by enhancing margins. The stone is not visualized. (*From* the Armed Forces Institute of Pathology/American Registry of Pathology; with permission.)

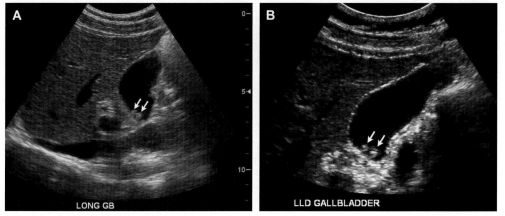

*Fig. 15.* Cholesterol polyps. (*A*) Initial longitudinal ultrasound shows two nondependent and non-shadowing 5-mm moderately echogenic nodules (*arrows*) abutting the gallbladder wall. (*B*) Two years later the nodules are unchanged in size, appearance, and location (*arrows*).

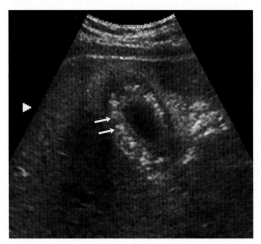

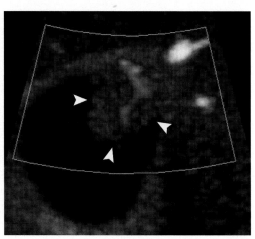

Fig. 16. Adenomyomatosis. Transverse ultrasound shows multiple discrete 1-mm echogenic cholesterol crystals in the intramural diverticula (Rokitansky-Aschoff sinuses) (*arrows*) within a thickened gallbladder wall in this asymptomatic patient who had adenomyomatosis. (*From* Harrow A. The gallbladder and biliary tree. In: Dogra V, Rubens D, editors. Ultrasound secrets. Philadelphia: Hanley and Belfus; 2004. p. 113–29; with permission.)

Fig. 17. Gallbladder adenoma. Transverse color Doppler ultrasound in a 67-year-old man presenting with a 2-week history of RUQ pain shows a 2-cm polypoid mass at the fundus with internal vascularity. Histology revealed a tubular villous adenoma with foci of carcinoma in situ. (*From* Harrow A. The gallbladder and biliary tree. In: Dogra V, Rubens D, editors. Ultrasound secrets. Philadelphia: Hanley and Belfus; 2004. p. 113–29; with permission.)

### Biliary ducts

Disease of the bile ducts usually is manifested by obstruction of the bile ducts with resultant dilatation of either the intrahepatic or extrahepatic ducts or both. Clinical presentation is varied and may include right upper quadrant or epigastric pain, fever, and jaundice. Biliary ductal dilatation may be attributable to multiple causes, including stones, intrinsic tumor, stricture, or compression by extrinsic masses. Ultrasound ideally is suited to screen both the intrahepatic and extrahepatic ducts for duct size and continuity. Either or both may be dilated, depending on the level of obstruction.

### Ultrasound diagnosis of biliary ductal dilatation

The extrahepatic common duct is measured from inner wall to inner wall at the level of the crossing of the right hepatic artery. The diameter at this level should not exceed 6 mm [1]. The diameter of the common duct is slightly greater distally as it approaches the pancreas, sometimes by as much

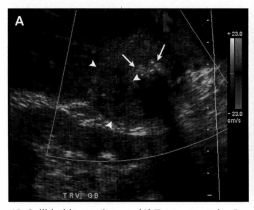

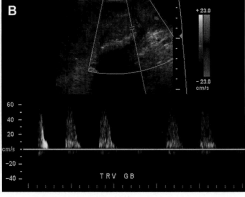

Fig. 18. Gallbladder carcinoma. (*A*) Transverse color Doppler image of the gallbladder shows stones (*arrows*) anterior to a 2-cm thickened hypoechoic wall with no discrete features but demonstrating some vascularity. (*B*) Spectral Doppler shows high-velocity arterial flow within the wall, concerning for tumor.

as 1 to 2 mm. There is still debate in the literature as to whether the bile duct dilates with age and whether it dilates postcholecystectomy [1,28]. Most laboratories consider a common bile duct (CBD) less than 6 mm normal, and a CBD that measures greater than or equal to 8 mm [1,29] abnormal. Clinically, if the patient has dilated ducts but no accompanying symptoms, such as elevated bilirubin, pain, sepsis, or elevated liver enzymes, including alkaline phosphatase, the dilated ducts are unlikely to be clinically relevant. Hence, the clinical scenario is of paramount importance when assessing the bile ducts. Intrahepatic bile ducts are normal if they measure 2 mm or less in the porta or no more than 40% of the diameter of the accompanying portal vein [1,30]. With the advent of newer equipment, however, it is now possible to see intrahepatic biliary ducts in normal

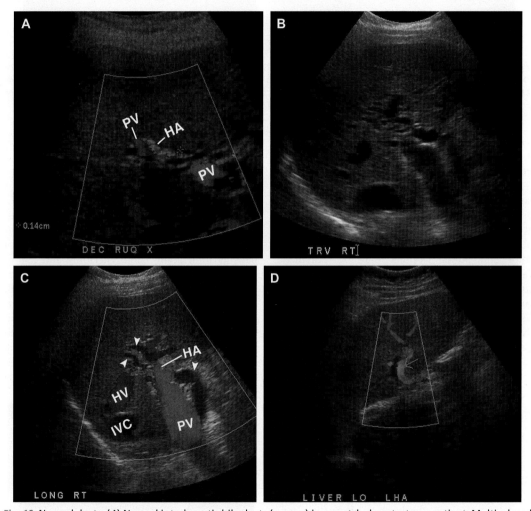

**Fig. 19.** Normal ducts. (A) Normal intrahepatic bile ducts (*cursors*) in a postcholecystectomy patient. Multicolored vessel in the center of the color box is the hepatic artery (*HA*), and dark red adjacent vessel is the portal vein (*PV*). (B & C) Patient who had abdominal pain, nausea, and jaundice 1 month postcholecystectomy. Note multiple anechoic irregularly branching tubes converging at the porta hepatis. Color Doppler image (*C*) confirms that some are avascular and represent ducts (*arrowheads*), whereas the portal veins (*red*), hepatic veins (*blue*), and hepatic arteries (*HA*) are correctly identified. The inferior vena cava (*IVC*) can be recognized by its anatomic position. (*From* Rubens D. Hepatobiliary imaging and its pitfalls. Radiol Clin North Am 2004:42:257–78; with permission.) (D) Grayscale image (not shown) demonstrated a dilated tubular structure. Sagittal color Doppler image shows antegrade flow in the tube (*arrow*) and no flow in the smaller adjacent tube. The larger tube was shown to be the hepatic artery with spectral Doppler and the adjacent tube is the portal vein. The bile ducts are not seen at all. (*From* Rubens D, Carson N. Doppler Evaluation of the Liver and Transjugular Intrahepatic Portovenous Shunts In: Dogra V, Rubens D, editors. Ultrasound Secrets. Philadelphia: Hanley and belfus; 2004. p. 403–19; with permission.)

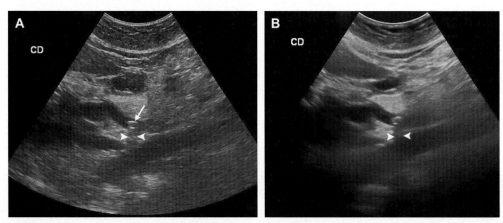

Fig. 20. Harmonic imaging of stones. (A) Standard longitudinal ultrasound imaging in the porta shows a dilated common duct obstructed by an incompletely visualized stone (*arrow*) with a faint posterior acoustic shadow (*arrowheads*) that is difficult to visualize. (B) Same view with harmonic imaging shows brighter, sharper echoes from the stone and a much sharper and darker shadow (*arrowheads*) posteriorly.

patients, especially when using harmonic imaging that significantly improves resolution [9] or high frequency transducers in slender patients (Fig. 19A). In general, intrahepatic biliary duct dilatation can be diagnosed when irregular angular branching, a central stellate configuration, and acoustic enhancement posterior to the ducts is observed (Fig. 19B) [1]. In addition, the use of color and power Doppler may be extremely valuable by demonstrating that dilated tubular structures in the liver are indeed ducts and not vascular structures (Fig. 19C). In the setting of cirrhosis, the hepatic arteries supply more blood to the liver and frequently dilate. As they also course parallel to the portal vein in the portal triads, they can be mistaken for dilated ducts (Fig. 19D).

## Diagnosis of biliary obstruction

Assuming the patient has a dilated common duct (≥6 mm) associated with clinical signs of obstruction, including elevated bilirubin or elevated alkaline phosphatase, how well does ultrasound identify the level and cause of obstruction? With good US technique, the level of obstruction can be defined in up to 92% of patients and the cause in up to 71% [1]. Important technical factors include patient positioning in the semierect right posterior oblique (RPO) or right lateral decubitus positions to minimize shadowing from overlying bowel gas in the gastric antrum or the duodenum, and the use of a transverse imaging plane to completely follow the duct to the level of the pancreas [1]. Additional technical improvements sometimes can be achieved by having the patient drink water to displace gas or by using a large footprint curvilinear transducer to compress bowel and bowel gas away from the distal duct.

## Causes of biliary obstruction

### Choledocholithiasis

Common duct stones are the most common disorder of the biliary tract, occurring in 8% to 20% of patients undergoing cholecystectomy and 2% to 4% of patients postcholecystectomy [30]. On ultrasound, stones are identified as echogenic foci with a distal acoustic shadow. They are easiest to see, however, when surrounded by anechoic bile in a dilated duct and when large enough to cast an acoustic shadow. Stones impacted in the distal duct may be difficult to recognize when their margins are inseparable from the adjacent duct

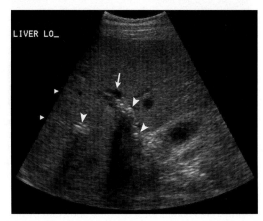

Fig. 21. Multiple intraductal stones. Longitudinal ultrasound shows a dilated duct (*arrow*) filled with multiple shadowing stones (*arrowheads*) in multiple ducts in this patient who had longstanding cholecystitis and cholangitis.

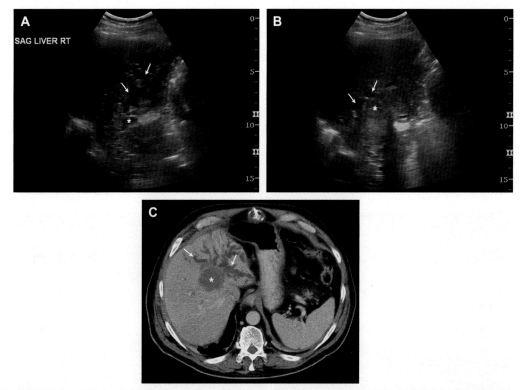

*Fig. 22.* Cholangiocarcinoma. (*A*) Longitudinal ultrasound image through the right lobe shows multiple dilated ducts (*arrows*) anterior to the portal vein (*asterisk*) but no discrete mass. (*B*) More centrally a longitudinal image through the left lobe shows centrally dilated ducts (*arrows*) with contour deformity of the ducts and the posterior margin of the liver by an ill-defined space-occupying lesion (*asterisk*) at the level of the caudate lobe. No discrete margins are identified. (*C*) Axial CT at the level of the caudate lobe shows a discrete low attenuation mass (*asterisk*) with obstruction and dilatation of the ducts of the left lobe. The adjacent liver parenchyma is atrophied slightly, especially anteriorly, where it abuts the diaphragm. Localization of the tumor and recognition of atrophy are much more apparent on CT than on ultrasound.

walls and surrounding echogenic fat. Additionally, small (<5 mm) stones may not cast an acoustic shadow, especially if they are deep in the abdomen or if spatial compounding is used. Harmonic imaging that decreases speckle and improves

visualization of the acoustic shadow is a key ingredient to successful imaging [9] (Fig. 20). Similarly, transducer compression, patient positioning, and the use of the liver or water-filled bowel as an acoustic window to avoid interference from bowel gas are

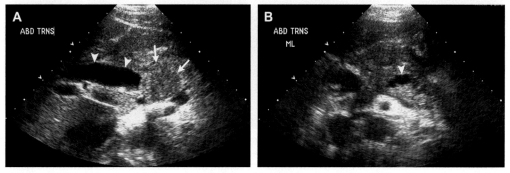

*Fig. 23.* Pancreatic carcinoma. (*A*) Transverse ultrasound image shows a markedly dilated common duct (*arrowheads*) that terminates abruptly at the level of a slightly hypoechoic, rounded mass (*arrows*). (*B*) Transverse image through the body of the pancreas shows a dilated pancreatic duct (*arrowhead*), indicating that the level of obstruction is in the pancreatic head.

important maneuvers to improve visualization of stones in the extrahepatic duct. With good technique, Laing and colleagues achieved an overall sensitivity of 75% for US in the detection of cholelithiasis, with visualization of 89% of proximal and 70% of distal calculi as compared to surgery [31].

Pitfalls include patients who are obstructed without dilatation. This can occur from intermittent obstruction from stones. As many as one third of common bile duct calculi are found in nondilated bile ducts (Fig. 1*B*) [1]. In this group of patients, ultrasound is insensitive and MRCP or endoscopic retrograde cholangiopancreatography (ERCP) should be considered. Although the vast majority of stones occur in the distal duct, stones may also be identified in the intrahepatic ducts and may be the clue to more distal obstruction (Fig. 21).

### Neoplasm

Benign neoplasms of the biliary tree are rare. The most common is the adenoma, which may be discovered incidentally at surgery or imaging or that may actually obstruct the biliary tree and present with pain or jaundice. On ultrasound these soft

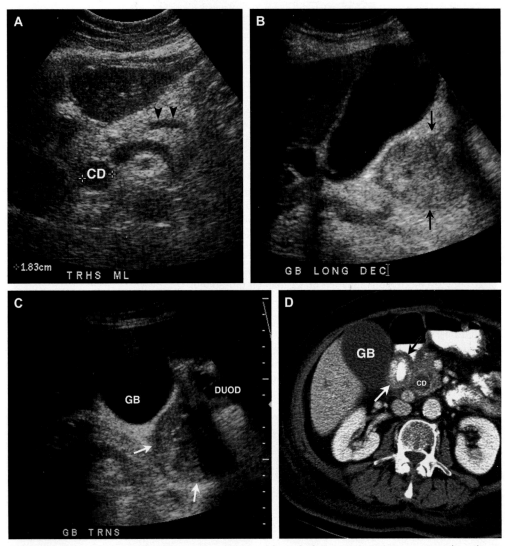

*Fig. 24.* Duodenal carcinoma with biliary, pancreatic, and bowel obstruction. Patient presented to the emergency department with nausea and jaundice. (*A*) Transverse ultrasound of the pancreas shows a 1.8-cm common duct (*CD*) and a dilated pancreatic duct (*arrowheads*). (*B*) Longitudinal ultrasound shows a distended gallbladder with a soft-tissue mass (*arrows*) behind it. (*C*) On transverse imaging, the mass (*arrows*) obstructs the duodenum (*Duod*), which has a fluid-filled proximal lumen. (*D*) CT confirms the circumferential duodenal tumor (*arrows*). Note distended gallbladder and common duct (*CD*). GB, gallbladder. (*From* Rubens D. Hepatobiliary imaging and its pitfalls. Radiol Clin North Am 2004;42:257–78; with permission.)

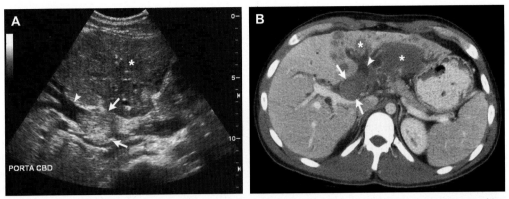

*Fig. 25.* Intraductal hepatocellular carcinoma with invasion of the biliary ducts. (*A*) Transverse ultrasound image at the porta shows an echogenic mass (*arrows*) obstructing the intrahepatic bile duct (*arrowhead*), which is markedly dilated. The echotexture of the left lobe of the liver is heterogeneous, nodular, and distorted (*asterisk*), lacking the normal vascular landmarks. (*B*) CT obtained at the same level shows the tumor (*arrows*) obstructing the intrahepatic duct (*arrowhead*). There is additional tumor (*asterisks*) involving the left lobe with multiple nodular metastases. The intraparenchymal extent of the tumor is much greater on CT than would be expected by the ultrasound images. Unlike the cholangiocarcinoma in **Fig. 22**, this tumor expands the left lobe.

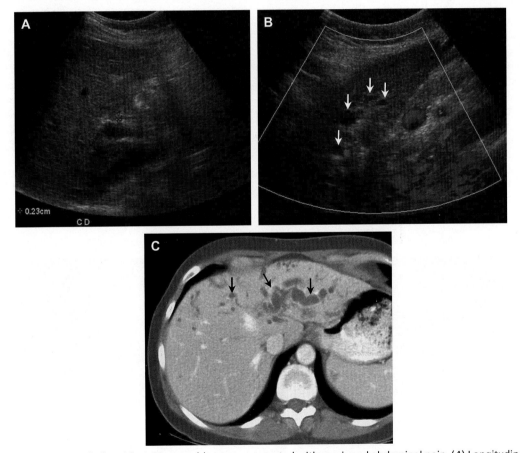

*Fig. 26.* Sclerosing cholangitis. A 50-year-old woman presented with sepsis and abdominal pain. (*A*) Longitudinal ultrasound of the right lobe is normal, with the common duct (*cursors*) measuring 2 mm. (*B*) Longitudinal ultrasound of the left lobe shows multiple markedly enlarged ducts (*arrows*). (*C*) CT shows asymmetrically enlarged ducts (*arrows*) with enhancing walls, indicating inflammation. No central obstructing mass is identified. Emergent biliary drainage was performed, which alleviated the patient's symptoms. (*From* Rubens D. Hepatobiliary imaging and its pitfalls. Radiol Clin North Am 2004;42:257–78; with permission.)

tissue masses are homogeneous, isoechoic to the liver parenchyma, and, if obstructing, cause proximal dilatation of the biliary tree [19]. Biliary cystadenomas are also rare and although benign histologically, tend to recur locally and may transform into cystadenocarcinomas [19]. They occur most commonly intrahepatically (83%) with the remainder in the extrahepatic bile ducts. These lesions tend to occur in middle-aged women and are large (3 to 40 cm), solitary cystic masses [19]. Ultrasound findings range from unilocular cyst to multilocular cysts sometimes with mural nodules and papillary projections. Calcification is common and may occur within the cyst wall or in the septations. Cystic fluid may be simple or complex, containing mucin, protein, or hemorrhagic debris. Differential diagnoses include echinococcal cysts, hemorrhagic cysts, cystic metastasis, and abscess.

Cholangiocarcinoma is the primary malignant neoplasm of the biliary tree. Risk factors include sclerosing cholangitis, choledochal cysts, and parasitic infection with liver flukes. Cholangiocarcinomas may arise anywhere along the biliary tree, but are most common at the hilum (50%–60%), otherwise known as a Klatskin tumors. Intrahepatic or peripheral cholangiocarcinomas comprise 10%, and extrahepatic or distal cholangiocarcinomas make up the remaining 30% [28,32]. Tumors are variable in their growth patterns and consequently in their ultrasound appearance. Tumor spread may be within or adjacent to the duct wall in a scirrhous pattern, leading to stricture and biliary ductal dilatation. This component of the tumor is fibrous. Walls of the ducts are thickened without a discrete tumor mass [33]. The tumor itself may not be directly visualized on US, only its resultant obstruction. However, careful imaging of the duct walls may reveal focal irregularity to establish a tumor diagnosis [34]. Lesions show decreased attenuation in comparison to the liver on the portal venous phase images of contrast-enhanced CT or MR imaging and are often much more apparent than on noncontrast ultrasound (Fig. 22). Glandular cells within the tumor produce mucin and contribute to greater mass effect than the stromal fibrous component [33]. Mass-like lesions are most common in the hilum or in the periphery of the liver. As the tumor extends outside the ducts and forms a mass, it may obstruct adjacent vessels, either the portal veins or hepatic arteries. As many as 50% of patients are reported to have associated portal venous involvement [34]. Chronic vascular obstruction caused by extrinsic compression or especially portal vein thrombosis may lead to lobar atrophy, a unique and common feature of peripheral cholangiocarcinoma [30,33]. The peripheral masses are large and present as indeterminate soft-tissue masses, indistinguishable on US from primary hepatocellular carcinoma or metastatic disease. Intraductal masses are uncommon within the liver and are more common in the extrahepatic duct, where they tend to be polypoid. A distal carcinoma may also be scirrhous and may locally thicken the duct wall, in which case it may be indistinguishable from the adjacent pancreas or ampulla. The echogenicity of cholangiocarcinomas is variable, ranging from hypoechoic to moderately echogenic.

Secondary malignant neoplastic involvement of the bile ducts occurs by extrinsic compression or direct extension. Causes of extrinsic compression

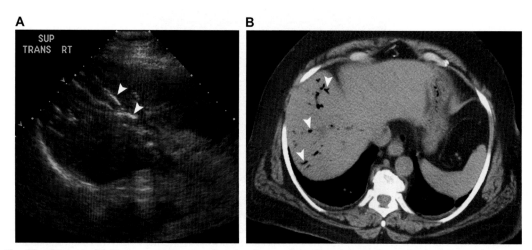

*Fig. 27.* Biliary air. (*A*) Transverse ultrasound at the dome of the liver in a patient who had acute cholecystitis shows smooth, linear echoes (*arrowheads*) with some posterior shadowing. (*B*) Corresponding axial CT through the same region confirms that the echoes on ultrasound represent air in the mildly dilated bile ducts (*arrowheads*).

are myriad and include hepatic metastases displacing the intrahepatic ducts or extrahepatic obstruction caused by pancreatic carcinoma (Fig. 23), lymphadenopathy, or tumors of the adjacent gastrointestinal tract (Fig. 24). Intrinsic biliary duct obstruction is usually the result of hepatocellular carcinoma, which has a propensity to invade the biliary tree and the adjacent vessels [30] (Fig. 25). Differentiation from cholangiocarcinoma is made on contrast enhanced CT or MR imaging, which demonstrates marked arterial phase enhancement of hepatocellular carcinoma versus only moderate early and sometimes more intense delayed phase enhancement of typical cholangiocarcinomas [30].

## Inflammatory disorders of the biliary ducts

Acute inflammatory processes include acute bacterial cholangitis, which occurs in concert with biliary

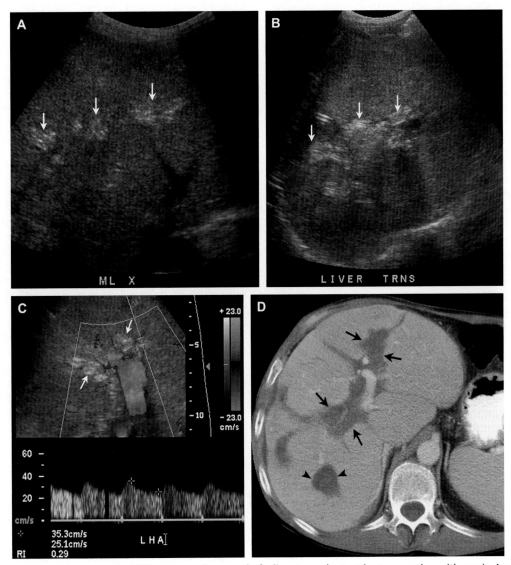

*Fig. 28.* Biliary duct necrosis. (*A*) Transverse ultrasound of a liver transplant patient presenting with sepsis. Amorphous echogenic debris (*arrows*) is seen on grayscale. (*B*) Two months later the process has progressed. The echogenic areas (*arrows*) are more confluent and linear and cast acoustic shadows that obscure the adjacent parenchyma. (*C*) Color Doppler image shows echogenic debris in a ductal distribution (*arrows*) and a low resistive index (<0.5) in the hepatic artery, signifying hepatic arterial stenosis or thrombosis. (*D*) The extensive biliary duct necrosis (*arrows*) and the resulting liver abscess (*arrowheads*) are documented by CT. The abscess was obscured on the ultrasound because of shadowing from air in the ducts. (*From* Rubens D. Hepatobiliary imaging and its pitfalls. Radiol Clin North Am 2004:42:257–78; with permission.)

obstruction in the presence of common duct stones. Clinical presentation is nonspecific, with fever, right upper quadrant pain, and jaundice. US is useful to determine the level, and if possible, the cause of obstruction. Duct walls are thickened and ducts may contain internal debris. The ducts are usually dilated and there may be associated hepatic complications, including liver abscess. Other inflammatory processes adjacent to the ducts may result in obstruction without infection. Mirizzi syndrome involves acute cholecystitis caused by an impacted cystic duct stone that also compresses, inflames, and obstructs the adjacent common duct. Inflammation from pancreatitis can also inflame and narrow the common bile duct causing obstruction and jaundice. Recurrent pyogenic cholangiohepatitis (also known as oriental cholangiohepatitis) is a disease of unknown etiology characterized by strictures, stasis, and stone formation. It is most common in people of Asian descent. It is characterized on ultrasound by dilated ducts filled with stones and debris. Stones are typically noncalcified and of soft-tissue attenuation. Recurrent obstruction may result in focal atrophy of the surrounding liver parenchyma, often a key to the diagnosis [35].

Sclerosing cholangitis may be primary (idiopathic or associated with inflammatory bowel disease) or secondary to prior biliary infection. The pathophysiology is of inflammation followed by segmental fibrosis that leads to strictures and areas of biliary stasis. The latter may result in abscess formation with acute presentation. Chronically, patients progress to cirrhosis and liver failure. Sclerosing cholangitis gives rise to segmental dilation of the bile ducts, often only in one portion of the liver (Figs. 26). Bile duct walls are thickened and irregular, and the segmental strictures give the ducts a beaded appearance on ultrasound. Because there is no mass causing the obstruction, sclerosing cholangitis is difficult to distinguish from an infiltrating form of cholangiocarcinoma. Unfortunately these patients are also at increased risk for cholangiocarcinoma, which occurs in 10% to 30% of patients [36]. AIDS cholangitis, an end-stage infection usually caused by cryptosporidium or cytomegalovirus, also causes strictures and bile duct thickening indistinguishable from primary sclerosing cholangitis [28,30].

### Biliary air and biliary necrosis

Air in the biliary tree may result from transient or prolonged communication with the gastrointestinal tract. Air from the duodenum is introduced into the bile duct as the sphincter of Oddi opens with passage of a stone (Fig. 27) or with ERCP. Sustained communication occurs following sphincterotomy,

an endobiliary stent placement, or biliary enteric fistula. Gas can also arise in the biliary tree as a result of infection, from reflux, emphysematous cholecystitis, or biliary necrosis with secondary abscess formation. On US biliary air gives a typical appearance of smooth, linear, bright echoes that are located adjacent to the portal veins. There may or may not be associated biliary ductal dilatation. Biliary duct necrosis is a critical complication that may occur following liver transplantation, usually secondary to ischemia from hepatic artery stenosis or thrombosis. If biliary necrosis occurs, the ducts become enlarged and filled with pus or necrotic debris. On ultrasound they may appear echogenic, irregular, and enlarged without the usual anechoic bile. Echoes are frequently nodular in appearance (Fig. 28). Shadowing may occur if gas is also present.

### Summary

US is currently recommended as the primary initial imaging modality for the evaluation of the gallbladder and bile ducts. Recent technical advances such as harmonic imaging and spatial compounding have improved detection of biliary stones, the most common disease of the biliary tract. Tumors and benign inflammatory conditions that mimic tumors may also be detected, but a specific diagnosis may not be readily apparent. If the margins of the gallbladder are indistinct, as in patients with gallbladder carcinoma or xanthogranulomatous cholecystitis, or if perforation or abscess are suspected in case of complicated cholecystitis, CT or MR imaging may be useful to assess the extent and character of the disease process. When the site or cause of biliary obstruction is not apparent, as in cholangiocarcinoma or distal common duct obstruction, further evaluation with contrast enhanced CT or MR imaging with MRCP also is indicated.

### References

[1] Laing FC. The gallbladder and bile ducts. In: Rumack CM, Wilson SR, Charboneau JW, editors. Diagnostic ultrasound. Vol. 1. St Louis: Mosby-Year Book; 1998. p. 175–223.

[2] Gore RM, Yaghmai V, Newmark GM, et al. Imaging benign and malignant disease of the gallbladder. Radiol Clin North Am 2002;40(6): 1307–23.

[3] Cooperberg PL, Gibney RG. Imaging of the gallbladder. Radiology 1987;163(3):605–13.

[4] Ralls PW, Colletti PM, Lapin SA, et al. Real-time sonography in suspected acute cholecystitis. Prospective evaluation of primary and secondary signs. Radiology 1985;155(3):767–71.

[5] Laing FC, Jeffrey RB Jr. Choledocholithiasis and cystic duct obstruction: difficult ultrasonographic diagnosis. Radiology 1983;146(2):475–9.

[6] Hough DM, Glazebrook KN, Paulson EK, et al. Value of prone positioning in the ultrasonographic diagnosis of gallstones: prospective study. J Ultrasound Med 2000;19(9):633–8.

[7] Choudhry S, Gorman B, Charboneau JW, et al. Comparison of tissue harmonic imaging with conventional US in abdominal disease. Radiographics 2000;20(4):1127–35.

[8] Hong HS, Han JK, Kim TK, et al. Ultrasonographic evaluation of the gallbladder: comparison of fundamental, tissue harmonic, and pulse inversion harmonic imaging. J Ultrasound Med 2001;20(1):35–41.

[9] Ortega D, Burns PN, Hope Simpson D, et al. Tissue harmonic imaging: is it a benefit for bile duct sonography? AJR Am J Roentgenol 2001; 176(3):653–9.

[10] Teefey SA, Baron RL, Radke HM, et al. Gangrenous cholecystitis: new observations on sonography. J Ultrasound Med 1991;10(11):603–6.

[11] Kalliafas S, Ziegler DW, Flancbaum L, et al. Acute acalculous cholecystitis: incidence, risk factors, diagnosis, and outcome. Am Surg 1998;64(5):471–5.

[12] Cornwell EE III, Rodriguez A, Mirvis SE, et al. Acute acalculous cholecystitis in critically injured patients. Preoperative diagnostic imaging. Ann Surg 1989;210(1):52–5.

[13] Blankenberg F, Wirth R, Jeffrey RB Jr, et al. Computed tomography as an adjunct to ultrasound in the diagnosis of acute acalculous cholecystitis. Gastrointest Radiol 1991;16(2):149–53.

[14] Habib FA, Kolachalam RB, Khilnani R, et al. Role of laparoscopic cholecystectomy in the management of gangrenous cholecystitis. Am J Surg 2001;181(1):71–5.

[15] Simeone JF, Brink JA, Mueller PR, et al. The sonographic diagnosis of acute gangrenous cholecystitis: importance of the Murphy sign. AJR Am J Roentgenol 1989;152(2):289–90.

[16] Takada T, Yasuda H, Uchiyama K, et al. Pericholecystic abscess: classification of US findings to determine the proper therapy. Radiology 1989; 172(3):693–7.

[17] Forsberg L, Andersson R, Hederstrom E, et al. Ultrasonography and gallbladder perforation in acute cholecystitis. Acta Radiol 1988;29(2):203–5.

[18] Bloom RA, Libson E, Lebensart PD, et al. The ultrasound spectrum of emphysematous cholecystitis. J Clin Ultrasound 1989;17(4):251–6.

[19] Levy AD, Murakata LA, Abbott RM, et al. From the archives of the AFIP. Benign tumors and tumorlike lesions of the gallbladder and extrahepatic bile ducts: radiologic-pathologic correlation. Armed Forces Institute of Pathology. Radiographics 2002;22(2):387–413.

[20] Rybicki FJ. The WES sign. Radiology 2000; 214(3):881–2.

[21] Roberts KM, Parsons MA. Xanthogranulomatous cholecystitis: clinicopathological study of 13 cases. J Clin Pathol 1987;40(4):412–7.

[22] Ootani T, Shirai Y, Tsukada K, et al. Relationship between gallbladder carcinoma and the segmental type of adenomyomatosis of the gallbladder. Cancer 1992;69(11):2647–52.

[23] Raghavendra BN, Subramanyam BR, Balthazar EJ, et al. Sonography of adenomyomatosis of the gallbladder: radiologic-pathologic correlation. Radiology 1983;146(3):747–52.

[24] Mainprize KS, Gould SW, Gilbert JM. Surgical management of polypoid lesions of the gallbladder. Br J Surg 2000;87(4):414–7.

[25] Yeh CN, Jan YY, Chao TC, et al. Laparoscopic cholecystectomy for polypoid lesions of the gallbladder: a clinicopathologic study. Surg Laparosc Endosc Percutan Tech 2001;11(3): 176–81.

[26] Albores-Saavedra J, Henson DE, Klimsta DS. Tumors of the gallbladder, extrahepatic bile ducts, and ampulla of vater. In: Atlas of tumor pathology. Fasc 27, ser 3. Washington DC: Armed Forces Institute of Pathology; 2000.

[27] Levy AD, Murakata LA, Rohrmann CA Jr. Gallbladder carcinoma: radiologic-pathologic correlation. Radiographics 2001;21(2):295–314; questionnaire, 549–55.

[28] Khalili K, Wilson SR. The biliary tree and gallbladder. In: Rumack CM, Wilson SR, Charboneau JW, et al, editors. Diagnostic ultrasound. St Louis, MO: Mosby; 2005. p. 171–212.

[29] Ralls PW, Jeffrey RB Jr, Kane RA, et al. Ultrasonography. Gastroenterol Clin North Am 2002; 31(3):801–25, vii.

[30] Baron RL, Tublin ME, Peterson MS. Imaging the spectrum of biliary tract disease. Radiol Clin North Am 2002;40(6):1325–54.

[31] Laing FC, Jeffrey RB, Wing VW. Improved visualization of choledocholithiasis by sonography. AJR Am J Roentgenol 1984;143(5):949–52.

[32] Nakeeb A, Pitt HA, Sohn TA, et al. Cholangiocarcinoma. A spectrum of intrahepatic, perihilar, and distal tumors. Ann Surg 1996;224(4): 463–73; discussion 473–5.

[33] Lim JH. Cholangiocarcinoma: morphologic classification according to growth pattern and imaging findings. AJR Am J Roentgenol 2003;181(3): 819–27.

[34] Hann LE, Greatrex KV, Bach AM, et al. Cholangiocarcinoma at the hepatic hilus: sonographic findings. AJR Am J Roentgenol 1997;168(4): 985–9.

[35] Hanbidge AE, Buckler PM, O'Malley ME, et al. From the RSNA refresher courses: imaging evaluation for acute pain in the right upper quadrant. Radiographics 2004;24(4):1117–35.

[36] MacFaul GR, Chapman RW. Sclerosing cholangitis. Curr Opin Gastroenterol 2006;22(3):288–93.

ELSEVIER
SAUNDERS

ULTRASOUND
CLINICS

Ultrasound Clin 2 (2007) 415–422

# Ultrasound of Acute Pancreatitis

Hisham Tchelepi, MD[a],*, Phil W. Ralls, MD[b]

- Pathophysiology and clinical presentation
- Sonographic features
  *Pancreatic findings*
  *Peripancreatic findings*

*Vascular findings*
- Summary
- References

Sonography is important in imaging patients with clinically suspected acute pancreatitis. All patients who present with acute pancreatitis for the first time should have sonography to evaluate the biliary tree for gallstones as a cause of pancreatitis. Sonography can also determine if bile duct dilatation, suggestive of obstruction, is present. However, the ability of sonography to visualize the pancreas in acute pancreatitis is sometimes limited. This limitation is often caused by the presence of ileus, sometimes a "sentinel loop" that precludes the ability of sonography to identify or delineate abnormalities of the parenchyma of the gland. Many times this limitation can be overcome by using compression techniques and scanning in various positions, such as left lateral decubitus or semierect positions. The diagnosis may be suspected when the typical ancillary findings of pancreatitis are noted in the retroperitoneal space, even if the gland itself is poorly seen.

Many times sonographic findings can facilitate the diagnosis of acute pancreatitis when it is clinically unsuspected. In addition, sonography may be helpful in identifying complications of known acute pancreatitis. Sonography may be helpful in selecting those patients who require CT scanning to evaluate for the possibility of pancreatic necrosis or in identifying those patients who would benefit from therapeutic endoscopic retrograde cholangiopancreatography (ERCP) when bile duct calculi are present.

## Pathophysiology and clinical presentation

Acute pancreatitis is an acute inflammatory process of the pancreas that may also involve the peripancreatic tissues, as well as more remote organ systems. The severity of the disease ranges from interstitial edema in mild disease to focal or diffuse

[a] Department of Radiologic Sciences, Wake-Forest University School of Medicine, Medical Center Boulevard, Winston-Salem, NC 27157-1088, USA
[b] Department of Radiology, Keck School of Medicine, University of Southern California, Los Angeles, CA, USA
* Corresponding author.
*E-mail address:* htchelep@wfubmc.edu (H. Tchelepi).

doi:10.1016/j.cult.2007.08.009

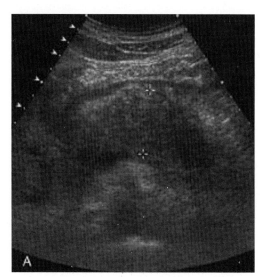

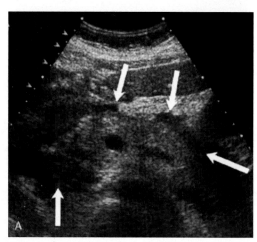

*Fig. 1.* Acute pancreatitis with pancreatic enlargement. Note: The criterion used for enlargement of the pancreas is 23 mm or greater antero-posterior (AP) dimension at the level of the superior mesenteric artery (SMA). This measurement is three standard deviations above the mean. In this patient with a clinical picture of pancreatitis, the pancreas is enlarged to 40 mm, hypoechoic and slightly heterogeneous. The ventral surface of the pancreas is indistinct.

*Fig. 3.* Acute pancreatitis, peripancreatic inflammation. The pancreas appears nearly normal. However, there is hypoechoic inflammation ventral to the body and head and dorsal to the head (*arrows*).

hemorrhage into, or necrosis of, the pancreatic parenchyma in its severe form.

There are many causes of acute pancreatitis, the most common being gallstones. Biliary sludge and alcohol abuse are other common causes. In addition, a variety of medications may cause pancreatitis. Pancreatic divisum, hypertriglyceridemia, and pancreatic carcinoma are also predisposing factors.

The diagnosis of acute pancreatitis is usually made when the serum amylase and lipase levels are elevated in the setting of abdominal pain. The severity of the disease is assessed based on clinical, laboratory, and imaging findings. Clinically, the Ranson and Atlanta classifications are

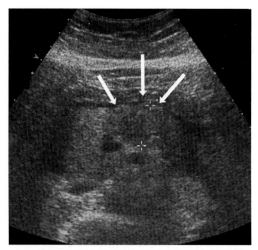

*Fig. 2.* Acute pancreatitis–focal hypoechoic mass. Focal hypoechoic mass (calipers), measuring 25 mm. Note the focal bulge in the ventral surface of the pancreas (*arrows*).

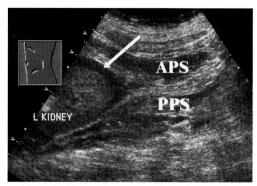

*Fig. 4.* Acute pancreatitis, inflammation in the left retroperitoneal spaces. Coronal oblique longitudinal image through the left flank. Notice that the inflammation (*arrow*) around the left kidney in the perirenal space is sonographically hypoechoic to anechoic. This makes distinction from fluid collections problematic in many cases. Multiple anatomic areas of inflammation are common in acute pancreatitis. Notice that three retroperitoneal spaces are affected in this patient: the anterior pararenal space (APS), the perirenal space (*arrow*) and the posterior pararenal space (PPS). L Kidney is the left kidney.

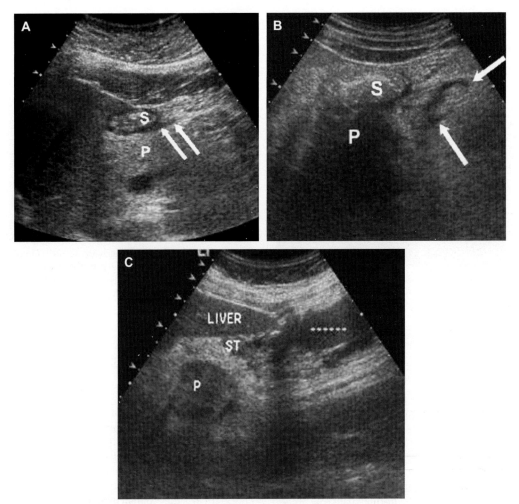

*Fig. 5.* Acute pancreatitis, inflammation of the transverse mesocolon in three patients. (*A*) Longitudinal image through the stomach (S) and pancreas (P). There is subtle inflammation of the lesser omentum (*arrows*). (*B*) Longitudinal image through the stomach (S). Note inflammation in the lesser omentum (*arrows*). There is also considerable inflammation in the pancreas and peripancreatic region (P). (*C*) Longitudinal image through the stomach (ST) and pancreas (P). There is an inflammatory mass in the lesser omentum (*asterisks*). A fluid collection might look like this, but there no fluid was obtained on aspiration.

commonly used to grade the severity of acute pancreatitis and to predict prognosis. Since pancreatic necrosis is neither easily nor accurately detected by sonography, ultrasound is not recommended as an appropriate imaging modality for assessing the severity of pancreatitis. CT is the best means of detecting pancreatic necrosis and the full extent of peripancreatic and retroperitoneal inflammatory changes; therefore, for this purpose contrast enhanced CT remains the imaging modality of choice.

## Sonographic features

The sonographic findings in acute pancreatitis can be classified into three major groups: changes affecting the pancreatic gland, peripancreatic abnormalities, and miscellaneous associated findings [1,2].

### *Pancreatic findings*

Features that should be assessed during the evaluation of the pancreatic gland include the thickness of the gland, parenchymal echogenicity relative to liver parenchyma, glandular heterogeneity, focal regions of altered echogenicity, focal gland abnormalities (masses), visualization of the pancreatic duct, and whether the ventral gland margin is distinct or indistinct. While the thickness (anterior to posterior) of the pancreas varies widely, published measurements for the thickness of the body of the

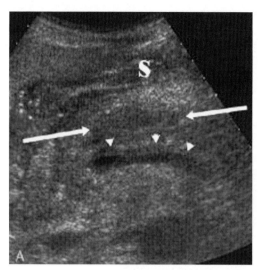

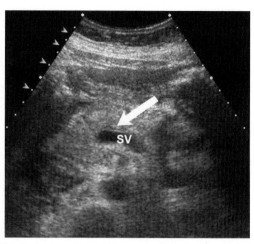

*Fig. 6.* Acute pancreatitis, peripancreatic and perivascular inflammation. Transverse sonogram shows a large region of inflammation ventral to the pancreas (*arrows*), behind the stomach (S). There is more subtle perivascular inflammation ventral to the splenic vein (*arrowheads*).

*Fig. 7.* Acute pancreatitis, perivascular inflammation. Transverse sonogram of the pancreatic body shows a small, linear area of hypoechoic inflammation (*arrow*) ventral to the splenic vein (SV) near the SV/SMV confluence.

normal pancreas in 261 adults was 10.1 mm plus or minus 3.8 mm, with a range of 4 mm to 23 mm [3]. At the authors' institution a measurement over 23 mm is considered abnormal. This measurement is made at the level of the superior mesenteric artery in the transverse plane (Fig. 1). The echogenicity of the gland is compared with that of the liver. The echogenicity of the normal pancreas should

be similar or increased in comparison to the liver [4]; however, the presence of fatty infiltration of the liver can make such comparison useless, resulting in descriptions of spuriously "decreased" pancreatic echogenicity, so-called "pseudopancreatitis." In addition, the normal pancreas should be homogeneous in echotexture. The gland is considered abnormal if the parenchymal echogenicity is

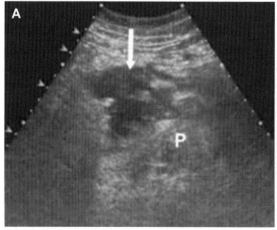

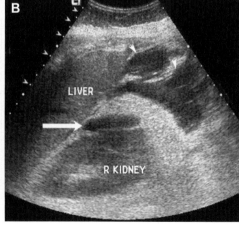

*Fig. 8.* Acute pancreatitis associated fluid collections in two patients. (*A*) Oblique sonogram showing a fluid collection (*arrow*) in a patient with acute pancreatitis ventral to the pancreatic head (P), which is very hypoechoic. (*B*) There are three acute pancreatitis-associated fluid collections in the right retroperitoneum, one of which is in the perirenal space (*arrow*). The other two retroperitoneal collections are ventral to the perirenal space collection (*arrowheads*).

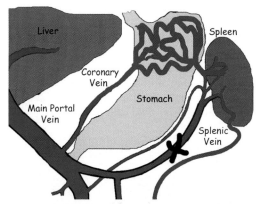

*Fig. 9.* Sinestral portal hypertension. Hepatopetal collaterals bypass the splenic vein clot "X" via the short gastric veins, resulting in isolated gastric varices and ultimately with hepatopetal flow in the coronary (left gastric) vein.

heterogeneous or if there are focal hypoechoic areas. The mass-like changes encountered in acute pancreatitis are almost always hypoechoic (Fig. 2). Occasionally these inflammatory masses may be difficult to distinguish from solid tumors, such as pancreatic adenocarcinomas. Although this distinction may be difficult, the presence of associated peri- and extrapancreatic imaging findings helps establish the diagnosis of a pancreatitis-associated mass rather than a tumor. Occasionally in acute pancreatitis, the gland may appear normal in echogenicity and size. In such cases the diagnosis is made when peripancreatic inflammation is present (Fig. 3).

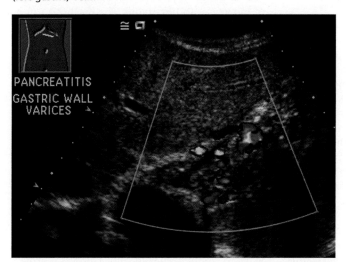

*Fig. 10.* Gastric wall varices from isolated thrombosis of the splenic vein in acute pancreatitis. Transverse color Doppler image of the stomach, demonstrating multiple dilated gastric varices in this patient with acute pancreatitis. The patient also had an enlarged spleen (not shown).

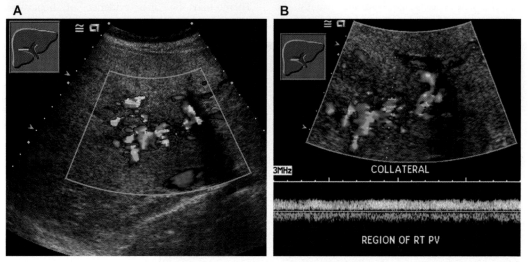

*Fig. 11.* Acute pancreatitis, main and right portal vein thrombosis with collaterals. (*A*) Transverse color Doppler sonogram at the level of the right portal vein. There is clot in the right portal vein with hepatopetal venous collaterals around the thrombosed vessel. (*B*) Spectral wave Doppler interrogation proved that these vessels were veins.

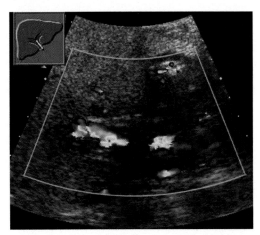

*Fig. 12.* Cavernous transformation of the portal vein. Multiple venous collaterals in the region of the thrombosed main portal vein in the porta hepatis.

## Peripancreatic findings

The most common peripancreatic abnormalities seen in patients with acute pancreatitis are retroperitoneal inflammation (slightly more than 60%) and fluid collections (about 25%). The presence of extra-pancreatic disease is associated with worse prognosis [5,6]. These changes can be seen in the peripancreatic retroperitoneum, the anterior and posterior and posterior pararenal spaces (Fig. 4), the perirenal spaces, and the transverse mesocolon (Fig. 5). When the pancreas is adequately visualized inflammation can be seen ventral to the pancreas (Fig. 6), along the transverse mesocolon and less commonly in the omental fat. Perivascular inflammation is another feature that can be seen in patients with acute pancreatitis (Fig. 7). The vessels involved are usually the splenic and superior mesenteric veins [7,8]. Inflammation is typically hypoechoic to anechoic and may be visualized as linear stranding. Larger areas can even be mass-like. Fluid collections in acute pancreatitis occur in the same areas as inflammation, but are less common (Fig. 8). It may be difficult or impossible to distinguish inflammation from fluid collections.

## Vascular findings

Acute pancreatitis is associated with thrombosis of the portal vein and splenic vein. Such thrombosis is the most common vascular complication seen in patients with acute pancreatitis [9]. It may be difficult to identify short segment clots in the splenic vein because of the long course of the vein and difficulty in visualizing the entire length of the vein with ultrasound. The diagnosis can be established with both grayscale and color Doppler.

Isolated splenic vein thrombosis usually results in so-called "sinestral" (left sided) portal hypertension (Fig. 9). Hepatopetal collaterals bypass the splenic vein clot via the short gastric veins, then result in isolated gastric varices, and ultimately cause hepatopetal flow in the coronary (left gastric) vein (Fig. 10). Portal vein thrombosis may be partial, focal or diffuse-involving the whole portal system (Fig. 11). Often, the collaterals associated with splenic vein clot are the key diagnostic findings in patients with splenic vein thrombosis, rather the identification of the clot itself.

Extensive thrombosis of the main portal vein results in cavernous transformation of the portal vein, which is readily seen with color Doppler (Fig. 12). There may be also evidence of hepatopetal

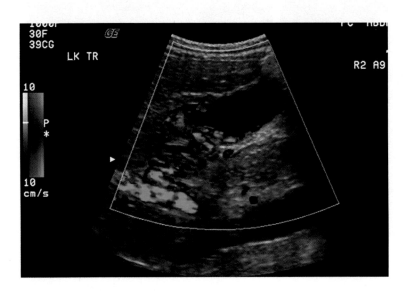

*Fig. 13.* Gallbladder wall varices. Color Doppler sonogram of the gall bladder demonstrating varices in the gallbladder wall in this patient with acute pancreatitis and portal vein thrombosis.

A                                             B

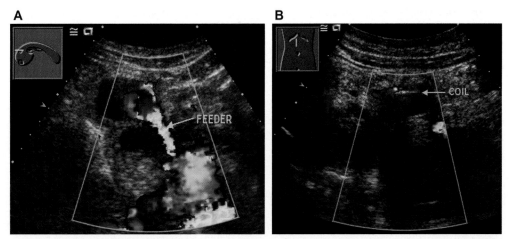

*Fig. 14.* Arterial pseudoaneurysm of the gastroduodenal artery in acute pancreatitis. (A) Transverse color Doppler sonogram identifies a pseudoaneurysm arising from the gastroduodenal artery with characteristic "Ying-Yang" pattern. Color Doppler also shows the feeding vessel (neck) to the aneurysm (*arrow*). Note that the pseudoaneurysm is partially thrombosed. (B) Same patient following embolization of the pseudoaneurysm. Color Doppler image demonstrates persistent blood flow within the aneurysm beyond the coil (*arrow*). This is usually the result of newly recruited vessels by the pseudoaneurysm. The patient was re-embolized and subsequent color Doppler evaluation showed no evidence of blood flow to the pseudoaneurysm.

gallbladder wall varicosities associated with the thrombosed portal vein (Fig. 13).

Another rare vascular complication is the formation of arterial pseudoaneurysms that may bleed and result in increased patient morbidity. Color Doppler is an ideal tool for diagnosing

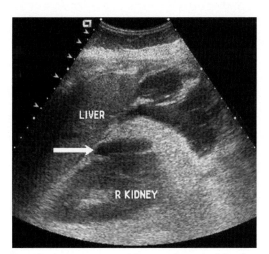

*Fig. 15.* Acute pancreatitis, extrahepatic bile duct stone. This oblique longitudinal sonogram of the common (extrahepatic) bile duct (calipers) shows a distal stone (*arrow*). This duct is dilated to 12 mm. The main reason to do ultrasound in patients with acute pancreatitis is to diagnose gallstones as a cause of the disease. Finding common duct dilatation or duct stones should prompt retrograde cholangiography to remove the stone, and hopefully ameliorate the clinical course of the disease.

pseudoaneurysms and, following embolization, for determining if further treatment is necessary (Fig. 14A). At our institution, postembolization color Doppler ultrasound examinations of all pseudoaneurysms are routinely performed to check for the presence of persistent or recurrent blood flow to the pseudoaneurysm. Despite the initial success of embolization, many pseudoaneurysms will recruit new vessels in a very short period of time and, if that is the case, re-embolization is performed with additional follow up by Doppler ultrasound to confirm successful embolization (Fig. 14B).

## Summary

Ultrasound plays an important role in the imaging and management of patients with acute pancreatitis. First and foremost, sonography can diagnose gallstones and sludge as causes of acute pancreatitis and detect biliary obstruction (Fig. 15). Sonography must be performed even in known alcoholics to exclude gallstones as a cause of pancreatitis. If biliary obstruction is noted, referral to ERCP is indicated. Recent studies have shown that ultrasound can detect pancreatic abnormalities much more frequently than older studies have suggested [10].

However, the most sensitive prognostic indicator in patients with acute pancreatitis is quantification of pancreatic gland necrosis, which currently cannot be accurately assessed with ultrasound. Glandular necrosis is evaluated in clinically severe cases using contrast enhanced CT. This may change in the future, once intravenous bubble ultrasound contrast agents become available in the United States.

## References

[1] Freise J. Evaluation of sonography in the diagnosis of acute pancreatitis. In: Beger HG, Buchler M, editors. Acute pancreatitis. Berlin: Springer-Verlag; 1987. p. 118–31.

[2] Jeffrey RB Jr. Sonography in acute pancreatitis. In: Freeny PC, editor. Radiology of the pancreas, Radiol Clin North Am, 27. Philadelphia: WB Saunders; 1989. p. 5–17.

[3] Guerra M, Gutierrez L, Carrasco R, et al. Size and echogenicity of the pancreas in Chilean adults: echo tomography study in 261 patients. Rev Med Chil 1995;123:720–6.

[4] Cotton PB, Lees WR, Vallon AG, et al. Gray-scale ultrasonography and endoscopic pancreatography in pancreatic diagnosis. Radiology 1980; 134:453–9.

[5] Balthazar EJ. Acute pancreatitis: assessment of severity with clinical and CT evaluation. Radiology 2002;223:603–13.

[6] Vernacchia FS, Jeffrey RB Jr, Federle MP, et al. Pancreatic abscess: predictive value of early abdominal CT. Radiology 1986;162:435–8.

[7] Jeffrey RB Jr, Laing FC, Wing VW. Extrapancreatic spread of acute pancreatitis: new observations with real-time US. Radiology 1986;159: 707–11.

[8] Jeffrey RB, Federly MP, Laing FC. Computed tomography of mesenteric involvement in fulminant pancreatitis. Radiology 1983;147: 185–8.

[9] Dorffel T, Wruck T, Ruckert RI. Vascular complications in acute pancreatitis assessed by color duplex ultrasonography. Pancreas 2000;21(2): 126–33.

[10] Finstad TA, Tchelepi H, Ralls PW. Sonography of acute pancreatitis: prevalence of findings and pictorial essay. Ultrasound Q 2005;21(2): 95–104.

ELSEVIER
SAUNDERS

ULTRASOUND
CLINICS

Ultrasound Clin 2 (2007) 423–435

# Ultrasound Imaging of Pancreatic Transplantation

Keyanoosh Hosseinzadeh, MD[a],*, Jade Wong-You-Cheong, MD[b]

- Types of pancreatic transplantation
- Surgical techniques
  - *Arterial anastomosis*
  - *Venous Management*
  - *Duct management*
- Role of ultrasound
- Complications
  - *Rejection*

- *Vascular complications*
- *Pancreatitis*
- *Intra-abdominal fluid collections*
- *Post-transplantation lymphoproliferative disorder*
- Summary
- References

Type 1 diabetes mellitus is the leading cause of end-stage renal disease (ESRD) in the United States. Diabetes also results in severe, debilitating vascular complications, such as retinopathy, the leading cause of blindness in young and middle aged adults, and in coronary artery and peripheral vascular disease. Vascularized parenchymal pancreatic transplantation was initially developed to restore endogenous insulin secretion responsive to normal feedback controls and is currently the only therapy that reliably establishes a long-term insulin-independent euglycemic state with normalization of glycosylated hemoglobin levels.

The first vascularized pancreatic transplantation was performed in 1966 [1]. Since then there have been many refinements in the surgical technique, accompanied by advances in immunosuppression and patient selection, with a steady increase in success rates. According to the International Pancreas Transplant Registry (IPTR) data, as of 2004 more

than 23,000 pancreas transplants had been reported to the IPTR, with 17,000 performed in the United States and almost 6000 outside of the United States [2]. Long- and short-term patient survival rates have improved consistently over the years and 1-year survival rates are now more than 95% for all categories of transplants performed in 2002 and 2003. Five-year patient survival rates spanning the 1998 and 1999 to 2002 and 2003 interval have also improved significantly and are now more than 80% for all the different types of pancreatic transplantation. Notwithstanding the progress made in recent years, complications do occur in the immediate and late post-operative period, and include graft rejection, pancreatitis, vascular thrombosis, exocrine leaks, perigraft collections, hemorrhage, and post-transplantation lymphoproliferative disorder.

Imaging of pancreas transplant recipients is performed for signs and symptoms such as pain, fever, abdominal distension or leukocytosis, and when

[a] Department of Radiology, Division of Abdominal Imaging, University of Pittsburgh School of Medicine, University of Pittsburgh Medical Center (Presbyterian Campus), 200 Lothrop Street, Room 3950 CHP MT, Pittsburgh, PA 15213, USA
[b] Department of Radiology, Section of Abdominal Imaging, University of Maryland School of Medicine, University of Maryland Medical Center, 22 South Greene Street, Baltimore, MD 21201-1595, USA
* Corresponding author.
*E-mail address:* hosseinzadehk@upmc.edu (K. Hosseinzadeh).

doi:10.1016/j.cult.2007.08.001

there is clinical concern for graft dysfunction based on abnormal serologic or urinary indices. Sonography is considered the primary imaging modality of choice for the detection of early and late postoperative complications of the pancreatic allograft. Radiologic imaging should be performed with close communication between the radiologist and surgeon, including specific details of the type of duct and vascular management, time interval since transplantation, and any clinical evidence of graft dysfunction. Knowledge of the transplantation technique, postoperative imaging anatomy, and any complications is necessary for effective interpretation of the sonographic findings. Knowledge of the limitations of sonography is also important, however, so that alternative imaging modalities can be considered in order to solve specific problems.

This article will begin by describing the different types of pancreas allograft transplantation, including the various forms of duct management and venous drainage. Sonographic technique and common sonographic findings are described. The role of sonography in the effective diagnosis and treatment of allograft disorders is emphasized. Limitations of sonography in the workup of these patients are discussed, together with the incorporation of alternative and complementary imaging modalities.

## Types of pancreatic transplantation

There are three types of pancreatic transplantation: simultaneous pancreas–kidney transplantation (SPK), pancreas after kidney transplantation (PAK), and pancreas transplantation alone (PTA). Between 1987 and June 2004, according to the IPTR, approximately 78% of all pancreatic transplants performed in the United States were SPK procedures, 16% were PAK procedures, and 7% were PTA [2].

The SPK procedure is reserved for patients who have severe type 1 diabetes mellitus and uremia. In most cases the pancreas and kidney are derived from the same cadaver donor, although increasingly, because of organ shortages, simultaneous transplantation of a cadaver pancreas allograft and a living donor renal transplant is performed when possible. The PAK procedure is performed either in type 1 diabetic patients with a functioning kidney transplant or recipients of SPK with failure of the pancreas allograft but a normally functioning renal transplant. While the SPK procedure is more commonly performed than solitary pancreas transplants, there is an increasing emphasis on performing renal transplantation early in uremic diabetic patients to preempt the need for

dialysis. Hence, the number of PAK procedures has increased significantly in recent years. In 2003, of the 1328 pancreas transplants performed in the United States, 338 were PAK (25%). One main advantage of PAK transplantation is the ability to use the kidney from a living donor with its higher graft survival rates. Patient survival rates are also higher at 1 and 2 years for those recipients with a living donor kidney compared with those with a cadaveric kidney [2]. There has been a significant change in the percentage of recipients whose kidney was provided by a living donor from 37% for the years 1988 and 1989 to 69% for the years 2002 and 2003 [2]. Pancreas transplant alone, PTA, the least commonly performed type of pancreatic transplantation, is considered in young patients who have non-uremic brittle type 1 diabetes mellitus with rapidly progressive diabetic complications.

Between 2000 and 2004, the overall patient survival rate for primary cadaveric donor pancreas transplants was highest in the PTA category, but was greater than or equal to 95% at 1 year and greater than or equal to 88% at 3 years for all recipient categories (SPK, PAK, and PTA). The 1- and 3-year graft survival rate was significantly higher in the SPK than the PAK and PTA categories; 85%, 78%, and 76%, respectively, at 1 year, and a 3-year graft survival rate greater than or equal to 62% in all three recipient categories. The rate of early technical graft loss was highest in the PTA category, with graft venous thrombosis being the major cause of graft loss. In technically successful SPK, PAK, and PTA transplants, immunologic graft failure rates for the period 2000 to 2004 were 2%, 8%, and 10%, respectively, at 1 year [2].

## Surgical techniques

In most centers the whole pancreas is harvested from the cadaver donor and transplanted within the peritoneal cavity.

### Arterial anastomosis

The harvested pancreas graft, attached to a small segment of duodenum containing the ampulla of Vater, should have a full length splenic artery and the proximal superior mesenteric artery including the inferior pancreaticoduodenal artery. The donor common iliac artery bifurcation becomes the arterial conduit for the Y graft. The donor Y-iliac artery is used to form an end-to-end anastomosis with the donor splenic and superior mesenteric artery: the splenic artery being anastomosed to the donor internal iliac artery limb and the superior mesenteric artery to the external iliac artery limb. The revascularization of the pancreas allograft is performed in

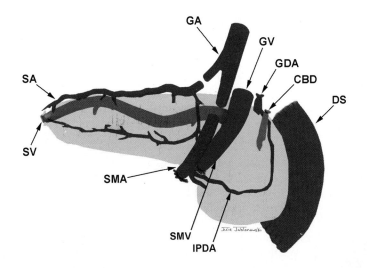

**Fig. 1.** Schematic illustration of the back-table reconstruction of the normal arterial anastomosis of the harvested pancreas allograft. Splenic (*SA*) and superior mesenteric artery (*SMA*) are anastomosed to the recipient external or common iliac artery by way of a Y-graft artery (*GA*). The head of the pancreas is supplied by the inferior pancreatic duodenal artery (*IPDA*), which arises from the SMA. The gastroduodenal (*GDA*) artery is ligated. The donor portal/graft vein (*GV*) is mobilized during procurement to the confluence of the splenic vein (*SV*) and superior mesenteric vein (*SMV*). Note ligated distal common bile duct (*CBD*) and duodenal stump (*DS*).

an end-to-side fashion ideally to the right common iliac or external iliac artery, mainly because of ease of mobilization of the right external iliac vasculature (Fig. 1). There is a higher incidence of graft thrombosis with locations other than the right iliac vessels [3].

### Venous management

The preferred method of venous drainage remains controversial. Systemic venous drainage in which the donor portal/graft vein is anastomosed to the recipient common or external iliac vein is used in 80% of cases and has excellent long-term results (Fig. 2). One disadvantage of this technique is peripheral hyperinsulinemia, however, which is associated with insulin resistance, altered lipid metabolism and advanced arteriosclerosis. A more physiologic approach that eliminates hyperinsulinemia by allowing insulin to circulate through the liver before the systemic circulation is anastomosis of the donor portal vein in an end-to-side fashion to the recipient's infrapancreatic superior mesenteric vein (Fig. 3).

### Duct management

There are two forms of duct management for drainage of exocrine secretions: bladder versus enteric drainage. In bladder drainage, the pancreas allograft is positioned laterally in the pelvis with the duodenal segment/pancreatic head oriented caudally so that the duodenum can be anastomosed to the bladder dome (see Fig. 2). In enteric drained pancreas allografts, the head of the pancreas is oriented cephalad and the duodenum is anastomosed to the jejunum (see Fig. 3).

Bladder drainage has revolutionized the safety of pancreas transplantation. It is, however, limited almost exclusively to grafts that have systematic

venous drainage to iliac veins. Bladder drainage has the advantage that a decrease in urinary lipase and amylase can serve as markers for rejection, acute surgical complications are fewer, and overall improved control of arterial hypertension has been noted. However, bladder drainage results in unique complications, such as dehydration,

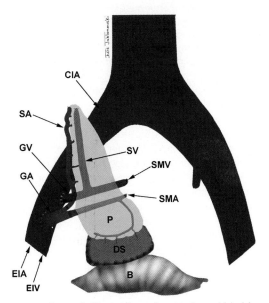

**Fig. 2.** Schematic illustration of systemic and bladder drainage. The Y graft artery (*GA*) is anastomosed to the recipient external (*EIA*) or common iliac artery (*CIA*). The donor portal/graft vein (*GV*) is attached to the recipient external iliac vein (*EIV*). The pancreas (*P*) attached to the oversewn duodenal stump (*DS*) is anastomosed to the bladder (*B*) in a side-to-side fashion, creating a duodenocystostomy. SA, splenic artery; SMA, superior mesenteric artery; SMV, superior mesenteric vein; SV, splenic vein.

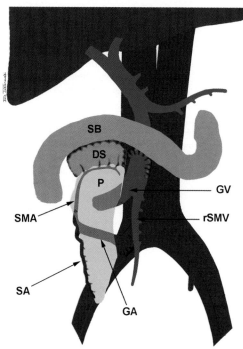

*Fig. 3.* Schematic illustration of portal–enteric drainage. The Y graft artery (*GA*) is anastomosed to the recipient external (*EIA*) or common iliac artery (*CIA*). The donor portal/graft vein (*GV*) is anastomosed to the recipient superior mesenteric vein (*rSMV*) in an end-to-side anastomosis. The pancreas attached to the oversewn duodenal stump (*DS*) is anastomosed in a side-to-side fashion to the recipient small bowel (*SB*). SA, splenic artery; SMA, superior mesenteric artery.

metabolic acidosis, graft pancreatitis, recurrent urinary tract infections, and urethral complications such as strictures, erosions, and fistulae [4]. Consequent to these complications, 15% to 25% of patients who have bladder drainage require conversion to enteric drainage [5,6]. As a result of improvements in immunosuppression, primary enteric drainage of exocrine secretions is now increasingly used, resulting in fewer metabolic and urologic complications. Enteric drainage is achieved by direct side-to-side anastomosis to the recipient small bowel and less frequently by anastomosis to diverting Roux-en-Y limb. In most of all types of transplants, enteric drainage is used for duct management (81% of SPK, 67% of PAK, and 56% of PTA cases) [2]. Despite the evolution in enteric drainage, the proportion of patients undergoing portal venous drainage has remained low, representing between 20% and 28% of cases for all three recipient categories [2]. The benefit of combined portal-enteric drainage appears to be related mostly to lower urological complication rates rather than to improved rejection and diabetes control, and this appears mainly due to enteric drainage.

The impact of portal venous drainage remains controversial. Despite the immunologic or technical benefit of the portal-enteric drained technique, no significant benefit in overall graft survival has been demonstrated between enteric versus bladder drainage and for systemic versus portal drainage in pancreatic transplants [7–10].

## Role of ultrasound

Ultrasound plays an important role in the evaluation of the pancreatic allograft and vasculature and is the first-line imaging modality used in most institutions. Ultrasound evaluation of the pancreatic allograft is indicated in situations in which there is clinical suspicion for graft dysfunction based on abnormal urinary and serologic markers, fever, abdominal pain, ileus and hematuria. Typically a 3.5 to 5 MHz curvilinear or sector probe is used to obtain images parallel to the long and short axis of the allograft. Evaluation includes assessment of allograft size, morphology, echotexture, vasculature, and surrounding ascites or fluid collections. However, unlike renal transplants, sonography of the pancreatic allograft is technically more demanding and complex [11–13]. As the graft is intraperitoneal in location, visualization can be impeded by the presence of overlying bowel gas, especially for enterically drained grafts in which the head of the pancreas is situated more cranially. Additionally, the absence of a firm capsule renders the borders of the allograft indistinct, and differentiation of the allograft from surrounding edematous tissues and bowel is more difficult. The normal pancreatic allograft appears as a soft-tissue mass surrounded by echogenic mesenteric or omental fat and has an

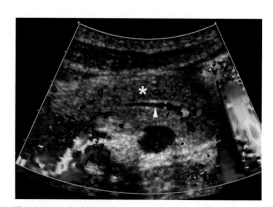

*Fig. 4.* Enteric drained pancreatic allograft. Longitudinal color flow Doppler ultrasound image oriented along the head and body of an enteric drained pancreatic transplant (*asterisk*) shows a nondilated pancreatic duct (*arrowhead*). Note normal parenchymal echogenicity and echotexture.

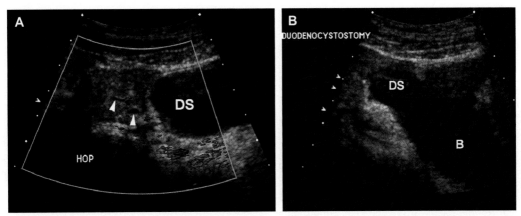

**Fig. 5.** Bladder drained pancreatic allograft. (*A*) Longitudinal ultrasound image with power Doppler through the head of the pancreas transplant with normal flow. The tortuous pancreatic duct (*arrowhead*) and fluid-filled duodenal stump (*DS*) are visible. (*B*) Longitudinal ultrasound image through the duodenocystostomy demonstrating duodenal stump (*DS*) and bladder (*B*).

echogenicity closer to muscle than the more echogenic native pancreas (Fig. 4). For a bladder drained allograft, moderate but incomplete distention of the bladder improves visualization of the pancreatic head, which is situated along the superolateral margin of the bladder dome with the tail positioned superiorly (Fig. 5).

Identification of the pancreatic allograft may be aided by spectral and color flow Doppler imaging. Specific vascular Doppler evaluation is critical for assessment of intraparenchymal and extraparenchymal vessels, including the anastomotic pedicle. The Y graft arterial anastomosis, donor portal/graft vein (Fig. 6), and splenic artery and vein can be readily identified (Fig. 7). The donor superior mesenteric artery and vein, however, are often too small to be recognized, and thus indirect evidence of patency can be inferred by the presence of arterial and venous Doppler waveforms within the head of the allograft (Fig. 8). Normal graft arterial waveforms display a low resistance, antegrade-only, continuous flow pattern that should also be present in the parenchyma of the body and tail of the allograft. Venous flow is low velocity and mono- to minimally biphasic, similar to the signal from the portal vein [14].

## Complications

### Rejection

Rejection can be acute or chronic. Rejection is common following pancreatic transplantation and is the largest single cause of graft failure, despite improved antirejection regimens. Repeated undiagnosed or partially treated episodes of acute rejection may progress to chronic rejection, the

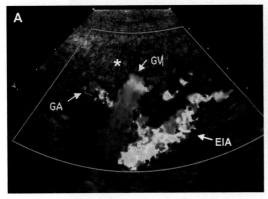
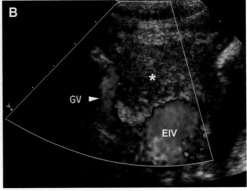

**Fig. 6.** Pancreatic allograft with normal graft artery and systemic venous drainage. (*A*) Transverse color flow Doppler image through the pancreatic head (*asterisk*) demonstrates the graft artery (*GA*) originating from the external iliac artery (*EIA*) and graft vein (*GV*). (*B*) Transverse color Doppler image through the graft vein (*GV*) of systemic venous drained pancreatic transplant (*asterisk*). The graft vein is anastomosed to the external iliac vein (*EIV*).

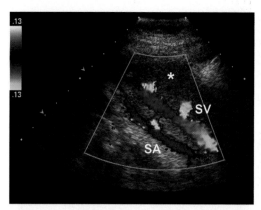

Fig. 7. Normal splenic artery and vein. Longitudinal color flow Doppler image through the body and tail of the pancreas allograft (*asterisk*). The splenic artery (*SA*) and vein (*SV*) are well visualized.

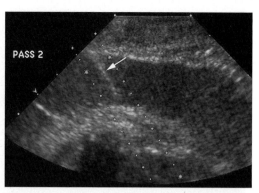

Fig. 9. Ultrasound of a guided biopsy through the tail of a pancreatic transplant. The needle (*arrow*) is seen through the borders of the needle guide. Note normal parenchymal echogenicity and echotexture.

hallmark of which is an obliterative vasculopathy involving the major pancreatic arteries and medium and small sized branches leading to parenchymal fibrosis and gland atrophy [15]. The incidence of chronic rejection increases over time and accounts for 20% to 30% of all graft failures after one year [2]. Abnormal serologic markers raising suspicion for acute rejection are hyperamylasemia, hyperlipasemia, and hyperglycemia. However, hyperglycemia has been noted with development of insulin resistance and islet-cell toxicity and is often a late manifestation of acute rejection. In bladder drained patients, lowered urinary amylase is a more specific marker. For SPK transplants, rejection typically involves both grafts, and serum creatinine level is the most sensitive marker for rejection. However, the laboratory parameters used to evaluate pancreatic allograft dysfunction have low sensitivity and specificity and patients rarely present with symptoms. No single biochemical marker has allowed acute rejection of a pancreas graft to be accurately distinguished from vascular thrombosis and pancreatitis. Imaging may therefore play a role in earlier detection.

Gray-scale imaging characteristics of acute rejection are nonspecific and include enlargement of the gland secondary to edema, which cannot be differentiated from acute pancreatitis or vascular compromise [16-18]. In acute rejection the gland is enlarged with focal or diffuse decreased echogenicity but without pancreatic ductal dilatation. With

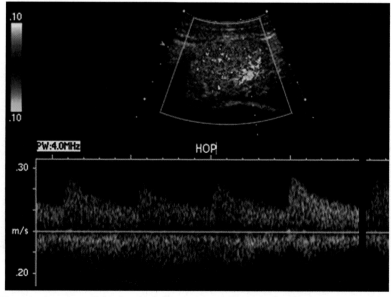

Fig. 8. Normal Doppler imaging of the head of the pancreas allograft. Duplex Doppler waveforms obtained in the head of the pancreas. There is low resistance arterial flow and an undulating venous waveform.

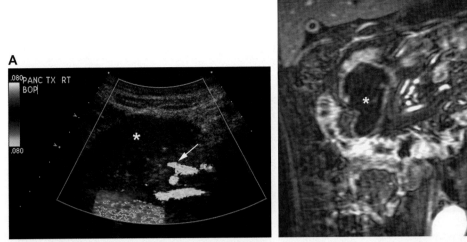

*Fig. 10.* Acutely infarcted enteric drained pancreatic allograft 7 days post-SPK transplantation. (*A*) Longitudinal color flow Doppler through pancreatic allograft demonstrates mildly enlarged hypoechoic pancreas (*asterisk*) with occluded graft artery stump (*arrow*) and absent parenchymal flow. (*B*) Coronal dynamic contrast-enhanced 3D MR angiography demonstrates nonenhancing allograft (*asterisk*). Pancreatectomy confirmed thrombosed graft artery and infarcted allograft.

chronic rejection the gland becomes atrophic and hyperechoic. Although it has been shown that renal parenchymal edema and obliterative vascular changes can cause a reduction in diastolic flow and a corresponding increase in parenchymal resistive index that can predict rejection in the transplanted kidney, this is not a reliable feature of rejection in the pancreatic allograft [13]. The pancreatic allograft does not have the investing capsule that surrounds the kidney, and, therefore swelling from allograft rejection does not cause increased intraparenchymal pressure and elevation of the resistive index. No reliable resistive index measurement has been determined to be of value in patients who have suspected rejection. Elevated resistive indices within parenchymal arteries can be associated with chronic or severe acute rejection of the pancreatic allograft or vascular thrombosis. Many patients who have mild or moderate acute rejection, however, may show no change in vascular resistance [19,20]. Given the insensitivity of gray-scale and Doppler ultrasound, the accepted standard of reference for determining pancreatic rejection is percutaneous ultrasound-guided biopsy. Recent large-scale

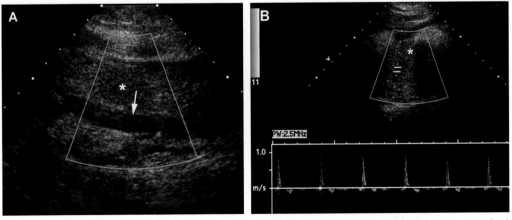

*Fig. 11.* Splenic vein thrombosis and allograft infarction 1 day post-SPK transplantation. (*A*) Power Doppler image through the body of pancreas shows an enlarged hypoechoic pancreas (*asterisk*) with thrombus in a distended splenic vein (*arrow*) and lack of flow within the parenchyma and vessel. (*B*) Duplex Doppler waveform through the head of the pancreas (*asterisk*) shows very high resistance arterial flow. No venous flow could be detected. Transplant pancreatectomy confirmed venous thrombosis and allograft infarction.

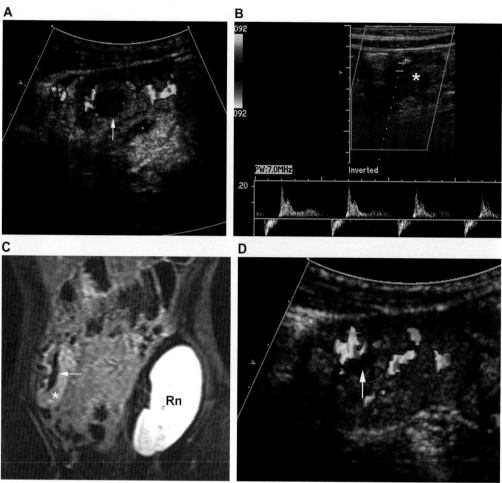

*Fig. 12.* Splenic vein thrombosis 6 days post-SPK transplantation with resolution following anticoagulation therapy. (*A*) Transverse color flow Doppler image through the tail of the pancreas demonstrates a distended splenic vein (*arrow*) with intraluminal echoes consistent with acute thrombus and without intraluminal color flow. (*B*) Duplex Doppler tracing from the tail of the pancreas (*asterisk*) demonstrating an abnormal arterial waveform with reversed diastolic flow. (*C*) Coronal dynamic contrast enhanced 3D MR angiography confirms the thrombus within the splenic vein (*arrow*). Enhancement of the pancreas (*asterisk*) was uniform and other major vessels were patent (not shown). Note left lower quadrant renal allograft (*Rn*). (*D*) Transverse color Doppler image through the tail of the pancreas 10 days after systemic anticoagulant therapy shows decrease in the amount of splenic vein thrombus (*arrow*) that eventually resolved completely.

series have revealed a low incidence of significant post-biopsy complications (1.2%–2.8%) (see below) and a high yield (89%–96%) of diagnostic samples [21,22]. Biopsies are best performed under local anesthesia. Real-time ultrasound guidance is preferred in the authors' institutions, but CT guidance may be used if the sonographic window is optimal. Typically an 18-gauge needle biopsy device is advanced through the peritoneum into the allograft and at least one core biopsy sample is obtained for histologic analysis (Fig. 9). Color Doppler imaging can aid in recognizing and avoiding any large extra- and intraparenchymal vessels. Following the biopsy an ultrasound is obtained to search for any immediate biopsy-related complication, specifically

perigraft hematoma. Other complications that have been described include peripancreatic and intraperitoneal hemorrhage, pancreatitis, infection, pancreatic fistula formation, arteriovenous fistula, pseudoaneurysm formation, and severe pain. Failed biopsies result from poor visualization of the allograft secondary to bowel, patient habitus, or a small pancreatic allograft, although a repeat ultrasound may reveal an adequate acoustic window for biopsy if overlying bowel is the causative factor.

### Vascular complications

Vascular thrombosis is the second most common cause of pancreatic graft loss after rejection, and if not recognized early it can result in propagation

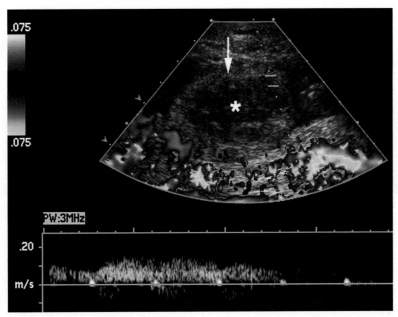

*Fig. 13.* Delayed graft thrombosis 4 years status post-PTA. Longitudinal duplex Doppler of the head and body of the allograft demonstrates an enlarged and heterogeneous gland with hypoechoic parenchyma centrally (*asterisk*) surrounded by a thick echogenic rim (*arrow*) with peripheral flow.

of thrombus within graft vessels, hemorrhagic pancreatitis, parenchymal necrosis, and infection. Allograft necrosis results in pancreatectomy in most cases. Thrombosis is heralded by a sudden rise in blood glucose and low urinary amylase in a bladder drained allograft. Vascular thrombosis can be acute or chronic [23]. Acute graft thrombosis, the most commonly observed complication, usually occurs soon after transplantation and is attributed to surgical technical factors or injury caused by pancreatitis. Venous thrombosis is more common than arterial thrombosis, especially in the early postoperative period. Given the variety of vascular anastomoses that are used for the arterial and venous systems, proper interpretation of cross-sectional imaging or angiography requires clear communication between surgeons and radiologists as to details of the vascular anastomoses. The imaging modality of choice for evaluation of suspected vascular complications is sonography with color flow and spectral Doppler imaging. The infarcted pancreatic transplant is enlarged, hypoechoic, and heterogeneous with complete absence of color flow and absence of duplex Doppler arterial or venous waveforms (Fig. 10). Evidence of vascular thrombosis is demonstrated by absence of arterial or venous Doppler tracings within donor splenic or graft vessels in addition to direct visualization of occlusive intraluminal echogenic material [24,25]. The intraluminal echogenic clot occluding a vessel, however, is not always visualized. Decreased or absent color flow must be confirmed by spectral Doppler analysis (Fig. 11).

Care should be used when diagnosing segmental venous thrombosis, because slow venous flow can be difficult to detect unless Doppler technique is optimized. If the donor graft or splenic veins are not visualized, then the absence of venous tracings in the parenchyma of the allograft in combination with arterial resistive indices greater than or equal to 1.0 has been shown to be highly suggestive of venous thrombosis in the first 12 days after transplantation [25]. The loss of diastolic flow is caused by the increased resistance to antegrade arterial blood flow. Segmental isolated splenic vein thrombosis can be treated with anticoagulants, and ultrasound can be used to monitor the therapeutic effects of anticoagulation therapy (Fig. 12) [26]. Delayed graft thrombosis is an autoimmune phenomenon believed to be caused by small parenchymal vessel arteritis resulting in occlusion of small parenchymal vessels progressing to proximal vessel occlusion and eventually to involve the donor graft artery and possibly graft vein (Fig. 13) [27].

Spectral Doppler is also useful in the diagnosis of anastomotic stenosis and pseudoaneurysm formation, which can be further evaluated by computed tomographic angiography (CTA) or magnetic resonance (MR) angiography. Arterial stenosis is rare and is identified by turbulent flow with increased peak systolic velocities at the site of stenosis [14]. Arterial pseudoaneurysms at or near the anastomosis may occur, either as a result of biopsy or when there is adjacent infection or inflammation, made worse by the digestive action of exocrine secretions.

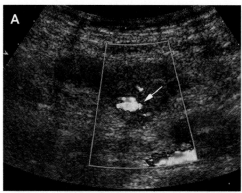
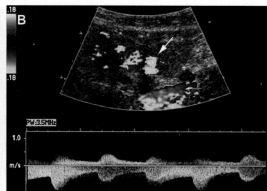

Fig. 14. Arteriovenous fistula 7 days post-percutaneous biopsy of a pancreatic allograft that revealed acute rejection. (*A*) Transverse color flow Doppler image through the tail of the pancreatic transplant showing a focal area of increased velocity (*arrow*); color settings have been optimized for the focal lesion. (*B*) Duplex Doppler waveform shows the characteristic high-velocity, low-resistance pattern of an arteriovenous fistula (*arrow*).

The characteristic to-and-fro spectral Doppler flow pattern and associated color flow features indicate an arterial pseudoaneurysm [28]. Arteriovenous fistulae are rare but can occur within the parenchyma, usually following a biopsy (Fig. 14) [29]. The feeding artery is not always identified but a characteristic high-velocity, low-resistance turbulent waveform is detected in a small focal area of increased color flow, often with aliasing.

As stated, sonographic evaluation of a pancreatic allograft can be technically challenging. Detailed assessment of the graft viability and vasculature of the graft can be difficult in the presence of overlying bowel gas and when the patient has an adverse body habitus. In contrast, CTA and MR imaging in combination with MR angiography are not limited by surrounding bowel gas and can demonstrate vascular anatomy, presence and extent of graft thrombosis, and graft enhancement [23,30–33]. Although CTA is technically less challenging, MR angiography is increasingly used over conventional angiography and CTA, because the contrast agents used in MR angiography are less nephrotoxic. MR imaging and MR angiography have the distinct advantage of having higher relative contrast and dynamic range than CTA. Both modalities are capable of mapping the entire arterial and venous anatomy of the pancreatic allograft, including the superior mesenteric artery and vein, which are infrequently seen on ultrasound. Graft viability is more accurately assessed by MR imaging [23,27,30,34,35]. If there is strong clinical suspicion for vascular compromise and the ultrasound examination yields a positive or indeterminate study, MR imaging / MR angiography is liberally used at the authors' institutions to further evaluate graft viability and vascularity, even in the immediate postoperative period. In a few situations, if clinical suspicion is high, MR imaging and MR angiography can be pursued even in the setting of a normal sonogram. MR

imaging and MR angiography are increasingly used to monitor anticoagulation therapy in patients who have splenic venous stump thrombosis, providing accurate delineation of the thrombus and its resolution [34]. Conventional angiography has limited use in the diagnosis of vascular complications in pancreatic transplant recipients, being reserved for therapy such as embolotherapy, angioplasty, or thrombolysis.

### Pancreatitis

Self-limiting edematous pancreatitis is common, particularly during the early postoperative period,

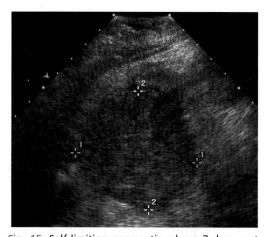

Fig. 15. Self-limiting pancreatic edema 7 days post-PTA. Patient presented with small bowel obstruction. Transverse gray-scale ultrasound shows an enlarged slightly heterogeneous head of pancreas (*outlined by calipers*). This appearance is nonspecific and can be a manifestation of postoperative edema, pancreatitis, acute rejection, or infection. At surgery performed for small bowel adhesions, the pancreas was edematous but showed no signs of rejection at biopsy.

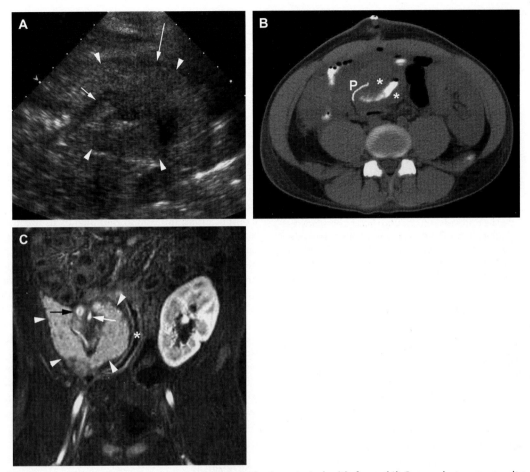

**Fig. 16.** Allograft pancreatitis 3 weeks post-PTA. Patient presented with fever. (*A*) Gray-scale transverse ultrasound shows an edematous heterogeneous allograft (*arrowheads*) with peripancreatic edema (*long arrow*). Central vascular pedicle has a curvilinear configuration (*short arrow*). (*B*) CT scan performed with oral contrast confirms infiltration of fat around the swollen allograft (*P*) and a thickened duodenal stump (*asterisk*). (*C*) Coronal dynamic contrast-enhanced 3D MR angiography demonstrates homogenous enhancement of the enlarged allograft (*arrowheads*) with patent splenic vein (*black arrow*) and artery (*white arrow*). Note the thickened duodenal stump (*asterisk*). Exploratory laparotomy and biopsy was performed for suspicion of rejection which revealed no evidence of infection or rejection.

with clinical parameters stabilizing within 1 week of surgery (Fig. 15). Acute pancreatitis is usually attributed to transplant procurement, preservation, and reperfusion injury. Patients typically present with abdominal pain or localized graft tenderness with non-specific elevations of serum amylase and lipase or decreased urinary amylase (bladder drained grafts). Gray-scale ultrasound often demonstrates nonspecific gland enlargement with overall decreased echogenicity (Fig. 16) and perigraft fluid. Complications associated with graft pancreatitis include pseudocyst formation, peripancreatic fluid collections, abscess formation, pancreatic necrosis and psuedoaneurysms. Ultrasound has a useful role in biopsy of the allograft to establish the diagnosis given the overlap of clinical and biochemical markers with acute rejection and vascular

compromise and for image-guided drainage of pseudocysts (Fig. 17). However, given the larger field of view, CT more effectively delineates the extent of associated fluid collections [36].

## Intra-abdominal fluid collections

Fluid collections are the most common complication detected by imaging and can represent seromas, hematomas, lymphoceles, abscesses, or pseudocysts. The character of the fluid cannot be determined by appearance alone. However, percutaneous sonographic and CT-guided aspirations and catheter placements are useful in diagnosis as well as therapeutic intervention. CT is more sensitive than ultrasound in the detection of anastomotic leaks and abdominal infection.

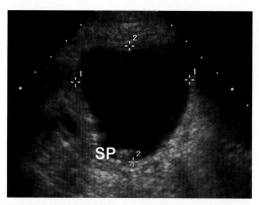

**Fig. 17.** Pseudocyst 8 years post-SPK transplantation. Gray-scale transverse ultrasound shows a peripancreatic pseudocyst (*outlined by calipers*) with a dependent echogenic structure representing an extruded silicone plug (*SP*). The silicone was used to occlude the pancreatic duct; this technique is not currently performed.

## Post-transplantation lymphoproliferative disorder

Post-transplantation lymphoproliferative disorder (PTLD) can occur in any transplantation setting. The disease represents a spectrum ranging from polyclonal hyperplasia to monoclonal malignant lymphoma. In most cases, the disorder results from Epstein-Barr virus (EBV)-induced B-cell proliferation of lymphocytes. PTLD may develop in approximately 1% to 2% of recipients of solid organ transplants. There is limited description available of the imaging features of PTLD in pancreas transplant recipients. A recent study retrospectively reviewed 337 pancreas transplant recipients and documented eight patients (2.4%) who developed PTLD. The majority had diffuse involvement of the allograft [37]. The pancreatic allograft is typically enlarged and heterogeneous, although uncommonly a focal mass is visualized. The imaging appearance may be indistinguishable from the typical imaging findings of acute pancreatitis or allograft rejection, because diffuse allograft involvement is the most common presentation. Extra-allograft involvement was less common including lymphadenopathy and hepatomegaly. The diagnosis of PTLD should be considered in pancreas transplant recipients who fail to respond to anti-inflammatory or antirejection therapy or if there are extra-allograft masses with involvement of either solid organs or lymphadenopathy. Tissue biopsy is necessary for final diagnosis.

## Summary

Ultrasound is the accepted primary imaging modality for assessment of pancreatic graft dysfunction and allows noninvasive, portable, inexpensive evaluation of the pancreas transplant. Ultrasound is an excellent modality for detection and image-guided drainage of perigraft collections. The addition of color flow and spectral Doppler imaging is essential for evaluating vascular integrity and vascular complications, especially in the immediate postoperative period. However, MR imaging/MR angiography and CTA should be considered to more completely assess parenchymal viability and vascular anatomy if the sonographic findings are indeterminate, or clinical suspicion remains high. Although the sensitivity and specificity of ultrasound is high in the detection of graft vascular complications, ultrasound is limited by its inability to distinguish rejection from pancreatitis. Sonographic findings should be interpreted in conjunction with the clinical history and serologic and urinary indices with the caveat that appropriate management may require further evaluation with CT or MR imaging. Currently no imaging modality can accurately diagnose or stage the severity of rejection, and ultrasound-guided biopsies are the standard of care. The optimal diagnosis and management of pancreas transplant recipients requires close communication between the radiologist and surgeons and good understanding by the radiologist of the surgical technique including the type of vascular and ductal management.

## References

[1] Kelly WD, Lillehei RC, Merkel FK, et al. Allotransplantation of the pancreas and duodenum along with the kidney in diabetic nephropathy. Surgery 1967;61(6):827–37.

[2] Gruessner AC, Sutherland DE. Pancreas transplant outcomes for United States (US) and non-US cases as reported to the United Network for Organ Sharing (UNOS) and the International Pancreas Transplant Registry (IPTR) as of June 2004. Clin Transplant 2005;19(4):433–55.

[3] Troppmann C, Gruessner AC, Benedetti E, et al. Vascular graft thrombosis after pancreatic transplantation: univariate and multivariate operative and nonoperative risk factor analysis. J Am Coll Surg 1996;182(4):285–316.

[4] Del Pizzo JJ, Jacobs SC, Bartlett ST, et al. Urological complications of bladder-drained pancreatic allografts. Br J Urol 1998;81(4):543–7.

[5] West M, Gruessner AC, Metrakos P, et al. Conversion from bladder to enteric drainage after pancreaticoduodenal transplantations. Surgery 1998;124(5):883–93.

[6] Sollinger HW, Odorico JS, Knechtle SJ, et al. Experience with 500 simultaneous pancreas–kidney transplants. Ann Surg 1998;228(3):284–96.

[7] Gaber AO, Shokouh-Amiri MH, Hathaway DK, et al. Results of pancreas transplantation with

portal venous and enteric drainage. Ann Surg 1995;221(6):613–22 [discussion: 622–4].

[8] Petruzzo P, Da Silva M, Feitosa LC, et al. Simultaneous pancreas–kidney transplantation: portal versus systemic venous drainage of the pancreas allografts. Clin Transplant 2000;14(4 Pt 1):287–91.

[9] Stratta RJ, Gaber AO, Shokouh-Amiri MH, et al. A prospective comparison of systemic-bladder versus portal-enteric drainage in vascularized pancreas transplantation. Surgery 2000;127(2):217–26.

[10] Philosophe B, Farney AC, Schweitzer EJ, et al. Superiority of portal venous drainage over systemic venous drainage in pancreas transplantation: a retrospective study. *Ann Surg* 2001;234(5): 689–96.

[11] Letourneau JG, Maile CW, Sutherland DE, et al. Ultrasound and computed tomography in the evaluation of pancreatic transplantation. Radiol Clin North Am 1987;25(2):345–55.

[12] Patel B, Markivee CR, Mahanta B, et al. Pancreatic transplantation: scintigraphy, US, and CT. *Radiology* 1988;167(3):685–7.

[13] Nikolaidis P, Amin RS, Hwang CM, et al. Role of sonography in pancreatic transplantation. Radiographics 2003;23(4):939–49.

[14] Low RA, Kuni CC, Letourneau JG. Pancreas transplant imaging: an overview. AJR Am J Roentgenol 1990;155(1):13–21.

[15] Papadimitriou JC, Drachenberg CB, Klassen DK, et al. Histological grading of chronic pancreas allograft rejection/graft sclerosis. Am J Transplant 2003;3(5):599–605.

[16] Yuh WT, Wiese JA, Abu-Yousef MM, et al. Pancreatic transplant imaging. Radiology 1988;167(3): 679–83.

[17] Gilabert R, Fernandez-Cruz L, Bru C, et al. Duplex-Doppler ultrasonography in monitoring clinical pancreas transplantation. Transpl Int 1988;1(3):172–7.

[18] Snider JF, Hunter DW, Kuni CC, et al. Pancreatic transplantation: radiologic evaluation of vascular complications. Radiology 1991;178(3):749–53.

[19] Aideyan OA, Foshager MC, Benedetti, et al. Correlation of the arterial resistive index in pancreas transplants of patients with transplant rejection. AJR Am J Roentgenol 1997;168(6):1445–7.

[20] Wong JJ, Krebs TL, Klassen DK, et al. Sonographic evaluation of acute pancreatic transplant rejection: morphology-Doppler analysis versus guided percutaneous biopsy. AJR Am J Roentgenol 1996;166(4):803–7.

[21] Atwell TD, Gorman B, Larson TS, et al. Pancreas transplants: experience with 232 percutaneous US-guided biopsy procedures in 88 patients. Radiology 2004;231(3):845–9.

[22] Klassen DK, Weir MR, Cangro CB, et al. Pancreas allograft biopsy: safety of percutaneous biopsy—results of a large experience. Transplantation 2002;73(4):553–5.

[23] Krebs TL, Daly B, Wong JJ, et al. Vascular complications of pancreatic transplantation: MR evaluation. Radiology 1995;196(3):793–8.

[24] Heyneman LE, Keogan MT, Tuttle-Newhall JE, et al. Pancreatic transplantation using portal venous and enteric drainage: the postoperative appearance of a new surgical procedure. J Comput Assist Tomogr 1999;23(2):283–90.

[25] Foshager MC, Hedlund LJ, Troppmann C, et al. Venous thrombosis of pancreatic transplants: diagnosis by duplex sonography. AJR Am J Roentgenol 1997;169(5):1269–73.

[26] Kuo PC, Wong J, Schweitzer EJ, et al. Outcome after splenic vein thrombosis in the pancreas allograft. Transplantation 1997;64(6):933–5.

[27] Krebs TL, Daly B, Wong-You-Cheong JJ, et al. Acute pancreatic transplant rejection: evaluation with dynamic contrast-enhanced MR imaging compared with histopathologic analysis. Radiology 1999;210(2):437–42.

[28] Tobben PJ, Zajko AB, Sumkin JH, et al. Pseudoaneurysms complicating organ transplantation: roles of CT, duplex sonography, and angiography. Radiology 1988;169(1):65–70.

[29] Delis S, Dervenis C, Bramis J, et al. Vascular complications of pancreas transplantation. Pancreas 2004;28(4):413–20.

[30] Hagspiel KD, Nandalur K, Burkholder B, et al. Contrast-enhanced MR angiography after pancreas transplantation: normal appearance and vascular complications. AJR Am J Roentgenol 2005;184(2):465–73.

[31] Freund MC, Steurer W, Gassner EM, et al. Spectrum of imaging findings after pancreas transplantation with enteric exocrine drainage: Part 2, posttransplantation complications. AJR Am J Roentgenol 2004;182(4):919–25.

[32] Freund MC, Steurer W, Gassner EM, et al. Spectrum of imaging findings after pancreas transplantation with enteric exocrine drainage: Part 1, posttransplantation anatomy. AJR Am J Roentgenol 2004;182(4):911–7.

[33] Dachman AH, Newmark GM, Thistlethwaite JR Jr, et al. Imaging of pancreatic transplantation using portal venous and enteric exocrine drainage. AJR Am J Roentgenol 1998;171(1): 157–63.

[34] Dobos N, Roberts DA, Insko EK, et al. Contrast-enhanced MR angiography for evaluation of vascular complications of the pancreatic transplant. Radiographics 2005;25(3):687–95.

[35] Eubank WB, Schmiedl UP, Levy AE, et al. Venous thrombosis and occlusion after pancreas transplantation: evaluation with breath-hold gadolinium-enhanced three-dimensional MR imaging. AJR Am J Roentgenol 2000;175(2):381–5.

[36] Patel BK, Garvin PJ, Aridge DL, et al. Fluid collections developing after pancreatic transplantation: radiologic evaluation and intervention. Radiology 1991;181(1):215–20.

[37] Meador TL, Krebs TL, Wong-You-Cheong JJ, et al. Imaging features of posttransplantation lymphoproliferative disorder in pancreas transplant recipients. AJR Am J Roentgenol 2000;174(1): 121–4.

ELSEVIER
SAUNDERS

ULTRASOUND
CLINICS

Ultrasound Clin 2 (2007) 437–453

# Sonographic Evaluation of the Abdominal Aorta

Shweta Bhatt, MD[a], Hamad Ghazale, MS, RDMS[b],
Vikram S. Dogra, MD[a],*

- Sonographic anatomy and technique
- Abdominal aortic aneurysm
- Screening
  - *Screening tests*
  - *Selective screening*
  - *Effectiveness of screening*
- Making the diagnosis
  - *Classification of abdominal aortic aneurysm*
- Aneurysm rupture
  - *Predictors of aneurysm rupture*
  - *Sonographic findings*

- *Inflammatory abdominal aortic aneurysm*
- *Mycotic abdominal aortic aneurysm*
- *Pseudoaneurysm*
- Endograft evaluation
  - *Endoleak detection*
- Aortic dissection
- B-flow imaging
- Limitations of sonography for evaluation of abdominal aortic aneurysm and rupture
- Summary
- References

Abdominal aortic aneurysm (AAA) is a disease of aging, and the prevalence is expected to increase as the population of elderly patients grows. AAAs are associated with high mortality, as rupture of an AAA is the tenth leading cause of death in the United States. AAA can be diagnosed with CT, magnetic resonance imaging (MR imaging), and ultrasonography (US). US has nearly 100% sensitivity in detecting AAA and is readily available for routine and emergency evaluation [1]. In addition, there are no risk factors associated with US examination of the aorta as there are with CT and MR imaging, including exposure to ionizing radiation, risks associated with intravenous contrast, expense, and perhaps most important, time delay in performing the study. This review describes the sonographic technique for evaluation of the abdominal aorta (AA) and associated pathologies of the AA, including AAA.

## Sonographic anatomy and technique

The AA is a continuation of the thoracic aorta, beginning at the aortic hiatus in the diaphragm (thoracic vertebra level 12) and ending at the fourth lumbar vertebra, where it divides into the common iliac arteries. It descends in the midline, anterior to the vertebral column and to the left of the inferior vena cava. The normal luminal diameter of the infrarenal AA varies with age and gender. In young patients who do not have vascular disease, the infrarenal AA measures 2.3 cm in males and 1.9 cm

a Department of Imaging Sciences, University of Rochester Medical Center, University of Rochester School of Medicine, 601 Elmwood Avenue, Box 648, Rochester, NY 14642, USA
b Diagnostic Medical Sonography Program, Rochester Institute of Technology, 153 Lomb Memorial Drive, Rochester, NY 14623, USA
* Corresponding author.
E-mail address: vikram_dogra@urmc.rochester.edu (V.S. Dogra).

1556-858X/07/$ – see front matter © 2007 Elsevier Inc. All rights reserved.
ultrasound.theclinics.com

doi:10.1016/j.cult.2007.06.001

in females [2]. It increases in diameter with age. In one study, men who had a mean age of 70.4 years who did not have AAA had an average luminal diameter of 2.8 cm [3].

Abdominal aortic ultrasound is preferably performed after 8 to 12 hours of fasting. Fasting reduces bowel gas, which helps provide a better view of the AA. The standard protocol for scanning the AA consists of obtaining longitudinal and transverse images from the level of the diaphragm to the level of bifurcation of the AA, where the common iliac arteries are visualized like binoculars in the transverse view (Fig. 1). Abdominal aortic diameter is recorded at the proximal, mid, and distal aorta, along with measurement of the common iliac arteries just distal to the bifurcation. The inferior vena cava is also evaluated to document normal flow.

Sonographic evaluation of the AA is performed in a supine position or right and left lateral decubitus or right and left posterior oblique positions. Images are obtained in coronal and transverse planes. Placing the patient in the left lateral position and imaging in a coronal scan plane allows for better visualization of both iliac arteries in one image (Fig. 2). Application of gentle pressure or compression and changing the transducer angle may also help displace bowel gas and improve visualization of the aorta. The patient's body habitus plays an important role in determining the optimal type of transducer and frequency to be used. Usually 2.5 to 5 MHz sector, curvilinear array transducers provide optimal visualization of the aorta.

Sonographically the normal aorta has an anechoic echo-free lumen with echogenic walls. Artifactual intraluminal echoes may result from increased gain and slice-thickness or reverberation artifacts (Fig. 3). These types of echoes can be confused with thrombus or intraluminal tumor. The sonographer must change the patient's position or angulation of the transducer and correct the gain to see if these echoes can be eliminated. If these echoes disappear, they most likely represent an artifact.

The anteroposterior (AP) diameter of the aorta should be measured from a longitudinal image, because this allows correct placement of the calipers perpendicular to the long axis of the vessel. The

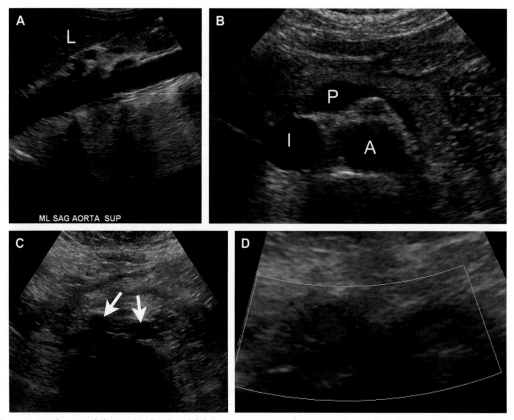

Fig. 1. Normal aorta. (*A*) Longitudinal and (*B*) transverse gray scale sonogram demonstrates the normal appearance of the proximal abdominal aorta (A, abdominal aorta; IVC, inferior vena cava; P, portal vein; L, liver). (*C, D*) Transverse gray scale and corresponding power Doppler sonograms of aortic bifurcation into common iliac arteries (*arrows*) are seen as "binocular" in appearance.

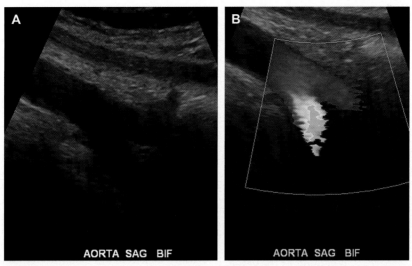

*Fig. 2.* Aortic bifurcation. (*A*) Longitudinal gray scale and (*B*) color flow Doppler images demonstrate the normal aortic bifurcation.

measurement should be taken from outer wall to outer wall and should not exceed 3 cm in diameter [4]. The diameter of the aorta decreases as it courses inferiorly. Consequently the AP measurement varies from one segment of the aorta to another and is also depends on age and the presence or absence of disease. When an aneurysm is observed, the operator must obtain the maximum true length, width, and transverse dimensions of the aneurysm and must measure the true lumen. The shape and location of the aneurysm should be determined. The exact relationship of the AAA to the origin of the renal arteries and the bifurcation should be noted. Involvement (ie, dilatation) of the common iliac arteries should also be documented.

Color flow Doppler is helpful in determining the patency and direction of blood flow in the aorta. The color box should be kept small, which improves the frame rate and enhances the color resolution. The color Doppler gain should be set at less than noise level and a low pulse repetition frequency (PRF) should be avoided to prevent aliasing. Methods of optimization of color flow Doppler are given in Table 1 [5].

Normal blood flow in the aorta is laminar. The flow pattern in the aorta is considered a

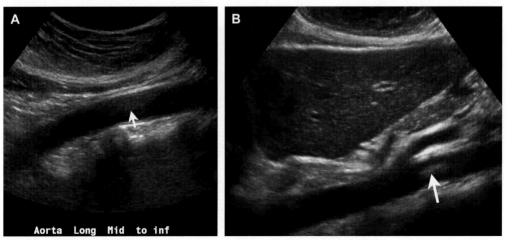

*Fig. 3.* (*A*) Longitudinal gray scale sonogram of the proximal aorta demonstrates a hypoechoic area of low level echoes along the anterior wall (*arrow*), mimicking a thrombus. This is an artifact secondary to partial volume averaging. (*B*) Longitudinal gray scale sonogram of the proximal aorta demonstrates a luminal echogenic focus (*arrow*), mimicking an intraluminal thrombus, arising secondary to a reverberation artifact.

| **Table 1:** Optimization of color flow Doppler | |
|---|---|
| Color box | Keeping the color box small results in improved frame rate and better color resolution |
| Doppler gain | Just below the noise level |
| Color scale (PRF) | Low PRF is more sensitive to low volume and low velocity flow but may lead to aliasing |
| Beam steering | Adjust to obtain satisfactory vessel angle |
| Gate size (sample volume) | Set the sample volume to a correct size, usually two thirds of the vessel lumen |
| Wall filter | A higher filter cuts out the noise and but also the slower velocity flow; keep the filter at 50–100 Hz |
| Focal zone | Color flow image is optimized at the level of the focal zone |

(*From* Bhatt S, Dogra V. Doppler imaging of the uterus and adnexae. Ultrasound Clinics 2006;1:201–21; with permission.)

high-resistance pattern. The proximal aorta normally demonstrates a biphasic waveform with reversal of flow in early diastole. The distal aorta demonstrates a triphasic waveform with a small component of forward flow in late diastole (Fig. 4) [6].

## Abdominal aortic aneurysm

An aortic aneurysm is defined as a focal dilation of the aorta with a diameter of at least 1.5 times that of the expected normal diameter of that given aortic segment; in the AA, enlargement of the aortic diameter of more than 3 cm is usually considered aneurysmal. Alternatively an AAA can be defined as a ratio of infrarenal to suprarenal aortic diameter of 1.2, or a history of AAA repair [7]. Prevalence of AAA has been estimated at 1.2% to 12.6% for men in the sixth to ninth decades, with almost two thirds of AAAs involving only the AA [8]. Overall, up to 13% of all patients in whom an aortic aneurysm is diagnosed have multiple aneurysms, with 25% to 28% of patients who have thoracic aortic aneurysms having concomitant AAAs [9]. Published data from the National Vital Statistics Report on deaths from the year 2000 showed that AAAs and aortic dissection were the tenth leading cause of death in white men of 65 to 74 years of age and accounted for nearly 16,000 deaths overall [10]. The high mortality associated with AAAs has led to an increase in the need to identify risk factors so that appropriate screening procedures can be undertaken for early diagnosis. AAA is most commonly a sequelae of atherosclerosis; therefore, predisposing risk factors for atherosclerosis, such as older age, smoking, and hypertension, are strongly associated with the development of AAA [11,12]. Although moderate alcohol consumption has been found to have a beneficial effect on coronary artery disease because of its positive effect on high-density lipoproteins, Wong and colleagues [13] found that higher alcohol consumption (>2 drinks per day) increased the risk for aortic aneurysmal disease in

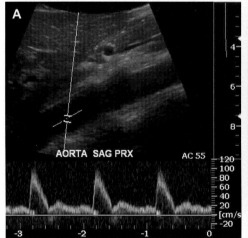 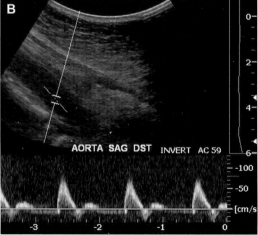

*Fig. 4.* Spectral Doppler waveform of the (*A*) proximal and (*B*) distal aorta demonstrate a high resistance monophasic waveform proximally and a triphasic waveform distally.

men who did not have pre-existing cardiovascular disease.

Predisposing factors for AAA are listed in Box 1.

## Screening

Most AAAs are asymptomatic until there is a rapid expansion of the aneurysm or rupture. The classic clinical triad of hypotension, back pain, and pulsatile abdominal mass is observed in only approximately 50% of patients presenting with a ruptured AAA [14]. Most patients who have AAA, however, present for the first time with abdominal pain. Pain may or may not be accompanied by hypovolemia and shock and is often mistaken for other more common causes of abdominal pain, such as a renal colic or diverticulitis [15]. Failure or delay to diagnose ruptured AAA on clinical presentation contributes to the high mortality rate. This emphasizes the need for an appropriate AAA screening method to identify and repair AAAs before they rupture. Schilling and colleagues were the first to begin screening for AAA in 1964 [16], but it has been justified for regular use only recently [17].

Lee and colleagues [18] analyzed the cost effectiveness of ultrasound screening for AAA and proposed that all men older than age 60 years should be screened for AAA and that this screening should be adopted and reimbursed by Medicare and other insurers. Effective January 1, 2007 the Centers for Medicare and Medicaid Services (CMS) approved Medicare reimbursement for a one-time AAA screening by abdominal US for men between the ages of 65 and 75 years who have ever smoked or who have a first-degree family history of AAA. Women who manifest other risk factors in a beneficiary category recommended for screening by the United States Preventive Services Task Force regarding AAA may also be eligible for receiving this reimbursement. Individualization of care, however, is recommended in the case of a woman seeking reimbursement for screening. For example, a healthy female smoker in her early seventies who has a first-degree family history for AAA that required surgery may be an eligible beneficiary [19].

### Screening tests

Although abdominal palpation was the original method of AAA screening, ultrasound is currently considered the preferred method of screening. Ultrasound has several advantages, such as accuracy (nearly 100% sensitivity and specificity for AAA), low cost, patient acceptance, no radiation exposure, short length of examination time (a quick screening takes less than 5 minutes [18]), and easy availability. CT of the abdomen is often obtained preoperatively for exact measurement and assessment of the geometry of the AAA, especially if the patient is being considered for stent graft placement, but it is not currently recommended for screening purposes.

### Selective screening

There are three important risk factors that are definitely associated with AAA, and patients who have these risk factors are therefore considered for selective screening. They include gender (males are 3–6 times more likely than women to have AAA) [20], age (most AAAs occur in patients older than 65 years) [21], and a history of smoking (smokers are 3–5 times more likely than nonsmokers to have AAA) [22]. Because of the high prevalence of AAA in these categories, limiting screening to a sub-selected population based on these criteria is useful. Besides these criteria, positive association with AAA is also seen with a positive family history, white race, a history of occlusive vascular disease, and the absence of diabetes [22].

### Effectiveness of screening

Various studies have demonstrated a significant reduction in mortality rates from AAA as a result of screening for aortic aneurysm. Four randomized trials [23–26] of AAA screening, including more than 125,000 men, have now reported results for up to 5 to 10 years of follow-up, and all four trials documented a reduction in AAA-related mortality, ranging from 21% to 68% [17].

### Making the diagnosis

US is the most commonly used screening modality for AAA, with an accuracy of almost 100% [18]. Sonographically the most common appearance of AAA is of a dilated vessel with associated atherosclerotic changes, such as an irregular wall with calcifications or echogenic mural thrombus, located circumferentially or eccentrically (Fig. 5). Measurement of the aorta is critical to make a diagnosis of

---

**Box 1: Predisposing risk factors for abdominal aortic aneurysm**

1. Smoking
2. Age; more common after the sixth decade
3. Hypertension
4. Hyperlipidemia
5. Atherosclerosis
6. Moderate alcohol consumption; >2 drinks per day
7. Gender; men are 10 times more likely to have AAA than women
8. Positive family history
9. Congenital disorders such as Marfan and Ehlers Danlos syndrome

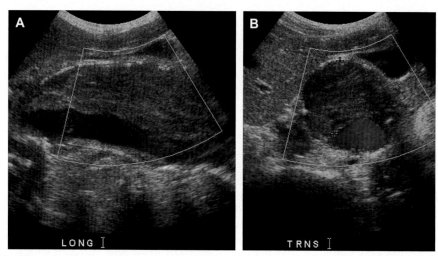

Fig. 5. AAA. (A) Longitudinal and (B) transverse color flow Doppler images demonstrate an infrarenal AAA with a thrombus that occludes approximately two thirds of the lumen.

AAA. Criteria for making the diagnosis of AAA on the basis of measurement have been mentioned, and include: (1) focal dilatation of the AA more than 3.0 cm, (2) increase in the aortic diameter to 1.5 times the normal expected diameter, and (3) ratio of infrarenal to suprarenal aortic diameter more than or equal to 1.2. There may be variations in measurement of the aneurysm size depending on technique. The aneurysmal sac should be measured from outer wall to outer wall from a longitudinal image. The transverse diameter should be measured perpendicular to the long axis of the aorta (Fig. 6). This is particularly important in ectatic aortas, in which a transverse measurement may give an erroneously high number, because it is actually an oblique rather than true transverse measurement. Sometimes the presence of concentric thrombus may make the aortic diameter look smaller. Three-dimensional (3D) US is a useful technique for assessment of AAA, allowing measurements to be made with multiplanar reconstructions from the 3D volume data. An attempt should also be made to visualize the abdominal aortic branches and to demonstrate whether or not they are also aneurysmally dilated.

Color flow Doppler evaluation should follow the gray scale examination of the aorta. Sudden change in the aortic lumen diameter causes turbulent flow within the aneurysmal sac. This turbulent flow may give rise to the "pseudo yin-yang" sign (Fig. 7) and must not be mistaken for a pseudoaneurysm. Flow within the AAA may also be turbulent because of the presence of mural thrombus [27].

### Classification of abdominal aortic aneurysm

AAAs can be classified according to location, morphologic shape, and etiology. See Fig. 8 and Table 2 [28] for details.

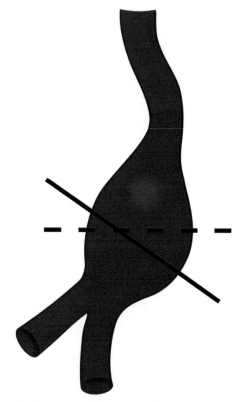

Fig. 6. Diagrammatic representation of measurement of an AAA in an ectatic aorta. The correct method of measuring an AAA is perpendicular to the long axis of the aorta as shown by the continuous line. The dotted line shows that a transverse image relative to the patient yields an oblique incorrect measurement that exaggerates the diameter of an ectatic aorta.

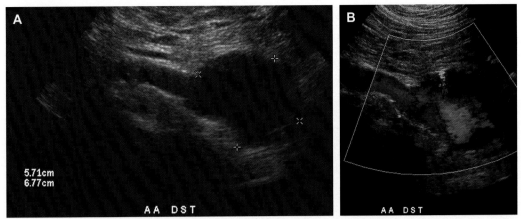

*Fig. 7.* Pseudo yin-yang sign. (*A*) Longitudinal gray scale sonogram of the distal AA demonstrates a fusiform aneurysm. (*B*) Corresponding color flow Doppler evaluation demonstrates a pseudo yin-yang pattern (*blue and red*) of color flow within the aneurysm.

## Aneurysm rupture

The high mortality rate associated with AAAs is secondary to rupture of the aneurysm leading to exsanguination. Spontaneous rupture of an AAA (>6 cm) has a mortality rate ranging from 66% to 95%. Of patients who have AAA rupture, 40% to 50% die before they reach the hospital, and the overall mortality rate of a ruptured AAA is greater than 90% [29].

The most important role of ultrasound, therefore, is to assess the size of the aneurysm and its rate of enlargement, which are the two most important factors in predicting the likelihood of rupture. AAAs do not conform to the law of Laplace, however, and there is growing evidence that aneurysm rupture involves a complex series of biologic changes in the aortic wall [30] and is not just related to diameter.

The most frequent site of aortic rupture is in the left retroperitoneum [31,32]. Rupture also most commonly involves the middle one third of the aneurysm, where the aneurysmal diameter is the largest [32]. In an autopsy series of AAA, aneurysm ruptures were found to occur more frequently in the posterior wall (67%) and in the inferior portion (61%) [33].

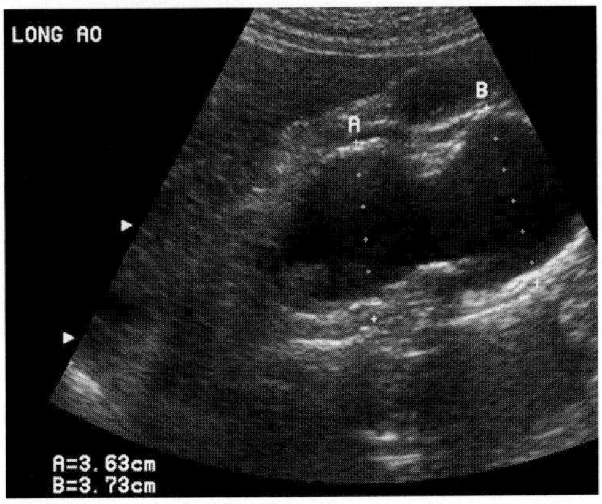

## Predictors of aneurysm rupture

### Maximum diameter

Size of the aneurysm refers to the maximum cross-sectional diameter of the aorta. The best predictor of rupture risk for an AAA is the size at the most recent ultrasound. Because of a higher variability in the measurement of the transverse diameter of the aorta, measurement of the anteroposterior diameter is the preferred method for measuring an AAA by ultrasound [3]. The risk for rupture increases sharply for aneurysms 6 cm or greater in size [34]. In a 15-year study by Brown and colleagues [35], AAAs measuring 5.0 to 5.9 cm had a risk for rupture of 1% per year. If the AAA measured 6 cm or more in maximal diameter, however, risk for rupture increased to 14% per year. Women who had similarly sized AAAs had a fourfold higher risk for rupture [35]. Newer studies, however, have reported that the "maximum diameter criterion" is not reliable in predicting aneurysm rupture because of the lack of a physically sound theoretic basis. Biomechanical factors such as wall stress and strain also play a major role in predicting the risk for aneurysm rupture [36].

*Fig. 8.* Hourglass aorta. Longitudinal gray scale sonogram of the AA demonstrates an hourglass appearance caused by two discontinuous focal segments of aneurysmal dilatation. The aortic diameter in between is normal in caliber.

**Table 2:** Classification of abdominal aortic aneurysms

| According to location | Suprarenal |
| --- | --- |
| | Above the origin of the renal arteries |
| | Very rare |
| | Juxtarenal |
| | AAA involving the part of the abdominal aorta in which the renal arteries originate |
| | Often involves the renal arteries |
| | Infrarenal |
| | Most common location |
| According to morphology | Fusiform |
| | Appears as a symmetric enlargement of the AA secondary to a circumferential weakness in the aortic wall |
| | Saccular |
| | Localized dilatation with eccentric outpouching of the aortic wall |
| | Usually a pseudoaneurysm secondary to trauma or enlargement of a penetrating ulcer and infection |
| | Hourglass (Fig. 8) |
| | Two noncontiguous areas of focal dilatation of aorta separated by normal caliber aorta |
| According to etiology | Atherosclerotic |
| | Most common type of AAA |
| | Inflammatory [50] |
| | 5% to 10% of all AAA |
| | Younger age group |
| | Three distinct features: |
| | − Marked thickening of aneurysm wall |
| | − Fibrosis of adjacent retroperitoneum |
| | − Rigid adherence of adjacent structures to anterior aneurysm wall |
| | Mycotic [28] |
| | Less than 1% of all aortic aneurysms |
| | Atypical location and age group should raise suspicion of mycotic AAA. |
| | Commonly saccular |
| | Common causative organisms: *Salmonella* spp and *Staphylococcus aureus* |
| | High mortality rate |
| | Patients are often septic, with positive blood cultures. |

*Expansion rate*

Mean growth rate of AAAs in men is 3.2 mm per annum and in women it is 2.6 mm per annum. The risk for rupture was first attributed to expansion rate by Limet and colleagues [37]. This association of increased rate of expansion with aortic rupture was further confirmed by Lederle and colleagues [38] and Brown and colleagues [35]. Cronenwett [39], however, found that expansion rate depended on current AAA diameter rather than a fixed rate, and this was further supported by Vega de Ceniga and colleagues [40]. Expansion rate is approximately 2.2 mm per annum for an AAA of less than 3 cm and 6.4 cm for an AAA of greater than 5 cm in diameter. Other factors reported to be associated with expansion rate are pulse pressure, systolic and diastolic blood pressure, and smoking. Diabetes, for unknown reasons, has a negative correlation with growth of AAAs.

*Mural thrombus*

Other factors associated with rupture are the presence of mural thrombus and calcifications. Siegel and colleagues [41] in a retrospective study demonstrated that aneurysms that ruptured had less mural thrombus and calcification than AAAs that did not rupture, stating that mural thrombus has a protective effect on the AAA by cushioning the pulsations of flowing blood and thus preventing its rupture. Results obtained by Simao da Silva and colleagues [33], however, who found mural thrombus at the site of aortic rupture in 80% of autopsy specimens they studied, contradicted the concept of mural thrombus as being protective. There is a possibility, however, that these thrombi may have formed post-rupture. This theory was further supported by Fontaine and colleagues [42], who concluded that mural thrombus acts as a source of proteases in aneurysms and thus increases the likelihood of enlargement and rupture.

### Gender

Female sex is another independent factor for rupture of AAAs, with evidence of a more rapid growth rate of aneurysms in females [43]. AAAs are less common among women than men, but when present they rupture three times more frequently and at a smaller aortic diameter (mean, 5 cm versus 6 cm) [44].

### Abdominal aortic wall strain

Recently biomechanical factors such as abdominal aortic wall stress and wall strength have been suggested as more reliable parameters in predicting the risk for rupture, rather than the maximum diameter of AAA [36]. AAA rupture occurs when the stresses acting on an AAA exceed its wall strength. Current ultrasound modalities do not allow for assessment of these biomechanical factors, and measurements of biomechanical stress factors are still in the experimental stage. Long and colleagues [45] have described the usefulness of tissue Doppler imaging (TDI) in the measurement of compliance parameters in AAAs, including dilation, wall strain, and wall stiffness. TDI has been proposed as a simple and reliable method for aortic compliance measurement during routine ultrasound examination.

## Sonographic findings

With current state-of-the-art technology, ultrasound can be used successfully to triage patients when an AAA rupture is clinically suspected. Although at the authors' institution ultrasound is not used as a diagnostic modality for AAA rupture, rupture may be incidentally noted while a patient is being screened for AAA. It helps, therefore, to be aware of the possible ultrasound findings in AAA rupture.

The most common ultrasound findings of AAA rupture include retroperitoneal hematoma, which appears as an echogenic retroperitoneal fluid collection, particularly in periaortic location, and hemoperitoneum [46]. Other less common sonographic findings that can be seen in AAA rupture include morphologic deformation of the AA, hypoechoic or anechoic areas within the thrombus or abrupt interruption of the thrombus, floating thrombus within the aortic lumen, and a break in the continuity of the abdominal wall with or without the paraaortic hypoechoic area [46]. Hemorrhage into the psoas muscle has also been described. Contrast-enhanced CT is considered superior for the detection of ruptured AAAs, and these US findings often need to be confirmed by a follow-up CT scan, except in hypotensive patients. In rare instances, the presence of an active leak can also be demonstrated on ultrasound as a focal discontinuity in the aortic wall, with blood leaking through the break in the aortic wall on color Doppler (Fig. 9). Contrast-enhanced sonography (CES) is potentially useful for assessment of aortic aneurysmal rupture, with comparable efficacy as CT and with the added advantages of easy bedside availability and relative cost-effectiveness [47]. Demonstration of active extravasation of contrast medium on CES has significant potential as an indicator for rupture of AAA

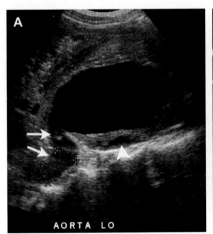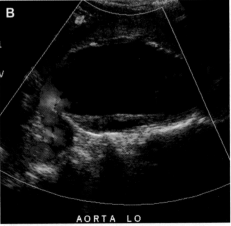

*Fig. 9.* Rupture of an AAA. A 62-year-old man presented with abdominal pain and hypotension. (*A*) Longitudinal gray scale sonogram of the AA demonstrates an AAA with peripheral thrombus. Posteriorly, at the upper end of the aneurysm, is a tubular hypoechoic structure (*arrows*), which is continuous with the lumen of the aneurysm sac. Also seen is a small hypoechoic area in the thrombus (*arrowhead*), which is a sequela of aortic wall rupture. (*B*) Corresponding color flow Doppler image demonstrates the presence of active bleeding. Such cases need no further imaging confirmation and the patient should be taken directly to the operating room without further delay. Surgery confirmed the sonographic findings.

with higher sensitivity and specificity [48]. The authors believe, however, that because of the urgency involved in diagnosing AAA rupture, contrast-enhanced US may not evolve as a preferred imaging modality because of the time factor.

Simplicity of ultrasound technique also enables emergency physicians to perform quick ultrasounds for immediate evaluation of aortic rupture [49]. At the authors' institution, however, a CT is preferred whenever an AAA rupture is clinically suspected.

### Inflammatory abdominal aortic aneurysm

Inflammatory AAAs account for 5% to 10% of all cases of AAAs and typically occur in a younger age group. Inflammatory AAAs usually present with back or abdominal pain and have three distinct features: (1) marked thickening of the aneurysm wall, (2) fibrosis of the adjacent retroperitoneum, and (3) rigid adherence of the adjacent structures to the anterior aneurysm wall [50].

### Mycotic abdominal aortic aneurysm

Mycotic AAAs (or infected AAAs) are rare entities (<1%) with a high mortality rate requiring early surgical intervention. If left untreated, they often lead to uncontrolled sepsis and catastrophic hemorrhage caused by rupture. Mycotic aneurysms can be classified into four types: (1) true mycotic aneurysms, (2) secondary mycotic aneurysms caused by bacterial arteritis, (3) infected pre-existing AAAs, and (4) post-traumatic infected pseudoaneurysms [51].

A high index of suspicion is required for diagnosis in the early stages. Clinical presentation of such aneurysms often includes fever, abdominal or back pain, leukocytosis, and expansile abdominal mass. In the pre-antibiotic era, bacterial endocarditis with *Streptococcus pyogenes* was the most common cause of mycotic aneurysms. Today *Staphylococcus aureus* and *Salmonella species* are the most commonly identified etiologic agents, most often secondary to arterial trauma or underlying immunodeficiency [52].

Mycotic aneurysms often develop at atypical locations in the AA, such as suprarenal, and in an atypical age group, ie, children [53]. They are typically smaller, eccentrically located, and saccular in shape.

Ultrasound findings in mycotic aneurysms have been rarely described. CT is the imaging modality of choice for diagnosis. Certain sonographic findings, however, can suggest the diagnosis. Mycotic aneurysms often present as a rapidly expanding aneurysm with lack of atherosclerotic changes within the aorta, such as absence of intimal calcification and thrombus. Occasionally air caused by infection may be identified in the wall of the AAA as echogenic foci with reverberation artifact. The presence of air is suggestive of an infective etiology [54]. Periaortic inflammatory changes such as retroperitoneal abscess and vertebral changes may be present. Ultrasound may be able to detect a large retroperitoneal abscess; however, detection of abnormalities in the bony cortex of the vertebral bodies is beyond the routine scope of ultrasound, and CT is required for evaluation of the adjacent vertebral bodies and disc spaces.

### Pseudoaneurysm

A pseudoaneurysm is a focal outpouching from the aorta resulting from disruption of one or more layers of the aortic wall. Pseudoaneurysms of the AA are rare and account for only 1% of all abdominal aneurysms [55]. Most commonly they develop secondary to trauma, which may be caused by blunt or penetrating injuries or may be iatrogenic secondary to vascular procedures [56]. They may also develop from penetrating atherosclerotic ulcers [57]. Rarely they can be mycotic in origin, such as tubercular [58]. Most reported cases of pseudoaneurysms have been seen in males, are associated with penetrating injuries, and involveg the suprarenal aorta [59,60]. They are usually saccular in shape with a narrow neck. These can be diagnosed with Doppler ultrasound by demonstrating a to-and-fro flow pattern of blood flow in the neck of the pseudoaneurysm [61,62] and a yin-yang pattern within the sac.

### Endograft evaluation

Currently endovascular aneurysm repair (EVAR) of an infrarenal AAA can be performed with Food and Drug Administration (FDA)-approved endografts that use either suprarenal or infrarenal fixation [63]. The Dutch Randomized Endovascular Aneurysm Management (DREAM) trial and the British Endovascular Aneurysm Repair (EVAR-1) trial showed favorable short-term results (reduced 30-day postoperative mortality) for endovascular repair of AAA. Recent study [64], however, which compared conventional (open repair) to endovascular treatment of AAAs over 2 years, demonstrated more deaths in the endovascular repair group of patients than in the open repair group, thus questioning its long-term effectiveness.

After graft placement, long-term follow-up is needed to determine whether the aneurysm sac has shrunk and also to monitor for the presence or absence of an endoleak. Endoleaks are defined as the persistence of blood flow outside the lumen of the endoluminal graft but within the aneurysm sac [65]. It is important to identify these endoleaks to prevent possible rupture of the aorta secondary to continued increase in size of the aneurysm. Endoleaks can be identified in 15% to 52% of patients after endovascular repair [66]. Endoleaks are classified into four types (Box 2) (Fig. 10). Type I and III endoleaks have been found to be associated with aneurysm rupture, whereas the risk for rupture of aneurysms with type II endoleaks and endotension appears small. Type I and III endoleaks should be corrected, preferably by endovascular means, because of the risk for rupture [67].

Contrast-enhanced CT (CECT) is the preferred imaging modality to assess the anatomy and migration of the graft and to assess for endoleaks. CEUS is an alternative in patients who have poor renal function [71]. Color Doppler imaging demonstrates blood flow between the endograft and the wall of the aortic aneurysm if an endoleak is present. The diameter of the aorta should be carefully measured to assess for interval growth. Type I leaks demonstrate high velocity flow at the site of the proximal attachment. Leaks at the distal limb attachment site demonstrate flow in the sac opposite the direction of flow in the lumen. IMA flow is antegrade in type I leaks. Type II leaks are characterized by slower flow within the aneurysm sac and retrograde flow in the IMA [72].

### Endoleak detection

CT is considered the gold standard for detection of endoleaks. MacLafferty and colleagues [73] demonstrated that color flow Doppler when compared

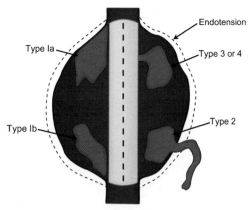

Fig. 10. Types of endoleaks. Diagrammatic representation shows the different types of endoleaks and endotension.

with CT had a sensitivity of 100%, specificity of 99%, positive predictive value of 88%, negative predictive value of 100%, and accuracy of 99% in the detection of endoleaks. Although color Doppler ultrasound is highly accurate in identifying the presence of an endoleak, it is not very accurate (66.7%) in distinguishing the type of endoleak [74]. Identification of an endoleak is based on the presence of color flow outside the endograft but within the aneurysm sac. Color Doppler ultrasound can serve as a useful adjunct to CT and is considered better for type II endoleak detection because of its real-time capability. It is also helpful in distinguishing "pseudo-endoleak" seen on CT caused by trapped perigraft contrast following AAA repair [75].

Color flow Doppler can also give false positive results secondary to the movement of clotted blood within the aneurysm sac. It is demonstrated as a color artifact secondary to transmitted pulsatile motion of the adjacent endograft. It is usually seen in the early postoperative period [69]. True endoleaks are identified as a uniform color Doppler appearance with demonstration of a peripheral flow waveform [69]. Demonstration of an arterial waveform confirms the continuity of the true endoleak with the vessel lumen and differentiates it from pulsating clotted blood. An increase in the diameter of the aneurysm sac by more than 0.5 cm is also an indication of endoleak or endotension.

CEUS has been reported to have 80% sensitivity, 100% specificity, and 100% positive predictive value in detecting endoleaks (Fig. 11) [76]. This may be superior in patients who have negative studies with CECT or in patients who have spinal hardware that may interfere with evaluation by CT [77,71].Further studies are needed, however, to determine the role of CEUS in evaluating patients who have endografts.

---

**Box 2:    Classification of endoleaks**

*White classification of endoleaks [68]*

Type I: Direct communication between the graft and aneurysm sac by way of an ineffective seal at the graft ends or attachment sites

Type II: Retrograde flow through lumbar arterials, the inferior mesenteric artery (IMA), or accessory renal arteries feeds into the aneurysm sac.

Type III: Seen in modular, multisegmental grafts. Leak occurs through deficiency in graft fabric and may be a result of altered hemodynamics secondary to aneurysm sac shrinkage.

Type IV: On contrast CT, appears as a blush of contrast outside the graft from contrast diffusion through the naturally porous graft fabric or through small defects in the fabric at the site of sutures or struts; may require angiography to distinguish from type III graft.

Endotension [69]. It is seen as a continued expansion in size of the aneurysm sac without evidence of endoleak. It is believed to be associated with high pressure inside the aneurysm sac and may potentially rupture if left untreated [70].

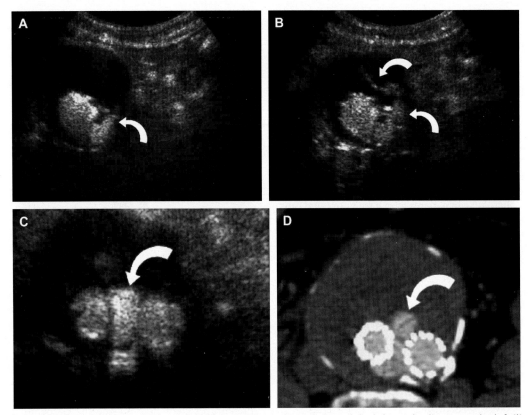

*Fig. 11.* (*A*) Type I endoleak . Axial arterial phase CEUS reveals a subtle endoleak (*arrow*) adjacent to the left iliac limb of the stent graft. (*B*) Axial CEUS image at the same level, acquired 2 minutes after injection, depicts a much larger endoleak (*arrows*) than appreciated in the arterial phase. (*C*) Type III endoleak. Arterial phase CEUS image demonstrates an endoleak (*arrow*) between the enhancing iliac limbs of the stent graft. (*D*) Corresponding axial arterial phase CT angiography images show exact concordance in endoleak depiction (*From* Dill-Macky MJ. Aortic endografts: detecting endoleaks using contrast-enhanced ultrasound. Ultrasound Q 2006;22:49–52; with permission).

## Aortic dissection

Abdominal aortic dissection is usually an extension of thoracic aortic dissection. The peak incidence of aortic dissection is in the sixth and seventh decades of life, with men affected twice as often as women [78]. Approximately three fourths of patients who have aortic dissection have a history of hypertension. The dissection is termed *acute* when it is diagnosed within 14 days after the first symptoms appear; it is termed *chronic* when it is diagnosed later [79].

Hypertension is believed to be a major risk factor for aortic dissection [78]. Atherosclerosis is not believed to be an independent risk factor for aortic dissection; however, an association between dissection and atherosclerosis may be found, which suggests increased incidence of aortic dissection in the presence of atherosclerosis [80,81]. Causes of aortic dissection are listed in Box 3.

Sonographically, aortic dissection can be diagnosed by the identification of an intimal flap. The intimal flap is visualized as a linear hyperechoic area within the aortic lumen, dividing the lumen into a true and false lumen (Fig. 12A–C). In acute dissection, the true and false lumens can be identified on color flow Doppler ultrasound as two parallel lumens with or without an entry point from the true into the false lumen (Fig. 12D). In chronic aortic dissections, there may be thrombosis of the false lumen with nonvisualization of the intimal flap. Such an appearance may mimic an AAA if the aorta is dilated and can be distinguished on ultrasound by the presence of intimal calcification in the inner wall of the thrombus.

Aortic dissection can be mimicked by the presence of layers of mural thrombi of varying echogenicities that may give a pseudo-appearance of two lumens within the aorta.

## B-flow imaging

B-flow is a new mode of imaging blood flow, introduced by General Electric Medical Systems in the a manner that it amplifies the particulate components of blood, giving the appearance of mobile, bright echoes in regions of flowing blood [83]. This mode has the advantage of an improved signal-to-noise ratio arising from binary coded transmissions, along with motion detection, to produce direct B-mode images of moving blood [84]. The purpose of introducing this modality was to overcome some of the disadvantages of color Doppler in vascular imaging, which include overwriting of the vessel wall (blooming or bleeding artifact), low frame rates, persistence, and angle dependency.

B-flow has high sensitivity in demonstrating intraluminal blood flow and the morphology of the blood vessel, such as the aortic wall thickness and atherosclerotic plaques. It can be particularly useful in imaging of ectatic aortas in which the angle dependency of Doppler imaging may result in erroneous measurement of peak systolic velocities.

late 1990s. It is a noninvasive, non-Doppler flow imaging tool that gives a gray scale morphologic display of intraluminal blood flow and tissue simultaneously (Fig. 13) [82]. It is based on a principle of coded excitation, wherein the digitally encoded ultrasound pulses are used in such

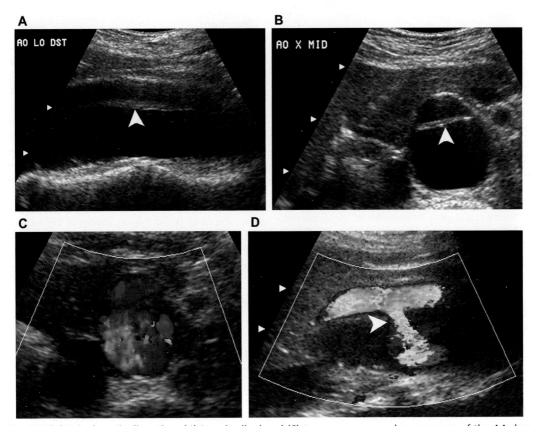

Fig. 12. Abdominal aortic dissection. (A) Longitudinal and (B) transverse gray scale sonograms of the AA demonstrate a linear echogenic band (*arrowhead*) traversing anteriorly within the lumen of the aorta. (C) Transverse color flow Doppler image demonstrates the false lumen anteriorly (*in blue*) and the true lumen posteriorly (*in red*). (D) Longitudinal color flow Doppler image demonstrates the entry point (*arrowhead*) of an intimal tear causing dissection. Gray scale finding of an aortic dissection may be mimicked by reverberation artifact and can be confirmed by changing the position of the transducer and obtaining transverse and longitudinal views. True dissection flap persists, whereas the artifact disappears with change in position of transducer.

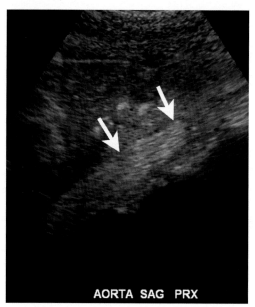

AORTA SAG PRX

*Fig. 13.* B-flow imaging of aorta. Longitudinal B-flow image of the normal proximal abdominal aorta (*arrows*).

Keeping in mind some of the limitations of B-flow listed in Table 3, this modality can serve as an important adjunct to color Doppler imaging for assessing the aorta and other abdominal vessels. Clevert and colleagues [85] compared B-flow, color Doppler, and power Doppler in arterial (carotid, vertebral, and abdominal aortic) dissection and found that B-flow had better accuracy for the diagnosis of arterial dissection compared with color Doppler and power Doppler. Flow within the true and false lumen, hypoechoic thrombi, intramural hematoma, and even movements of the dissection membrane are better distinguished with B-flow compared with color and power Doppler [85].

**Table 3: B-flow imaging advantages and disadvantages**

| Advantages | Disadvantages |
|---|---|
| No aliasing | No flow |
| No blooming | quantification |
| All velocities imaged | No aliasing |
| simultaneously | Limited |
| Angle-independent | penetration |
| Flow direction indicated | |
| Tissue and B-flow | |
| information are displayed | |
| simultaneously | |
| High spatial and time | |
| resolution | |

**Box 4:   Limitations of sonography**

1. Bowel gas, acute abdominal pain, or obesity may limit the exam.
2. The absence of free intraperitoneal fluid does not exclude rupture.
3. The presence of retroperitoneal hemorrhage cannot be reliably identified.
4. Small saccular aneurysms may be overlooked.
5. Oblique or angled imaging planes exaggerate the true aortic diameter.
6. Large para-aortic nodes may be confused with the aorta or may mimic AAA.

## Limitations of sonography for evaluation of abdominal aortic aneurysm and rupture

Although ultrasound is highly accurate in detecting AAA and aortic dissection, it is limited in several ways, as shown in Box 4.

## Summary

US is accurate in detecting AAAs and is readily available, inexpensive, and less time consuming than other imaging methods for screening patients for AAAs and for emergency evaluation for rupture of AAAs. Sonographic diagnosis of AAA is based on the maximum diameter of the aorta, and a diameter greater than 3 cm is considered an AAA. Sonography also helps in monitoring patients after endovascular repair and can detect endoleaks, although CT remains the gold standard. Sonography is also useful in detecting abdominal aortic dissection, because it can identify the intimal flap and sometimes even the entry point. Newer modes of US imaging such as B-flow imaging serves as an important adjunct to color Doppler imaging in assessment of the aorta and other abdominal vessels.

## References

[1] LaRoy LL, Cormier PJ, Matalon TA, et al. Imaging of abdominal aortic aneurysms. AJR Am J Roentgenol 1989;152:785–92.

[2] Pedersen OM, Aslaksen A, Vik-Mo H. Ultrasound measurement of the luminal diameter of the abdominal aorta and iliac arteries in patients without vascular disease. J Vasc Surg 1993;17: 596–601.

[3] Wanhainen A, Bergqvist D, Bjorck M. Measuring the abdominal aorta with ultrasonography and computed tomography—difference and variability. Eur J Vasc Endovasc Surg 2002;24: 428–34.

[4] Zwiebel WJ. Aortic and iliac aneurysm. Semin Ultrasound CT MR 1992;13:53–68.

[5] Bhatt S, Dogra V. Doppler imaging of the uterus and adnexae. Ultrasound Clinics 2006;1:201–21.

[6] Bluth EI, LoCascio L. Ultrasonic evaluation of the abdominal aorta. Echocardiography 1996; 13:197–206.

[7] Alcorn HG, Wolfson SK Jr, Sutton-Tyrrell K, et al. Risk factors for abdominal aortic aneurysms in older adults enrolled in The Cardiovascular Health Study. Arterioscler Thromb Vasc Biol 1996;16:963–70.

[8] Brunkwall J, Hauksson H, Bengtsson H, et al. Solitary aneurysms of the iliac arterial system: an estimate of their frequency of occurrence. J Vasc Surg 1989;10:381–4.

[9] Weisenberg D, Sahar Y, Sahar G, et al. Atherosclerosis of the aorta is common in patients with severe aortic stenosis: an intraoperative transesophageal echocardiographic study. J Thorac Cardiovasc Surg 2005;130:29–32.

[10] Ailawadi G, Eliason JL, Upchurch GR Jr. Current concepts in the pathogenesis of abdominal aortic aneurysm. J Vasc Surg 2003;38:584–8.

[11] Lederle FA, Johnson GR, Wilson SE, et al. Prevalence and associations of abdominal aortic aneurysm detected through screening. Aneurysm Detection and Management (ADAM) Veterans Affairs Cooperative Study Group. Ann Intern Med 1997;126:441–9.

[12] Reed D, Reed C, Stemmermann G, et al. Are aortic aneurysms caused by atherosclerosis? Circulation 1992;85:205–11.

[13] Wong DR, Willett WC, Rimm EB. Smoking, hypertension, alcohol consumption, and risk of abdominal aortic aneurysm in men. Am J Epidemiol 2007;165(7):838–45.

[14] Rohrer MJ, Cutler BS, Wheeler HB. Long-term survival and quality of life following rupturedabdominal aortic aneurysm. Arch Surg 1988;123:1213–7.

[15] Marston WA, Ahlquist R, Johnson G Jr, et al. Misdiagnosis of ruptured abdominal aortic aneurysms. J Vasc Surg 1992;16:17–22.

[16] Schilling FJ, Christakis G, Hempel HH, et al. The natural history of abdominal aortic and iliac atherosclerosis as detected by lateral abdominal roentgenograms in 2663 males. J Chronic Dis 1974;27:37–45.

[17] Lederle FA. Ultrasonographic screening for abdominal aortic aneurysms. Ann Intern Med 2003;139:516–22.

[18] Lee TY, Korn P, Heller JA, et al. The cost-effectiveness of a "quick-screen" program for abdominal aortic aneurysms. Surgery 2002;132:399–407.

[19] Screening for abdominal aortic aneurysm: recommendation statement. Ann Intern Med 2005;142:198–202.

[20] Lederle FA, Johnson GR, Wilson SE. Abdominal aortic aneurysm in women. J Vasc Surg 2001; 34:122–6.

[21] Scott RA, Vardulaki KA, Walker NM, et al. The long-term benefits of a single scan for abdominal aortic aneurysm (AAA) at age 65. Eur J Vasc Endovasc Surg 2001;21:535–40.

[22] Lederle FA, Johnson GR, Wilson SE, et al. The Aneurysm Detection and Management Study Screening Program: validation cohort and final results. Aneurysm Detection and Management Veterans Affairs Cooperative Study Investigators. Arch Intern Med 2000;160:1425–30.

[23] Lindholt JS, Juul S, Fasting H, et al. Hospital costs and benefits of screening for abdominal aortic aneurysms. Results from a randomised population screening trial. Eur J Vasc Endovasc Surg 2002;23:55–60.

[24] Ashton HA, Buxton MJ, Day NE, et al. The Multicentre Aneurysm Screening Study (MASS) into the effect of abdominal aortic aneurysm screening on mortality in men: a randomised controlled trial. Lancet 2002;360:1531–9.

[25] Scott RA, Wilson NM, Ashton HA, et al. Influence of screening on the incidence of ruptured abdominal aortic aneurysm: 5-year results of a randomized controlled study. Br J Surg 1995; 82:1066–70.

[26] Norman PE, Jamrozik K, Lawrence-Brown MM, et al. Population-based randomised controlled trial on impact of screening on mortality from abdominal aortic aneurysm. BMJ 2004;329:1259.

[27] Hermsen K, Chong WK. Ultrasound evaluation of abdominal aortic and iliac aneurysms and mesenteric ischemia. Radiol Clin North Am 2004;42:365–81.

[28] Chu P, Howden BP, Jones S, et al. Once bitten, twice shy: an unusual case report of a mycotic aortic aneurysm. ANZ J Surg 2005;75:1024–6.

[29] Beebe HG, Kritpracha B. Screening and preoperative imaging of candidates for conventional repair of abdominal aortic aneurysm. Semin Vasc Surg 1999;12:300–5.

[30] Choke E, Cockerill G, Wilson WR, et al. A review of biological factors implicated in abdominal aortic aneurysm rupture. Eur J Vasc Endovasc Surg 2005;30:227–44.

[31] Burger T, Meyer F, Tautenhahn J, et al. Ruptured infrarenal aortic aneurysm—a critical evaluation. Vasa 1999;28:30–3.

[32] Golledge J, Abrokwah J, Shenoy KN, et al. Morphology of ruptured abdominal aortic aneurysms. Eur J Vasc Endovasc Surg 1999;18: 96–104.

[33] Simao da Silva E, Rodrigues AJ, Magalhaes Castro de Tolosa E, et al. Morphology and diameter of infrarenal aortic aneurysms: a prospective autopsy study. Cardiovasc Surg 2000;8:526–32.

[34] Isselbacher EM. Thoracic and abdominal aortic aneurysms. Circulation 2005;111:816–28.

[35] Brown PM, Zelt DT, Sobolev B. The risk of rupture in untreated aneurysms: the impact of size, gender, and expansion rate. J Vasc Surg 2003;37:280–4.

[36] Vorp DA. Biomechanics of abdominal aortic aneurysm. J Biomech 2007;40(9):1887–902.

[37] Limet R, Sakalihassan N, Albert A. Determination of the expansion rate and incidence of rupture of abdominal aortic aneurysms. J Vasc Surg 1991;14:540–8.

[38] Lederle FA, Johnson GR, Wilson SE, et al. Rupture rate of large abdominal aortic aneurysms in patients refusing or unfit for elective repair. JAMA 2002;287:2968–72.

[39] Cronenwett JL. Variables that affect the expansion rate and rupture of abdominal aortic aneurysms. Ann N Y Acad Sci 1996;800:56–67.

[40] Vega de Ceniga M, Gomez R, Estallo L, et al. Growth rate and associated factors in small abdominal aortic aneurysms. Eur J Vasc Endovasc Surg 2006;31:231–6.

[41] Siegel CL, Cohan RH, Korobkin M, et al. Abdominal aortic aneurysm morphology: CT features in patients with ruptured and nonruptured aneurysms. AJR Am J Roentgenol 1994;163:1123–9.

[42] Fontaine V, Jacob MP, Houard X, et al. Involvement of the mural thrombus as a site of protease release and activation in human aortic aneurysms. Am J Pathol 2002;161:1701–10.

[43] Mofidi R, Goldie VJ, Kelman J, et al. Influence of sex on expansion rate of abdominal aortic aneurysms. Br J Surg 2007;94:310–4.

[44] Fillinger MF, Marra SP, Raghavan ML, et al. Prediction of rupture risk in abdominal aortic aneurysm during observation: wall stress versus diameter. J Vasc Surg 2003;37:724–32.

[45] Long A, Rouet L, Bissery A, et al. Compliance of abdominal aortic aneurysms: evaluation of tissue Doppler imaging. Ultrasound Med Biol 2004;30:1099–108.

[46] Catalano O, Siani A. Ruptured abdominal aortic aneurysm: categorization of sonographic findings and report of 3 new signs. J Ultrasound Med 2005;24:1077–83.

[47] Catalano O, Lobianco R, Cusati B, et al. Contrast-enhanced sonography for diagnosis of ruptured abdominal aortic aneurysm. AJR Am J Roentgenol 2005;184:423–7.

[48] Catalano O, Sandomenico F, Raso MM, et al. Real-time, contrast-enhanced sonography: a new tool for detecting active bleeding. J Trauma 2005;59:933–9.

[49] Knaut AL, Kendall JL, Patten R, et al. Ultrasonographic measurement of aortic diameter by emergency physicians approximates results obtained by computed tomography. J Emerg Med 2005;28:119–26.

[50] Walker DI, Bloor K, Williams G, et al. Inflammatory aneurysms of the abdominal aorta. Br J Surg 1972;59:609–14.

[51] Papadimitriou D, Tachtsi M, Koutsias S, et al. Mycotic aneurysm of the infrarenal aorta. Vasa 2003;32:218–20.

[52] Gomes MN, Choyke PL, Wallace RB. Infected aortic aneurysms. A changing entity. Ann Surg 1992;215:435–42.

[53] Millar AJ, Gilbert RD, Brown RA, et al. Abdominal aortic aneurysms in children. J Pediatr Surg 1996;31:1624–8.

[54] Naganuma H, Ishida H, Konno K, et al. Mycotic abdominal aneurysm: report of a case with emphasis on the presence of gas echoes. Abdom Imaging 2001;26:420–2.

[55] Bennett DE, Cherry JK. The natural history of traumatic aneurysms of the aorta. Surgery 1967;61:516–23.

[56] Cutry AF, Whitley D, Patterson RB. Midaortic pseudoaneurysm complicating extensive endovascular stenting of aortic disease. J Vasc Surg 1997;26:958–62.

[57] Tsuji Y, Okita Y, Sugimoto K, et al. Multiple penetrating atherosclerotic ulcers of the aorta: report of a case. Vasc Endovascular Surg 2006;40:495–8.

[58] Choudhary SK, Bhan A, Talwar S, et al. Tubercular pseudoaneurysms of aorta. Ann Thorac Surg 2001;72:1239–44.

[59] Miller JS, Wall MJ Jr, Mattox KL. Ruptured aortic pseudoaneurysm 28 years after gunshot wound: case report and review of the literature. J Trauma 1998;44:214–6.

[60] Borioni R, Garofalo M, Seddio F, et al. Posttraumatic infrarenal abdominal aortic pseudoaneurysm. Tex Heart Inst J 1999;26:312–4.

[61] Erturk H, Erden A, Yurdakul M, et al. Pseudoaneurysm of the abdominal aorta diagnosed by color duplex Doppler sonography. J Clin Ultrasound 1999;27:202–5.

[62] Gonzalez Llorente J, Gallego Gallego M, Martinez Arnaiz A. Chronic post-traumatic pseudoaneurysm of the abdominal aorta diagnosed by duplex Doppler ultrasonography. A case report. Acta Radiol 1997;38:121–3.

[63] Lalka S, Johnson M, Namyslowski J, et al. Renal interventions after abdominal aortic aneurysm repair using an aortic endograft with suprarenal fixation. Am J Surg 2006;192:577–82.

[64] Blankensteijn JD, de Jong SE, Prinssen M, et al. Two-year outcomes after conventional or endovascular repair of abdominal aortic aneurysms. N Engl J Med 2005;352:2398–405.

[65] White GH, Yu W, May J. Endoleak—a proposed new terminology to describe incomplete aneurysm exclusion by an endoluminal graft. J Endovasc Surg 1996;3:124–5.

[66] May J, White GH, Waugh R, et al. Life-table analysis of primary and assisted success following endoluminal repair of abdominal aortic aneurysms: the role of supplementary endovascular intervention in improving outcome. Eur J Vasc Endovasc Surg 2000;19:648–55.

[67] Heikkinen MA, Arko FR, Zarins CK. What is the significance of endoleaks and endotension. Surg Clin North Am 2004;84:1337–52 vii.

[68] Pacanowski JP Jr, Dieter RS, Stevens SL, et al. Endoleak: the Achilles heel of endovascular abdominal aortic aneurysm exclusion—a case report. WMJ 2002;101:57–8 63.

[69] Berdejo GL, Lipsitz EC. Ultrasound imaging assessment following endovascular aortic aneurysm repair. 5th edition. Philadelphia: Elsevier Saunders; 2005.

[70] Dubenec SR, White GH, Pasenau J, et al. Endotension. A review of current views on

pathophysiology and treatment. J Cardiovasc Surg (Torino) 2003;44:553–7.

[71] Pearce WH, Astleford P. What's new in vascular ultrasound. Surg Clin North Am 2004;84: 1113–26, vii.

[72] Greenfield AL, Halpern EJ, Bonn J, et al. Application of duplex US for characterization of endoleaks in abdominal aortic stent-grafts: report of five cases. Radiology 2002;225:845–51.

[73] McLafferty RB, McCrary BS, Mattos MA, et al. The use of color-flow duplex scan for the detection of endoleaks. J Vasc Surg 2002;36:100–4.

[74] Zannetti S, De Rango P, Parente B, et al. Role of duplex scan in endoleak detection after endoluminal abdominal aortic aneurysm repair. Eur J Vasc Endovasc Surg 2000;19:531–5.

[75] Lee WA, Rubin GD, Johnson BL, et al. "Pseudoendoleak"—residual intrasaccular contrast after endovascular stent-graft repair. J Endovasc Ther 2002;9:119–23.

[76] Dill-Macky MJ. Aortic endografts: detecting endoleaks using contrast-enhanced ultrasound. Ultrasound Q 2006;22:49–52.

[77] Napoli V, Bargellini I, Sardella SG, et al. Abdominal aortic aneurysm: contrast-enhanced US for missed endoleaks after endoluminal repair. Radiology 2004;233:217–25.

[78] Hagan PG, Nienaber CA, Isselbacher EM, et al. The International Registry of Acute Aortic Dissection (IRAD): new insights into an old disease. JAMA 2000;283:897–903.

[79] Pretre R, Von Segesser LK. Aortic dissection. Lancet 1997;349:1461–4.

[80] Hayashi H, Matsuoka Y, Sakamoto I, et al. Penetrating atherosclerotic ulcer of the aorta: imaging features and disease concept. Radiographics 2000;20:995–1005.

[81] Larson EW, Edwards WD. Risk factors for aortic dissection: a necropsy study of 161 cases. Am J Cardiol 1984;53:849–55.

[82] Weskott HP. B-flow—a new method for detecting blood flow. Ultraschall Med 2000;21: 59–65.

[83] Wachsberg RH. B-flow, a non-Doppler technology for flow mapping: early experience in the abdomen. Ultrasound Q 2003;19:114–22.

[84] Whittingham TA. Medical diagnostic applications and sources. Prog Biophys Mol Biol 2007; 93:84–110.

[85] Clevert DA, Rupp N, Reiser M, et al. Improved diagnosis of vascular dissection by ultrasound B-flow: a comparison with color-coded Doppler and power Doppler sonography. Eur Radiol 2005;15:342–7.

ELSEVIER
SAUNDERS

U L T R A S O U N D
C L I N I C S

Ultrasound Clin 2 (2007) 455–475

# Imaging Renal Artery Stenosis

Hicham Moukaddam, MD[a],*, Jeffrey Pollak, MD[b],
Leslie M. Scoutt, MD[b]

- Pathology and natural history
- Doppler ultrasound
  *Technique and normal findings*
  *Diagnostic criteria for renal artery*
  *stenosis*
- Computed tomographic angiography
- Magnetic resonance angiography
- ACE inhibitor scintigraphy
- Summary
- References

Hypertension affects up to 58.4 million people in the United States [1] and is one of the most common diseases worldwide with well known morbidity and mortality. The vast majority of patients who have hypertension, approximately 90% to 98%, have essential hypertension without structural lesions or other abnormalities identifiable by currently available imaging modalities. It is estimated that only 0.5% to less than 5% of all patients who have hypertension have true renovascular hypertension (RVH) [2,3], defined as hypertension secondary to renal artery stenosis (RAS). Many patients who have RVH also have some degree of associated essential hypertension, but nonetheless may benefit from treatment of the RAS. In addition to causing hypertension, RAS may also lead to renal insufficiency [2–7]. In fact, Scoble and Hamilton [8] have suggested that up to 40% of elderly hypertensive patients who have renal dysfunction and no known primary renal pathology have significant RAS. It is well known that medical treatment of RVH is less successful than pharmaceutical control of essential hypertension. Many studies have reported, however, that percutaneous or surgical revascularization may significantly improve hypertension in patients who have RAS, thereby reducing the morbidity associated with hypertension. Furthermore, revascularization may salvage or even improve renal function in some patients [3–5, 8–11].

Screening hypertensive patients at risk for RAS is therefore extremely important, because RAS is the most common potentially surgically curable cause of hypertension. Because of the high prevalence of hypertension in the general population and the low incidence of RVH among these patients (0.5%–5%) [2,3], however, screening all hypertensive patients is neither practical nor cost effective. Screening for RAS is thus recommended only for enriched patient populations considered to be at high risk for RAS. The clinical criteria most predictive of RAS are listed in Box 1. In such patient populations the prevalence of RVH increases to approximately 20% to 30% [12].

Although digital subtraction angiography (DSA) with measurement of the pressure gradient across a stenosis in the renal artery remains the gold standard examination for diagnosing RAS, it is an invasive, expensive study with potentially significant complications and morbidity, including infection, hemorrhage, vascular injury such as renal artery dissection or cholesterol plaque embolization,

[a] Department of Diagnostic Radiology, Yale New Haven Hospital, 20 York Street, New Haven, CT 06511, USA
[b] Yale University School of Medicine, Department of Diagnostic Radiology, 20 York Street, New Haven, CT 06511, USA
* Corresponding author.
*E-mail address:* hmoukaddam@hotmail.com (H. Moukaddam).

doi:10.1016/j.cult.2007.06.002

**Box 1:  Clinical risk factors for RVH**

- Abrupt onset of severe hypertension (diastolic blood pressure >120 mm Hg)
- Accelerated or malignant hypertension (grade III or IV retinopathy)
- Hypertension refractory to appropriate three-drug regimen
- Onset of hypertension before age 30 or after age 60 years
- Hypertension with rapidly progressive renal failure
- Renal failure that develops in response to ACE inhibitor
- Hypertension associated with an upper abdominal bruit
- Episodes of recurrent severe hypertension and pulmonary edema
- Lack of family history of hypertension

nephrotoxicity, and allergic reactions. Sampling of renin levels in the renal veins is also occasionally performed for diagnosis of RVH and to identify which kidney is responsible for the hypertension. Samples are usually obtained from the right and left main renal veins and from the inferior vena cava above and below the level of the renal veins. A renal vein renin level from one kidney greater than 1.5 times that of the other kidney is diagnostic of RVH. Renal vein renin sampling is also an invasive procedure with risks for hemorrhage and vascular injury and the risk associated with the use of iodinated contrast agents. The need for an accurate noninvasive screening technique is therefore clear. Scintigraphy, Doppler ultrasonography (DUS), computed tomographic angiography (CT angiography), and magnetic resonance angiography (MR angiography) of the kidneys and renal arteries have all been advocated as useful potential screening modalities for RAS. Although captopril renal scintigraphy provides physiologic information, it does not provide anatomic confirmation of abnormal physiology and is limited in evaluating patients who have bilateral RAS. CT angiography and MR angiography provide excellent anatomic evaluation of the renal arteries. Neither modality, however, provides physiologic confirmation of the clinical significance of an anatomic stricture. The physiologic significance of a stenosis is critical in clinical practice, because atherosclerotic lesions can coexist in patients who have essential hypertension without initiating the angiotensin cascade and causing RVH. In addition, CT angiography subjects the patient to the risks inherent with the administration of potentially nephrotoxic iodinated IV contrast, and the spatial resolution of MR angiography remains less than that of CT angiography or DSA, limiting anatomic

evaluation of the distal and accessory renal arteries. Doppler ultrasound has the potential to provide physiologic and anatomic information without the risk associated with IV contrast. The spatial resolution is inferior to CT angiography or MR angiography, however, and many examinations are technically limited, especially in the obese patient. This article describes these different modalities in the diagnosis of RAS with emphasis on DUS.

## Pathology and natural history

In the United States, atherosclerotic disease is the most common cause of RVH, particularly in patients older than age 50 years [3]. RAS caused by atherosclerosis is more common in men and in patients who have coronary artery and peripheral vascular atherosclerosis [3,13,14]. Atheromatous stenoses typically involve the proximal 1 cm of the main renal artery, the ostia, or branch points. The second most common cause of RAS is fibromuscular dysplasia. RAS secondary to fibromuscular dysplasia tends to occur in young to middle aged women, and the narrowing most often involves the middle to distal main renal artery. RAS caused by atherosclerosis or fibromuscular dysplasia may be bilateral in up to 50% of cases. Other rare causes of RVH include vasculitis (Takayasu's arteritis), neurofibromatosis, radiation injury, renal artery or aortic dissection, embolization, congenital abdominal aortic coarctation, or extrinsic compression by a mass or hematoma. Causes of RAS, however, are geographic in distribution, and there are significant variations in the etiology of RVH worldwide. In India, for example, Takayasu's arteritis is responsible for two thirds of all cases of RVH.

RAS is known to cause RVH by triggering excessive renin secretion by the ischemic kidney. Renin is transformed into angiotensinogen in the liver, which is then metabolized into angiotensin I. Angiotensin I is transformed in the lungs into angiotensin II, which causes increased aldosterone secretion by the kidneys, resulting in hypertension. Furthermore, if left untreated atherosclerotic RAS tends to progress, leading to worsening renal function and renal artery thrombosis [4,11,15]. For renal arteries with an atherosclerotic stenosis of 75% or greater diameter reduction, it is estimated that 12% to 20% occlude within 1 year. If the arterial diameter reduction is 50% or greater, 20% to 50% progress to more severe disease within a few years. In addition, renal length decreases by 1 cm or more per year in approximately 19% of patients who have a 60% arterial diameter reduction [16]. Textor and Wilcox [4] reported that 5% to 16% of untreated atherosclerotic lesions progress to complete occlusion.

## Doppler ultrasound

DUS is a noninvasive, inexpensive imaging technique without the risks for nephrotoxicity or allergic reaction that are associated with iodinated IV contrast agents or gadolinium. In addition, DUS provides physiologic and anatomic data. For these reasons, DUS has been explored since the 1980s as a screening method for diagnosing RAS.

A complete Doppler ultrasound examination to evaluate for RAS requires Doppler interrogation of the main renal arteries from origin to renal hilum and evaluation of waveforms of the intraparenchymal renal arteries. Gray scale imaging of the kidneys and the aorta is also performed. Examination of the full length of the main renal arteries is technically difficult, and in approximately 20% to 30% of adult patients, overlying bowel gas, obesity, and aortic calcifications impede visualization of the entire main renal artery on ultrasound examination [17]. Although Li and colleagues [18] published a recent study reporting a technically successful examination rate of 99%, the cause of this unusually high technical success rate was attributed to the fact the patients included in the study were Chinese and were overall much thinner than a typical Western patient population. Full evaluation of the intraparenchymal arteries, however, is much easier and can be accomplished in virtually any patient who can breathhold.

### Technique and normal findings

The kidneys and the aorta are first examined with gray scale imaging. The maximum renal length is measured from a longitudinal image and the echogenicity and thickness of the renal cortex is described. Note is made of renal masses, atrophy or cortical thinning, scarring, hydronephrosis, or renal calculi. The kidneys should be symmetric in length, cortical thickness, and echogenicity. Gray scale and color imaging of the abdominal aorta is also performed, because the presence of plaque, thrombus, dissection, or aneurysm should increase concern for atherosclerotic plaque involving the origin of the renal arteries.

DUS of the native kidneys is best performed with a 2.5- to 3-MHz curved array transducer and preferably by a dedicated, experienced sonographer, because the examination is operator-dependent and there is a slow learning curve. The patient should fast for 8 to 12 hours before the examination. Harmonic imaging and spatial compounding techniques should be used if available, and numerous scanning planes and acoustic windows are typically required for complete visualization of the main renal arteries. The main renal arteries originate laterally from the aorta just below the left

renal vein and are often best visualized using a transverse midline approach (Fig. 1). If visualization of the renal arteries is obscured by overlying bowel gas, coronal images through the aorta may occasionally demonstrate the origins of both renal arteries in thin patients. This has been called a "banana peel" view (Fig. 2). A parasagittal or coronal approach angling transversely through the renal hilum toward the aorta with the patient in a slight decubitus position may also be used to visualize the entire length of the main renal artery from renal hilum to the aorta (Fig. 3). Decubitus positioning with intercostal scanning may be necessary in some patients. The right renal artery can also usually be identified in cross section on coronal images of the inferior vena cava (IVC), because it is the only vessel to course laterally under the IVC (Fig. 4). In this projection, the right renal artery often slightly indents the IVC. Although accessory renal arteries are not typically identified on DUS because of their small size, they can sometimes be identified arising from the aorta on transverse or longitudinal views with meticulous scanning technique (Fig. 5). If two vessels are identified exiting the renal hilum at the upper and lower poles, the possibility of multiple renal arteries or early branching of a single renal artery should be suspected, and one should attempt to trace the vessels individually to the aorta (see Fig. 5C). CT angiography, MR angiography, and angiography are much more sensitive imaging modalities than ultrasound for the identification of multiple renal arteries. The intraparenchymal renal vessels are best visualized using a translumbar lateral approach. The segmental renal arteries lie within the echogenic renal hilum and branch into the interlobular arteries that course lateral to the renal pyramids. The arcuate vessels run behind the renal pyramids parallel to the renal cortex (Fig. 6).

Optimization of color and pulse Doppler imaging parameters is critical for performance of a successful ultrasound examination, and in most cases color Doppler imaging facilitates identification of the renal arteries. The color gain should be maximized until the image is degraded by color flash artifact from noise or patient motion. The use of power Doppler techniques increases sensitivity to low volume slow flow and is less angle-dependent. The use of color Doppler decreases the frame rate and spatial resolution. In patients who have difficulty holding their breath, it may actually be easier to visualize the main renal arteries using gray scale imaging alone without color Doppler (Fig. 7). The pulse repetition frequency (PRF) should be set for arterial flow: high enough to prevent "bleeding" of flow from adjacent veins over the arteries and to reduce speckle artifact (noise) from the arteries and patient motion, but low enough to identify color

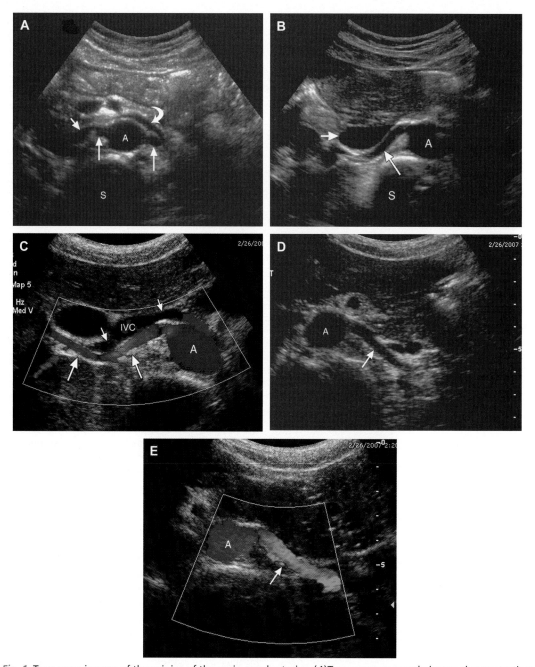

**Fig. 1.** Transverse images of the origins of the main renal arteries. (*A*)Transverse gray scale image demonstrating the origins of the right and left renal arteries (*long arrows*) from the aorta (*A*). Note left renal vein (*curved arrow*) anterior to the aorta, IVC (*short arrow*), and spine (*S*).(*B*) Transverse gray scale image of the proximal right renal artery (*long arrow*), inferior vena cava (*short arrow*), aorta (*A*),and spine (*S*). (*C*) Transverse color Doppler image of the right main renal artery (*long arrows*). Note IVC and renal veins (*short arrows*) anterior to the right renal artery and aorta (*A*). (*D*) Transverse gray scale image of the left main renal artery (*arrow*) and aorta (*A*). (*E*) Color Doppler image of the proximal left main renal artery (*arrow*) and aorta (*A*).

aliasing at the site of a stenosis. The pulse Doppler sample volume should just encompass the entire width of the renal artery. The optimal angle of insonation is between 30° and 60° and ideally should be kept constant on serial studies. An angle greater than 60° artifactually increases peak systolic velocity (PSV). The PRF should be set such that the Doppler waveform is large, filling the entire scale

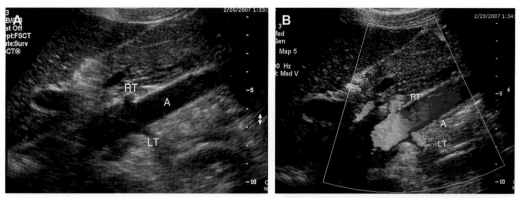

*Fig. 2.* Gray scale (*A*) and color Doppler (*B*) coronal "banana peel" image through the aorta (*A*) demonstrating the origins of the right (*RT*) and left (*LT*) main renal arteries.

(image) without causing aliasing. The wall filter should be kept low. Increasing the frame rate expands and widens the Doppler tracing and facilitates accurate measurement of the rate of systolic acceleration and acceleration time (Fig. 8).

PSV is measured in the aorta at the level of the origins of the renal arteries and is also measured every 1 to 2 centimeters along the length of the main renal arteries from the ostia to the renal hilum. At a minimum, PSV should be recorded in the main renal artery at the origin, mid, and hilum, and at any area of focal color aliasing. Waveforms from the interlobar or segmental intraparenchymal renal arteries at the upper and lower poles should be obtained to measure the acceleration index (AI), acceleration time (AT), and resistive index (RI). Optimally, three Doppler waveforms of the intraparenchymal renal arteries should be obtained

at each pole. The AI is derived by calculating the slope of the line from the onset of systole to the early systolic peak complex, and the AT is the length of time from the onset of systole to the early systolic peak complex. A schematic demonstrating how to measure the AI and AT is presented in Fig. 9. The early systolic peak complex does not always correspond to peak systole, because some normal renal artery waveforms may have an early systolic notch (Fig. 10B, C). In such patients, measuring to the point of PSV results in an incorrectly prolonged AI and AT. One should also visually inspect the pulse Doppler waveform to assess for a tardus parvus waveform, which is characterized by a low-velocity rounded systolic peak (see Fig. 9C). On pulse Doppler examination, the renal arteries normally have a low resistance waveform with continuous forward diastolic flow and a sharp systolic upstroke

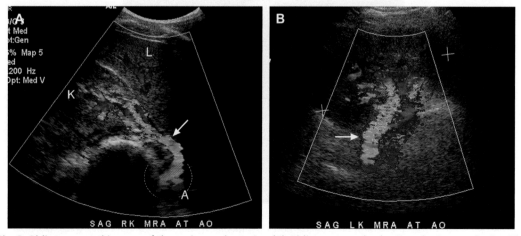

*Fig. 3.* Oblique coronal images of the main renal arteries. (*A*) Oblique coronal color Doppler image obtained by angling through the renal hilum toward the aorta, demonstrating the entire length of the right main renal artery (*arrow*). Segments of the renal vein are noted (*blue*). Kidney (*K*), liver (*L*), and aorta (*A*). (*B*) Oblique sagittal color Doppler image demonstrating the left main renal artery (*arrow*). The renal vein is adjacent and inferior (*blue*). Kidney (++).

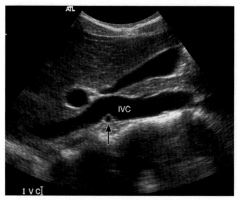

Fig. 4. Coronal gray scale image demonstrating the right renal artery in cross section (*arrow*) crossing under the inferior vena cava (IVC).

(Fig. 10). PSV typically is less than 100 cm/s in the main renal artery and decreases as the arterial tree is traced distally. The RI should be less than 0.7 in the intraparenchymal renal arteries [19], and the AT is normally less than 70 ms (see Fig. 10).

### Diagnostic criteria for renal artery stenosis

Anatomic evaluation of the main renal arteries is performed using gray scale and color images. Narrowing at the ostium with or without calcified plaque is suggestive of atherosclerotic stenosis (Fig. 11), whereas beading or even aneurysmal focal dilatation of the middle of the renal artery is suggestive of fibromuscular dysplasia (see Fig. 8). Post-stenotic dilatation may also be observed. On color Doppler interrogation, focal color aliasing or

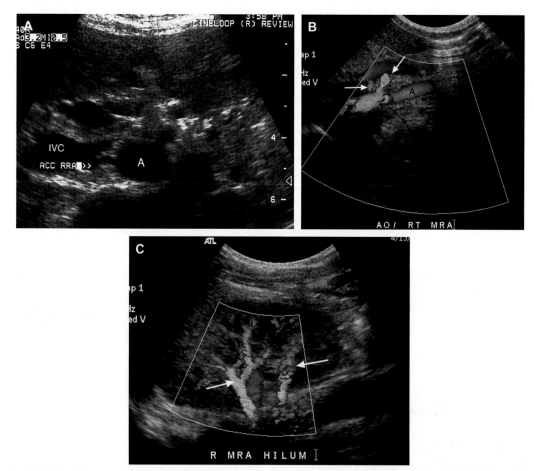

Fig. 5. Multiple/accessory renal arteries. (A) Transverse gray scale image demonstrating a small accessory right renal artery arising from the lateral wall of the aorta (A) medial to the inferior vena cava (IVC). (B) Oblique coronal color Doppler image depicting two right renal arteries (*arrows*) arising from the aorta (A). The more superior renal artery is smaller than the IVC (*blue*). (C) Note two renal arteries (*arrows*) at the level of the renal pelvis. In this patient, only one renal artery was initially identified arising from the aorta. Once the two vessels were noted in the renal pelvis, however, the sonographer was able to trace both vessels back to the aorta and thus identify the second renal artery.

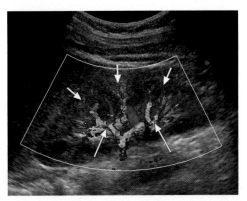

Fig. 6. Longitudinal color Doppler image of the kidney depicting the normal segmental (*long arrows*) and interlobar (*short arrows*) intraparenchymal renal arteries.

a "soft-tissue color bruit" (color artifact in the surrounding soft tissues) suggests an underlying stenosis with increased PSV (see Fig. 8; Fig. 12). Asymmetry of the renal length (>1.5 cm) and asymmetry of cortical thickness or echogenicity is also suggestive of underlying renal vascular pathology (Fig. 13A).

Physiologic information suggesting the clinical significance of an anatomic RAS may be determined on DUS using two approaches. It is well known that a hemodynamically significant stenosis causes a focal increase in PSV once the luminal diameter reduction exceeds 50%. The direct approach therefore depends on the identification of a focal increase in PSV at the anatomic site of a stenosis in the main renal artery. The second, or indirect, approach depends on the demonstration of a decrease in the rate of systolic acceleration within the intraparenchymal renal arteries, which occurs distal to

a more proximal hemodynamically significant stenosis in the main renal artery.

### Direct approach

PSV focally increases at the anatomic site of a hemodynamically significant stenosis in the main renal artery. On color Doppler, focal color aliasing, poststenotic turbulence, and poststenotic dilatation are also typically observed (see Fig. 11). Comparing the PSV at the origin of the main renal artery to the PSV of the aorta at the level of the renal arteries compensates for individual variations in cardiac output. This has been termed the RAR, the ratio of PSV in the main renal artery to the PSV in the aorta. Although there is some variation center to center, most investigators consider a PSV in the main renal artery greater than 180 or 200 cm/s and an RAR greater than 3.0 to 3.5 to be diagnostic of hemodynamically significant RAS, defined as a reduction in the diameter of the lumen by greater than 50% to 60% (see Figs. 11 and 12; Fig. 13) [17]. Using these criteria, the sensitivity of DUS to identify a hemodynamically significant RAS in the main renal artery has been reported to range from 79% to 91%, with specificities ranging from 73% to 97% [20,21]. A study by House and colleagues [20] found that lowering the threshold value for the RAR to 3.0 considerably improved the sensitivity with minimal adverse effects on specificity. A few investigators advocate using an RAR as low as 2.0 [18]. Li and colleagues [18] evaluated the accuracy and threshold values of various velocity parameters in the diagnosis of RAS (>50% luminal diameter reduction in this study). Four Doppler parameters, including PSV in the main renal artery and interlobar arteries, the RAR, and the ratio of PSV in the main renal artery to the PSV in the interlobar arteries (RIR)

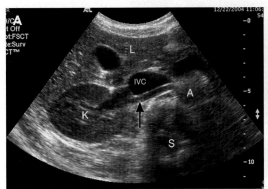
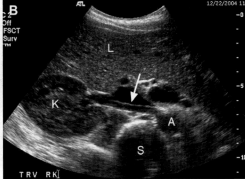

Fig. 7. (*A, B*) In this patient the entire right renal artery (*arrow*) is well visualized with gray scale imaging. Sometimes color flash artifact from patient motion may actually obscure visualization of the main renal arteries. Spatial resolution is better on gray scale images in comparison with color Doppler images, and the frame rate is also faster. Kidney (*K*), liver (*L*), aorta (*A*), spine (*S*), and inferior vena cava (*IVC*).

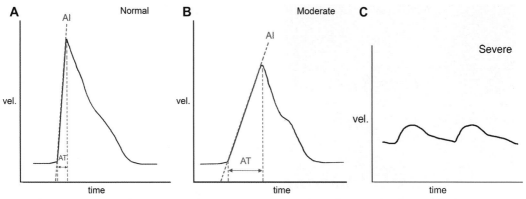

**Fig. 8.** Schematic diagrams demonstrating how to measure AI and AT. The AI is the slope of the line connecting the point of onset of systole and the early systolic peak (ESP) complex. The AT is the length of time (along the baseline) between these two points. (*A*) Normal renal artery waveform. (*B*) Abnormal waveform with a delay in systolic acceleration indicating a proximal stenosis in the main renal artery. (*C*) Tardus parvus waveform indicating a high-grade proximal stenosis.

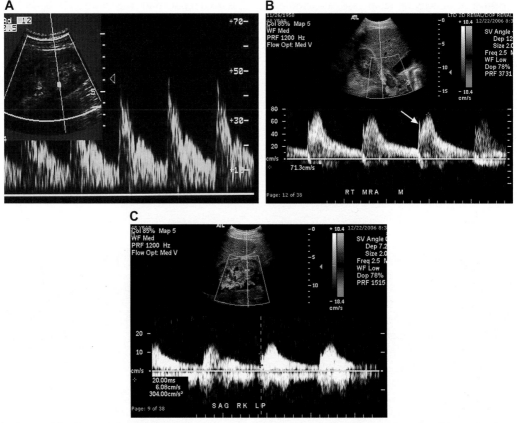

**Fig. 9.** Normal pulse Doppler waveforms of the renal arteries. (*A*) Pulse Doppler tracing of an intraparenchymal segmental renal artery demonstrates a sharp systolic upstroke and continuous forward diastolic flow. In this case the point of PSV is the same as the early systolic peak (ESP) complex. (*B*) Pulse Doppler tracing of a normal renal artery in another patient demonstrating an early systolic notch or ESP complex (*arrow*) before PSV (+) is reached. (*C*) Measurement of normal acceleration time (20 ms).

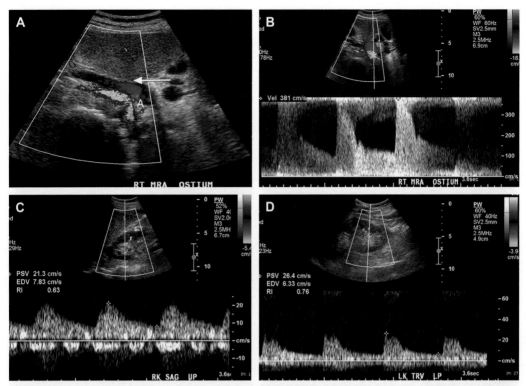

*Fig. 10.* RAS in a 61-year-old woman who had refractory hypertension. (*A*) Note narrowing (*arrow*) at the ostium of the right renal artery on color Doppler image. Poststenotic dilatation and color aliasing caused by the high velocity jet is noted. Aorta (*A*). (*B*) Pulse Doppler tracing reveals a PSV of 381 cm/s at the origin of the right renal artery. PSV in the aorta was 62 cm/s, yielding an RAR of >6.0. (*C*) Pulse Doppler tracing demonstrating delay in systolic acceleration (mild sloping of systolic upstroke) in the intraparenchymal right renal arteries consistent with the proximal stenosis. (*D*) In comparison, pulse Doppler interrogation reveals a normal sharp systolic upstroke in the left intraparenchymal renal arteries.

were measured. The RIR was determined to be the best parameter. Using threshold values of RIR greater than 5, main renal artery PSV greater than 150 cm/s, RAR greater than 2.0, and PSV less than 25 cm/s in the interlobar arteries, sensitivities were calculated to be 88%, 81%, 70%, and 74%, respectively [18]. An RIR greater than 5 and PSV less than 15 cm/s in the interlobar artery were found to provide the optimal combination of parameters, with sensitivity and specificity of 91% and 87%, respectively [18].

Multiple factors, however, may limit adequate visualization of the origins of the main renal arteries (which is where most renal artery stenoses occur), including obesity, dyspnea, overlying bowel gas, and shadowing from arterial calcifications. Cardiac arrhythmias or poor angle of Doppler insonation may also make estimates of PSV inaccurate. Direct evaluation of PSV in accessory renal arteries is also severely limited on ultrasound examination because of their small size [22–25]. It is estimated that accessory renal arteries occur in approximately 15% to 24% of patients [24–26]. Some

investigators believe, however, that the presence of a stenosis in an accessory renal artery is not associated with an increased risk for hypertension [27,28]. In a study performed by Bude and colleagues [28], a hemodynamically significant stenosis isolated to an accessory renal artery was found in only 1.5% of patients undergoing angiography for evaluation of RVH. This study concluded that failure to evaluate accessory renal arteries should not negatively affect the usefulness of a noninvasive study for detecting RVH [28].

*Indirect approach*

A decrease in the rate of systolic acceleration within the intraparenchymal renal arteries distal to a stenosis has also been reported to be an accurate method for diagnosing RAS. Several articles have shown excellent results with this indirect technique [29–31]. This approach has the potential to eliminate many of the technical and theoretic problems using the PSV of the main renal artery as the major diagnostic criterion for RAS, because intraparenchymal waveforms can be obtained in virtually all patients.

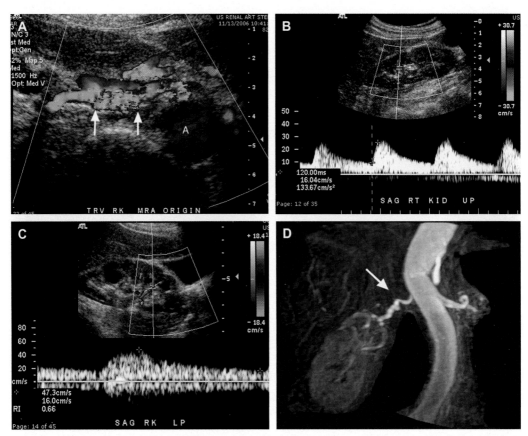

**Fig. 11.** Renal artery stenosis caused by fibromuscular dysplasia in a 43-year-old woman who had severe hypertension. (*A*) Color Doppler image reveals aliasing in the middle third of the right main renal artery (*arrows*), a typical location for stenosis caused by fibromuscular dysplasia. Aorta (*A*). (*B*) Intraparenchymal renal artery waveform demonstrating delay in systolic acceleration. AT = 120 ms. (*C*) Increasing the sweep speed widens or magnifies the tracing, making it easier to accurately measure AT and AI. (*D*) MRA demonstrates beading (*arrow*) of the middle third of the right main renal artery consistent with the diagnosis of fibromuscular dysplasia.

Stavros and colleagues [31] reported their results evaluating the AI, AT, and visual waveform inspection assessing for the tardus parvus waveform phenomenon as measures of the rate of systolic acceleration. The AI is the slope of the line from the beginning of systolic to the early systolic peak complex in meters per second squared (see Fig. 9). The AT is the time from the onset of systole to the early systolic peak complex (see Fig. 9). If the Doppler waveform shows more than one systolic peak, then the earliest (the early systolic peak complex) should be used for measurements of the AI and AT even if it is lower in amplitude than the second peak along the systolic curve. Stavros and colleagues [31] reported that an AI less than 3.0 m/s$^2$ had an accuracy of 85%, a sensitivity of 89%, and a specificity of 83% for detecting RAS. In their study, an AT of greater than or equal to 0.07 seconds was 89% accurate, 78% sensitive, and 94% specific (see Fig. 14) [31]. Although some interpreters rely

on these threshold measurements of the rate of systolic acceleration, many proponents of this indirect technique use a pattern recognition approach with visual inspection of the waveform, using identification of the tardus parvus pattern (rounding and flattening of the systolic peak) (see Fig. 9C) as sufficient evidence to differentiate normal from abnormal and to diagnose RAS (see Figs. 8 and 11). In the study of Stavros and colleagues [31], identification of a tardus parvus waveform pattern alone by visual inspection was 96% accurate, 95% sensitive, and 97% specific for diagnosing RAS. Observation of a delay in systolic acceleration in an intraparenchymal renal artery in one pole of the kidney when the other pole demonstrates a normal shape systolic upstroke can be used to diagnose RAS in one of multiple renal arteries or in a branch vessel, although the clinical significance of stenoses in accessory vessels remains controversial (see earlier discussion) (Fig. 15).

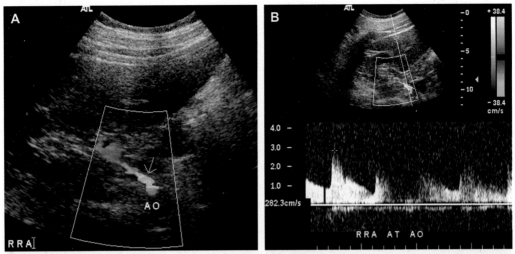

*Fig. 12.* RAS in a 66-year-old woman who had refractory hypertension. (*A*) Color Doppler image reveals aliasing (*arrow*) at the origin of the right renal artery. Aliasing occurs when blood flow velocity exceeds the Nyquist limit and helps guide where to place the Doppler cursor to maximize measurement of PSV. Aorta (*AO*). (*B*) Pulse Doppler tracing indicates that PSV is elevated to 282 cm/s at the site of the focal color aliasing, confirming the diagnosis of RAS.

These measures of the rate of systolic acceleration, however, are acknowledged to be less accurate for detecting moderate degrees of RAS (<70% diameter stenosis), which may still be amenable to surgical or percutaneous treatment [31]. Although Doppler interrogation of the intraparenchymal renal arteries can be performed by way of the translumbar approach in virtually all patients who can hold their breath, thus eliminating the problem of technically limited examinations associated with ultrasound assessment of PSV in the main renal artery, some theoretic issues remain unresolved. Collateral blood flow around a high-grade stenosis or occlusion may obscure the diagnosis of RAS. Other causes of decreased systolic acceleration may make this study nonspecific in certain patient populations. In children, for example, an abdominal coarctation (Fig. 16) or William syndrome (Fig. 17) may also result in delayed systolic acceleration and therefore may mimic RAS. Extrarenal factors, such as aortic/mitral valve disease, left ventricle dysfunction, or even cardiovascular medications such as after-load reducers, might decrease the rate of systolic acceleration also. Numerous factors, such as age, hypertension, and diabetes, also affect vessel compliance and peripheral vascular resistance, inhibiting or minimizing development of the tardus parvus waveform distal to a stenosis [32]. Such variables may explain why not all investigators report the same degree of success in identifying RAS using these measures of systolic acceleration, particularly in the elderly patient population [23]. Pre-administration of 25 mg of captopril 1 hour before Doppler ultrasound examination has been reported to exaggerate the tardus parvus waveform phenomenon in the intraparenchymal vessels of patients who have RAS, thereby increasing the sensitivity of DUS for the detection of RAS [33].

DUS can also be used to monitor patients following surgical or percutaneous revascularization to ensure that the kidney has adequate blood flow and that the graft, stent, or angioplastied vessel is patent and that restenosis has not occurred. In revascularized patients, absence of focal increase in PSV and redevelopment of a sharp systolic upstroke in the intraparenchymal renal arteries indicates a successful procedure (Fig. 18). An increase in PSV in the main renal artery or graft or the reappearance of an intraparenchymal tardus parvus waveform, however, suggests restenosis (Fig. 19).

Studies have also indicated that preoperative ultrasound examinations can predict which patients who have RAS will benefit from revascularization [34]. It is hypothesized that end organ damage may have already occurred in patients who have a small kidney with a thin, echogenic renal cortex or an RI greater than 0.8 in the intraparenchymal renal arteries, and that improvement of blood pressure or renal function is less likely following intervention in such patients [33–35]. Cohn and colleagues [35] report, in addition, that a diastolic to systolic ratio less than 0.3 correlates with lack of improvement in blood pressure and renal function following revascularization. On the other hand, Garcia-Criado and colleagues [36] concluded

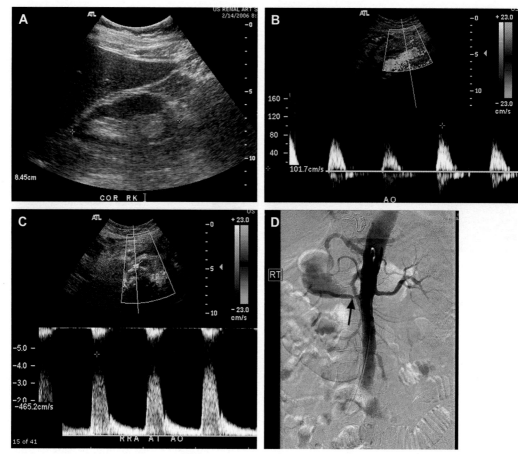

*Fig. 13.* RAS in a 56-year-old woman who had longstanding severe hypertension and renal failure. (*A*) Longitudinal gray scale image reveals that the right kidney (++) is small, measuring 8.4 cm. The renal cortex is thinned at the upper pole. The left kidney measured 10.1 cm in maximal longitudinal dimension. (*B*) Pulse Doppler tracing of the aorta demonstrates a PSV of 102 cm/s. (*C*) Pulse Doppler tracing of the origin of the main right renal artery reveals a PSV of 465 cm/s. The RAR is approximately 4.5. (*D*) These findings are consistent with a high-grade stenosis of the right renal artery, which was confirmed by angiography (*arrow*).

that an elevated RI should not preclude revascularization, because it was not a useful parameter in predicting improvement in renal function, although it was associated with poor blood pressure response.

The use of IV ultrasound contrast agents, not yet approved in the United States for this indication, improves visibility of the main renal arteries, making it easier to measure the PSV, thereby salvaging technically limited examinations (Fig. 20). Numerous studies have indicated that the use of IV ultrasound contrast agents increases the sensitivity and specificity of DUS for diagnosing RAS [37,38]. Although this technique holds much promise for the future, ultrasound contrast agents are not yet FDA approved, and false-positive examinations have been reported in clinical trials (D. Rubens, MD, personal communication, 1998).

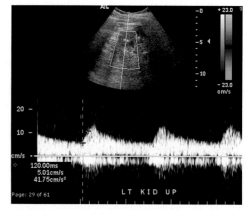

*Fig. 14.* Pulse Doppler tracing of an interlobar artery in the left kidney demonstrating delay in systolic acceleration indicated by a mild sloping of the systolic upstroke consistent with a proximal stenosis in a 73-year-old man who had refractory hypertension. The AT was 120 ms.

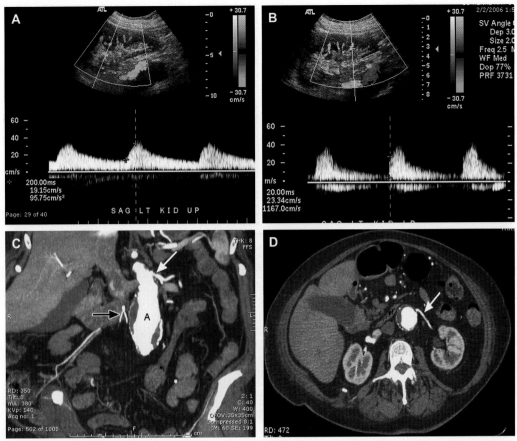

**Fig. 15.** RAS at the origin of one of two left main renal arteries in a 66-year-old woman who had refractory hypertension, renal failure, and an abdominal aortic aneurysm. (*A*) Pulse Doppler tracing reveals delayed systolic upstroke in a segmental vessel in the upper pole of the left kidney. The AT is markedly prolonged, 200 ms. The rate of systolic acceleration is normal in the lower pole, however (*B*), where a Doppler tracing of an interlobar artery reveals a sharp systolic upstroke and an AT of 20 ms. This discrepancy suggests that there are two renal arteries and that only the vessel to the upper pole of the left kidney is stenosed. Alternatively, a stenosis involving a branch vessel to the upper pole could result in the same findings. (*C*) CT angiography reveals a marked narrowing at the origin of the renal artery supplying the upper pole of the left kidney (*white arrow*). Note aortic aneurysm with intraluminal thrombus (*A*) and IVC filter (*black arrow*). (*D*) The smaller inferior renal artery (*arrow*), however, which supplies the lower pole of the left kidney is normal, without evidence of stenosis.

## Computed tomographic angiography

The introduction of spiral and multidetector computed tomography (CT) with three-dimensional post-processing techniques has made continuous data acquisition possible with a large volume during a single breath hold. Studies have reported a high correlation between the morphologic findings on spiral CT angiography and DSA, especially for evaluation of the renal arteries [39].

With this technique, axial slices with narrow collimation (1–3 mm) are obtained in the region of the renal arteries in the arterial phase before enhancement of the renal veins. A power injector is used to inject the contrast at a rate of 3 to 5 mL/s for a total volume of 100 to 150 mL. Accurate timing of the contrast bolus is important to achieve adequate opacification of the renal arteries. This is performed by manually calculating the delay time with a test injection, by automatically using the smart-prep technique (imaging starts when vascular enhancement reaches a certain predefined threshold, usually 150 HU), or by using an empiric delay of 20 to 25 seconds [40,41].

Reconstruction of secondary images from the primary data using algorithms such as shaded-surface display (SSD), maximum intensity projections (MIP), and volume rendering can be performed at a workstation (Fig. 21). Numerous studies have reported that CT angiography has a greater than 90% sensitivity and specificity for detection of ostial and proximal RAS as defined by a reduction in luminal

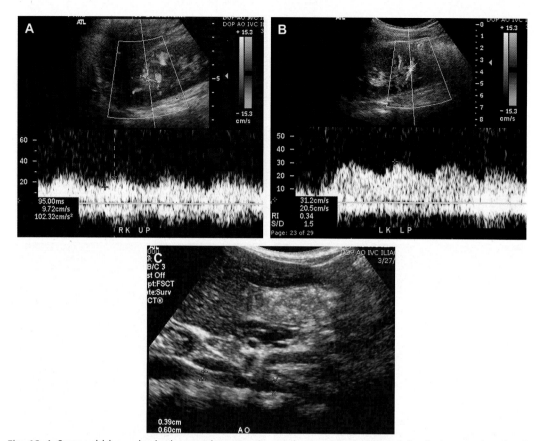

*Fig. 16.* A 6-year-old boy who had severe hypertension and coarctation of the abdominal aorta. (*A, B*) Pulse Doppler images reveal bilateral and symmetric tardus parvus waveforms indicating delay in systolic acceleration in the right and left segmental renal arteries. The AT on the right is 95 ms. Although this could indicate proximal bilateral RAS, this would be unusual. (*C*) Sagittal view of the aorta demonstrates severe narrowing of the abdominal aorta (++) at the level of the celiac axis and origin of the superior mesenteric artery (SMA), above the level of the renal arteries. No narrowing of the renal arteries was detected on MR angiography.

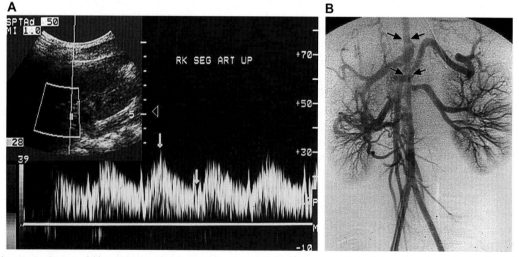

*Fig. 17.* An 8-year-old boy who had hypertension and William syndrome. (*A*) An intraparenchymal pulse Doppler waveform from the right kidney demonstrates a tardus parvus pattern. The arterial waveforms in the left kidney were similar. (*B*) Angiogram reveals diffuse narrowing of the abdominal aorta (*arrows*) above the origin of the renal arteries.

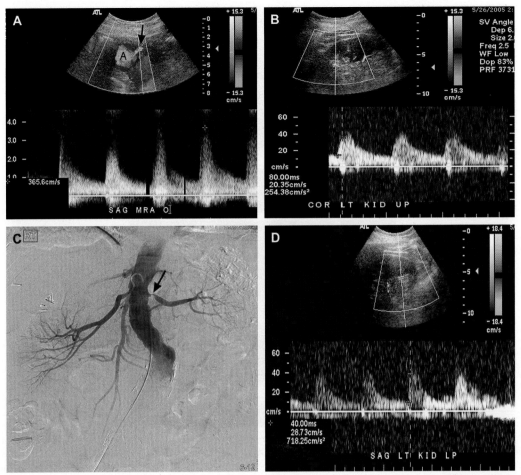

Fig. 18. A 72-year-old woman who had hypertension unresponsive to a three-drug regimen. (A) Pulse Doppler image of the origin of the left renal artery (*arrow*) demonstrates increased PSV at 366 cm/s; aorta (A). (B) Pulse Doppler image of a segmental artery in the upper pole of the left kidney demonstrating delayed systolic upstroke with an AT of 80 ms. (C) Angiogram confirming a tight stenosis at the origin of the left renal artery (*arrow*). (D) Following stenting of the left main renal artery, follow-up Doppler interrogation of the left kidney revealed no increase in PSV at the origin and normal intraparenchymal waveforms with a sharp systolic upstroke. The AT was 40 ms. There is thus no evidence of recurrent stenosis.

diameter of more than 50% to 60% [39,41,42] (Fig. 22). Secondary signs of RAS, such as poststenotic dilatation, decrease in renal size, cortical thinning, and decreased cortical enhancement, are also helpful in recognizing RAS on CT angiography. Patients who have fibromuscular dysplasia as a cause of RAS typically demonstrate narrowing in the middle third of the main renal artery, often over a long segment. A beaded appearance or true aneurysms may be noted. Up to 30% of patients have accessory renal arteries, and CT angiography has been shown to adequately identify these arteries [39,42–45]. A study comparing CT angiography to DSA in 82 patients (197 renal arteries examined, including 33 accessory arteries) reported that CT angiography was comparable to DSA in the detection of hemodynamically significant RAS (more than 50%

diameter reduction) with a sensitivity and specificity of 96% and 99%, respectively [39]. In addition, CT angiography depicted five adrenal masses and detected all accessory renal arteries. The study concluded by recommending CT angiography instead of DSA for evaluation of patients who have clinically suspected RVH [39].

In comparison to DSA, CT angiography has the additional advantage of clear visualization of calcified atherosclerotic plaques and has better spatial resolution than MR angiography. Multi-detector CT angiography, however, entails significant radiation exposure in addition to carrying the well known potential risks of IV iodinated contrast media, namely nephrotoxicity and allergic reaction. Mild atheromatous narrowing at the renal ostia or stenoses at branch points located in the smaller

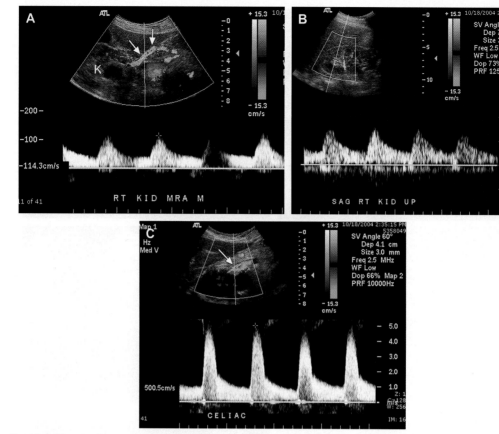

**Fig. 19.** A 59-year-old woman status-post (s/p) renal artery to gastroduodenal artery (GDA) bypass graft for treatment of RVH presenting with recurrent hypertension. (*A*) Duplex Doppler image demonstrates that the bypass graft (*arrows*) is widely patent with a normal PSV. Note slight delay in systolic acceleration. The origin of the graft with the GDA could not be visualized because of overlying bowel gas; kidney (*K*). (*B*) Pulse Doppler tracing of an intraparenchymal segmental artery in the right renal hilum reveals a mild tardus parvus pattern suggesting a proximal stenosis. (*C*) Pulse Doppler tracing of the origin of the celiac artery (*arrow*) from the aorta reveals a markedly elevated PSV >500 cm/s, indicating a tight stenosis that was confirmed angiographically and stented for control of the patient's hypertension.

vessels in the renal hilum are also more difficult to identify on CT angiography.

## Magnetic resonance angiography

Renal MR angiography allows accurate anatomic examination of the main renal arteries in patients suspected of having RAS without the risks associated with nephrotoxic iodinated contrast agents, ionizing radiation, or invasive arterial catheterization. In many institutions, MR angiography has replaced conventional angiography (DSA), unless DSA is performed in conjunction with an interventional procedure or coronary angiogram. Many investigators currently advocate using MR angiography as the primary noninvasive screening modality for RAS. Because FMD can be difficult to detect on MR angiography, however, there is some

controversy as to whether CT angiography, DSA, or Doppler ultrasound is preferable in young female hypertensive patients who are more likely to have FMD, because of the better spatial resolution of CT angiography and DSA (for evaluation of the smaller caliber distal renal artery or fibromuscular webs) and the ability of Doppler ultrasound to provide physiologic information.

Early MR angiography techniques were time consuming and images were degraded by respiratory artifacts. Modern gradient echo and parallel imaging techniques, however, allow MR angiography images to be acquired in a single breathhold. Images are obtained following the injection of IV gadolinium contrast (total dose = 0.2–0.3 mmol/Kg administered at an injection rate of 2–4 mL/s) and are timed for maximal enhancement of the renal arteries. Like the CT angiography technique, timing

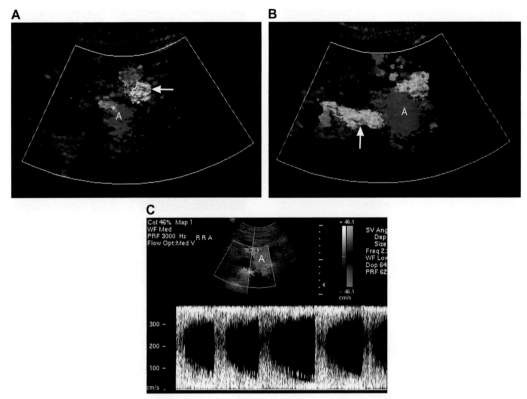

*Fig. 20.* Doppler ultrasound evaluation of the renal arteries using intravenous ultrasound contrast. (*A*) The right renal artery cannot be identified on baseline color Doppler transverse image of the aorta (*A*). Note color aliasing at origin of the SMA (*arrow*), indicating severe SMA stenosis in this patient who had known severe atherosclerotic disease and hypertension. (*B*) Following the administration of IV contrast, the origin from the aorta (*A*) and the first several centimeters of the right renal artery (*arrow*) are clearly visualized. Focal color aliasing suggests a significant underlying stenosis at the origin of the renal artery. The presence of aliasing helps guide placement of the pulse Doppler sample volume to detect the highest PSV. (*C*) Pulse Doppler image demonstrates aliasing of PSV over 300 cm/s, confirming severe stenosis of the right renal artery. In this patient, the use of IV contrast salvaged an otherwise nondiagnostic ultrasound examination. (*Courtesy of* J. Pellerito, MD, Manhassett, NY.)

is performed using a test bolus, a smart-prep technique, or a standard 20- to 25-second delay. Images are obtained in an oblique coronal plane to minimize the number of slices required to cover the renal arteries. This optimizes scan time and increases in-plane resolution. Typical scanning parameters are 36-cm field of view, 2-mm slice thickness, and a scan matrix of 320 × 192 for a resolution of 2 mm × 1.1 mm × 1.8 mm. MIP images and multiplanar projection images are created at a work station to provide an angiographic image (Fig. 23). The source images, however, should always be carefully reviewed [46].

Numerous series have reported excellent correlation between DSA and MR angiography for detection of RAS (50% or more diameter reduction), with sensitivities ranging from 88% to 100% and specificities exceeding 90% [46–52] (Fig. 24). MRI also allows evaluation of renal size and cortical thickness. The main limitations of MR angiography are spatial resolution and dependence of image quality on the patient's ability to breath-hold, which limits evaluation of smaller vessels, such as branch vessels in the hilum and the distal main renal artery, and detection of smaller accessory renal arteries that may arise anywhere along the abdominal aorta or iliac arteries in the pelvis [46]. The diagnosis of RAS secondary to FMD on MR angiography is thus difficult if the findings are subtle [46]. Also, in general MR angiography tends to overestimate the degree of stenosis [46]. In addition, MR angiography cannot evaluate the residual lumen within a metallic stent, which can be done with CT angiography, DSA, or Doppler ultrasound.

Several unconventional techniques have also been developed for evaluation of the potential functional or physiologic significance of a stenosis in the renal artery on MR angiography. In-flow

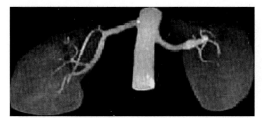

*Fig. 21.* Volume rendered MIP CT angiography of the renal arteries demonstrating bilateral normal renal arteries.

disease can be evaluated by analyzing the time curve or renal parenchymal enhancement assessing for delay or asymmetry of renal cortical enhancement [46].

The administration of IV gadolinium in patients who have abnormal renal function, however, may be limited in the future, because gadolinium is currently suspected to be a cause of a recently described but poorly understood nephrogenic fibrosing dermopathy, also called nephrogenic systemic fibrosis (NSF), which has been reported to have resulted in the death of some patients and severe debilitation in many others [53,54]. Noncontrast enhanced MR angiography techniques, such as cardiac- and respiratory-triggered balanced steady-state imaging, time of flight, and phase contrast MR angiography, are therefore being revisited in light of new evidence that gadolinium may not be safe in patients who have poor renal function.

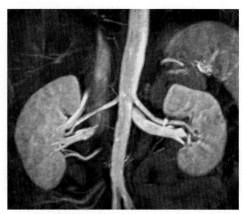

*Fig. 23.* Whole-volume MIP from an MR angiography demonstrating bilateral normal renal arteries. A smaller accessory renal artery is incompletely seen on the right inferiorly. Note left renal vein inferior to the left renal artery.

## ACE inhibitor scintigraphy

A kidney with RAS may exhibit impaired function during ACE inhibition. A decline in the glomerular filtration rate (GFR) of the affected kidney can be induced by ACE inhibition in patients who have unilateral RAS. Because the contralateral normal kidney is not affected, overall renal function is preserved. This decrease in renal function induced by ACE inhibition can be measured by renal scintigraphy, because the ACE inhibitor induces significant change in the time activity curves of the affected kidney when compared either with base

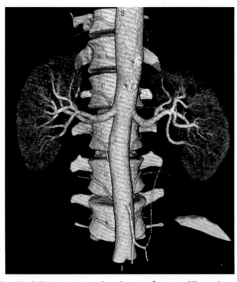

*Fig. 22.* 3-D reconstruction image from a CT angiography showing bilateral renal artery stenoses and an accessory right renal artery. There is minimal dilatation of the infrarenal abdominal aorta and the wall of the aorta is slightly irregular, consistent with atherosclerosis/plaque.

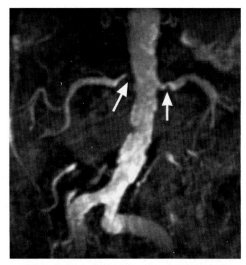

*Fig. 24.* Volume-rendered MIP from an MR angiography of the renal arteries showing bilateral RAS (*arrows*). Note diffuse irregularity of the aortic wall, indicating atherosclerosis.

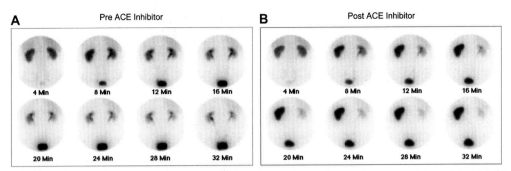

**A** Pre ACE Inhibitor       **B** Post ACE Inhibitor

*Fig. 25.* Captopril nuclear medicine study of a patient who had left RAS. (*A*) Before ingestion of ACE inhibitor, both kidneys demonstrate normal excretion of the radiopharmaceutical agent. (*B*) Following administration of the ACE inhibitor, the left kidney demonstrates persistent uptake and delayed excretion of the radiopharmaceutical. There is normal uptake and excretion on the right.

scintigraphy before ACE ingestion or with the contralateral normal kidney (Fig. 25). Specifically, ACE inhibitors induce renal retention of the radiopharmaceutical in patients who have RVH because of decreased urinary output secondary to reduced GFR.

ACE inhibitor scintigraphy is performed 1 hour after an oral dose of 25 mg of Captopril or 15 minutes after an IV dose of 0.04 mg/Kg of enalapril maleate [48]. Oral ACE inhibitors are withheld for 2 to 5 days before the examination. The most common radiopharmaceuticals currently used in the United States are Tc-99$^m$ mercaptoacetyltriglycine (MAG3 scan) or Tc-99$^m$ diethylenetriaminepentaacetic acid (DTPA scan). Sequential images and scintigraphy curves are obtained for 30 minutes after injection of the radiopharmaceutical.

In selected high-risk populations, ACE inhibitor scintigraphy is reported to be accurate in diagnosing RVH, with a reported sensitivity varying from 51% to 96% for detection of unilateral RAS (70% or more diameter reduction) [55]. Nuclear scintigraphy, however, is much less sensitive and specific in unselected patient populations. In addition, the sensitivity of ACE inhibitor scintigraphy is much lower in patients who have bilateral RAS, impaired renal function, or urinary obstruction and in patients who have taken ACE inhibitors over a long period of time [48]. In current clinical practice, ACE inhibitor scintigraphy is therefore considered to be less sensitive, and is therefore used much less frequently than other noninvasive examinations, such as DUS, CT angiography, or MR angiography to screen for RVH.

## Summary

Doppler ultrasound is an inexpensive, widely available, noninvasive screening method for diagnosing RVH. Doppler ultrasound examination uses physiologic and anatomic criteria for diagnosing RAS, as opposed to CT angiography and MR angiography, which provide only anatomic information, and nuclear scintigraphy, which relies on physiologic information alone to make the diagnosis of RAS. The main limitations of ultrasound are technical, resulting in poor visualization of the origins of the main renal arteries. In patients suspected of having RAS, the authors suggest the use of Doppler ultrasound as a first screening study, unless the patient is obese, dyspneic, or has heavy arterial calcifications. In such circumstances, screening with CT angiography or MR angiography is advisable because of the high rate of technical failure of DUS. If such patients have impaired renal function, however, CT angiography and MR angiography pose significant risks for nephrotoxicity and nephrogenic systemic fibrosis. and initial imaging with ultrasound may therefore be more appropriate. Furthermore, the use of IV ultrasound contrast agents is promising for the future and is predicted to increase the sensitivity and accuracy of RAS detection on ultrasound examination and to decrease the rate of technical failure.

## References

[1] Hajjar I, Kotchen TA. Trends in prevalence, awareness, treatment, and control of hypertension in the United States, 1988–2000. JAMA 2003;290:199–206.

[2] Mann SJ, Pickering TG. Detection of renovascular hypertension: state of the art: 1992. Ann Intern Med 1992;117:845–53.

[3] Garovic VD, Textor SC. Renovascular hypertension and ischemic nephropathy. Circulation 2005;112:1362–74.

[4] Textor SC, Wilcox CS. Renal artery stenosis: a common, treatable cause of renal failure? Annu Rev Med 2001;52:421–42.

[5] Cheung CM, Wright JR, Shurrab AE, et al. Epidemiology of renal dysfunction and patient

outcome in atherosclerotic renal artery occlusion. J Am Soc Nephrol 2002;13:149–57.

[6] Rimmer JM, Gennari FJ. Atherosclerotic renovascular disease and progressive renal failure. Ann Intern Med 1993;118:712–9.

[7] Fatica RA, Port FK, Young EW. Incidence trends and mortality in end-stage renal disease attributed to renovascular disease in the United States. Am J Kidney Dis 2001;137:1184–90.

[8] Scoble JE, Hamilton G. Atherosclerotic renovascular disease: remedial cause of renal failure in the elderly. BMJ 1990;300:1670–1.

[9] Zucchelli P, Chiarini C, Zuccala A, et al. Renal ischemia is the real problem in renovascular hypertension. In: Glorioso N, Laragh JH, Rappelli A, editors. Renovascular hypertension. New York: Raven Press; 1987. p. 273–80.

[10] Dorros G, Jaff MM, Mathia KL, et al. Four year follow-up of Palmaz-Schatz stent revascularization as treatment for atherosclerotic renal artery stenosis. Circulation 1998;98:642–7.

[11] Lewin A, Blaufox MD, Castle H, et al. Apparent prevalence of curable hypertension in the hypertension detection and follow-up program. Arch Intern Med 1985;145:424–7.

[12] Kaplan NM. Clinical hypertension. Baltimore (MD): Williams & Wilkins; 1990. p. 303–32.

[13] Landwehr DM, Vetrovec GW, Cowley MJ, et al. Association of renal artery stenosis with coronary artery disease in patients with hypertension and/or chronic renal insufficiency [abstract]. J Am Soc Nephrol 1983;33A.

[14] Missouris CG, Buckenham T, Cappuccio FP, et al. Renal artery stenosis: a common and important problem in patients with peripheral vascular disease. Am J Med 1994;96:10–4.

[15] Zierler RE, Berglin RO, Isaacson JA, et al. Natural history of atherosclerotic renal artery stenosis: a prospective study with duplex ultrasonography. J Vasc Surg 1994;19:250–8.

[16] Gutzman R, Zierler R, Isaacson J, et al. Renal atrophy and arterial stenosis: a prospective study with duplex ultrasound. Hypertension 1994;23:346–50.

[17] Lee HY, Grant EG. Sonography in renovascular hypertension. J Ultrasound Med 2002;21:431–41.

[18] Li JC, Wang L, Jiag YX, et al. Evaluation of renal artery stenosis with velocity parameters of Doppler sonography. J Ultrasound Med 2006;25(6):735–42.

[19] Gottleib RH, Luhmann K, Oates RP. Duplex ultrasound evaluation of normal native kidneys and native kidneys with urinary tract obstruction. J Ultrasound Med 1989;8:609–11.

[20] House MK, Dowling RJ, King P, et al. Using Doppler sonography to reveal renal artery stenosis: an evaluation of optimal imaging parameters. AJR Am J Roentgenol 1999;173:761–5.

[21] Kohler TR, Zierler RE, Martin RL, et al. Noninvasive diagnosis of renal artery stenosis by ultrasonic duplex scanning. J Vasc Surg 1986;4:450–6.

[22] Halpern EJ, Nazarian LN, Wechsler RJ, et al. US, CT and MR evaluation of accessory renal arteries and proximal renal arterial branches. Acad Radiol 1999;6:299–304.

[23] Kliewer MA, Tupler RH, Hertzberg BS, et al. Doppler evaluation of renal artery stenosis: interobserver agreement in the interpretation of waveform morphology. AJR Am J Roentgenol 1994;162:1371–6.

[24] Helenon O, Rody FE, Correas JM, et al. Color Doppler US of renovascular disease in native kidneys. Radiographics 1995;15:833–54.

[25] Berland LL, Koslin DB, Routh WD, et al. Renal artery stenosis: prospective evaluation of diagnosis with color duplex US compared with angiography. Radiology 1990;174:421–3.

[26] Geyer JR, Poutasse EF. Incidence of multiple renal arteries on aortography. JAMA 1962;182:120–5.

[27] Gupta A, Tello R. Accessory renal arteries are not related to hypertension risk: a review of MR angiography data. AJR Am J Roentgenol 2004;182:1521–4.

[28] Bude RO, Forauer AR, Caoili EM, et al. Is it necessary to study accessory arteries when screening the renal arteries for renovascular hypertension? Radiology 2003;226:411–6.

[29] Handa N, Funkunaga R, Etani H, et al. Efficacy of echo-Doppler examination for the evaluation of renovascular disease. Ultrasound Med Biol 1988;14:1–5.

[30] Patriquin HB, Lafortune M, Jequier JC, et al. Stenosis of the renal artery: assessment of slowed systole on the downstream circulation with Doppler sonography. Radiology 1992;184:479–85.

[31] Stavros AT, Parker SH, Yakes WF, et al. Segmental stenosis of the renal artery: pattern recognition of tardus and parvus abnormalities with duplex sonography. Radiology 1992;184:487–92.

[32] Bude RO, Rubin JM, Platt JF, et al. Pulsus tardus: its cause and potential limitations in detection of arterial stenosis. Radiology 1994;190:779–84.

[33] Qanadli SD, Soulez G, Therasse E, et al. Detection of renal artery stenosis: prospective comparison of captopril-enhanced Doppler sonography, captopril-enhanced scintigraphy, and MR angiography. AJR Am J Roentgenol 2001;177:1123–9.

[34] Radermacher J, Chavan A, Bleck J, et al. Use of Doppler ultrasonography to predict the outcome of therapy for renal artery stenosis. N Engl J Med 2001;344:410–7.

[35] Cohn EJ, Bejamin ME, Sandager GP, et al. Can intrarenal duplex waveform analysis predict successful renal artery revascularization? J Vasc Surg 1998;28:471–81.

[36] Garcia-Criado A, Gilabert R, Nicolau C, et al. Value of Doppler sonography for predicting clinical outcome after renal artery revascularization in atherosclerotic renal artery stenosis. J Ultrasound Med 2005;24:1641–7.

[37] Missouris CG, Allen CM, Balen FG, et al. Non-invasive screening for renal artery stenosis with ultrasound contrast enhancement. J Hypertens 1996;14:519–24.

[38] Blebea J, Zickler R, Volteas N, et al. Duplex imaging of the renal arteries with contrast enhancement. Vasc Endovascular Surg 2003;37: 424–36.

[39] Wittenberg G, Ken W, Tschammler A, et al. Spiral CT angiography of renal arteries: comparison with angiography. Eur Radiol 1999;9:546–51.

[40] Brink JA, Lim JT, Wang G, et al. Technical optimization of spiral CT for depiction of RAS: in vitro analysis. Radiology 1995;194:157–63.

[41] Urban BA, Ratner LE, Fishman EK. Three-dimensional volume-rendered CT angiography of the renal arteries and veins: normal anatomy, variants, and clinical applications. Radiographics 2001;21:373–86.

[42] Johnson PT, Halpern EJ, Kuszyk BS, et al. Renal artery stenosis: CT angiography—comparison of real-time volume rendering and maximum intensity projection algorithms. Radiology 1999; 211:337–43.

[43] Platt J, Ellis J, Korobkin M, et al. Helical CT evaluation of potential kidney donors: findings in 154 subjects. AJR Am J Roentgenol 1997;169: 1325–30.

[44] Rubin GD, Alfrey EJ, Drake MD, et al. Assessment of living renal donors with spiral CT. Radiology 1995;195:457–62.

[45] Smith PA, Ratner LE, Lynch FC, et al. Role of CT angiography in the preoperative evaluation for laparoscopic nephrectomy. Radiographics 1998; 18:589–601.

[46] Leung DA, Hagspiel KD, Angle JF, et al. MR angiography of the renal arteries. Radiol Clin North Am 2002;40:847–65.

[47] Bakker J, Beck FJ, Beutler JJ, et al. Renal artery stenosis and accessory renal arteries: accuracy of detection and visualization with gadolinium enhanced breath hold MR angiography. Radiology 1998;207:497–505.

[48] Soulez G, Olivia V, Turpin S, et al. Imaging of renovascular hypertension: respective values of renal scintigraphy, renal Doppler ultrasound and MR angiography. Radiographics 2000;20:1355–68.

[49] Prince MR, Narasimham DL, Stanley JC, et al. Breath-hold gadolinium-enhanced MR angiography of the abdominal aorta and its major branches. Radiology 1995;197:785–92.

[50] Hany TF, Debatin JF, Leung DA, et al. Evaluation of the aortoiliac and renal arteries: comparison of breath-hold, contrast-enhanced, three-dimensional MR angiography with conventional catheter angiography. Radiology 1997;204:357–62.

[51] Leung DA, Hoffman U, Pfammatter T, et al. Magnetic resonance angiography versus duplex sonography for diagnosing renovascular disease. Hypertension 1999;33:726–31.

[52] Thornton J, O'Callaghan J, Walshe J, et al. Comparison of digital subtraction angiography with gadolinium-enhanced magnetic resonance angiography in the diagnosis of renal artery stenosis. Eur Radiol 1999;9:930–4.

[53] Cowper SE. Nephrogenic fibrosing dermopathy: the first six years. Curr Opin Rheumatol 2003; 15:785–90.

[54] Streams BN, Liu V, Liegois N, et al. Clinical and pathologic features of nephrogenic fibrosing dermopathy: a report of two cases. J Am Acad Dermatol 2003;48:42–7.

[55] Prigent A. The diagnosis of renovascular hypertension: the role of captopril renal scintigraphy and related issues. Eur J Nucl Med 1993;20: 625–44.

ELSEVIER
SAUNDERS

# ULTRASOUND CLINICS

Ultrasound Clin 2 (2007) 477–492

# Ultrasound Assessment of the Mesenteric Arteries

Margarita V. Revzin, MD, MS, John S. Pellerito, MD

- Basic anatomy and collateral pathways
- Mesenteric hemodynamics
- Natural history of bowel ischemia
- Technique
- Examination protocol
- Diagnostic criteria

- Key points to successful evaluation
- Pitfalls
- Summary
- Acknowledgments
- References

Compromise of the mesenteric circulation is an uncommon cause of abdominal pain. Stenotic or occluded mesenteric arteries may not be able to provide sufficient blood supply to the bowel, resulting in ischemia or gangrene. Doppler ultrasonography is a valuable screening tool for evaluating the patency of the splanchnic (mesenteric) circulation in patients presenting with vague abdominal pain. Doppler ultrasonography can assess the degree of vessel lumen stenosis and the number of arteries affected, factors that are critical for patient management. Sonographic evaluation of the splanchnic circulation, however, is a technically challenging study that is operator- dependent and requires a thorough understanding of splanchnic anatomy and physiology and sonographic findings associated with arterial vascular disease. This article provides a review of general concepts, technical factors, and insights that allow for the successful evaluation of the mesenteric arteries.

## Basic anatomy and collateral pathways

A basic understanding of the mesenteric circulation provides a foundation for the interpretation of the sonographic examination. Normal mesenteric circulation can be compartmentalized into three major components: the major vessels (celiac artery [CA], superior mesenteric artery [SMA], and inferior mesenteric artery [IMA]), the intermediate vessels (arcades), and the microcirculation.

The CA arises from the anterior aspect of the proximal aorta, approximately at the level of the T12–L1 vertebral bodies. The length of the trunk does not exceed 1 to 3 cm, after which it branches into the splenic, hepatic, and left gastric arteries (Fig. 1) [1,2]. The celiac axis supplies solid visceral organs (ie, liver, pancreas, and spleen) and the stomach and proximal small bowel.

The SMA also arises from the anterior aspect of the abdominal aorta, just caudal to the origin of the CA, at the level of the L1 vertebral body (see Fig. 1). It courses ventrally and caudally over the uncinate process of the pancreas, following the mesentery of the small bowel into the right lower quadrant. Along its course, the SMA provides multiple branches that include the inferior pancreaticoduodenal artery, four to six jejunal branches, 9 to 13 ileal branches, the ileocolic artery, right colic artery, and middle colic artery. It supplies the intestine from the duodenum to the splenic flexure [1–4].

Division of US, CT and MRI, Department of Radiology, North Shore University Hospital, 300 Community Drive, Manhasset, NY 11030, USA
E-mail address: johnp@nshs.edu (J.S. Pellerito).

doi:10.1016/j.cult.2007.08.004

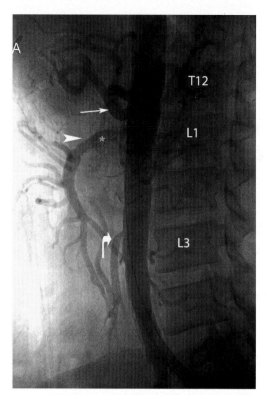

Fig. 1. Sagittal view of the aorta and its major branches on the aortogram. Relationship of the branches to the spine: CA (T12–L1) (*solid arrow*), SMA (L1) (*arrowhead*), IMA (L3) (*curved arrow*). Incidentally noted is a stent in the SMA (*asterisk*).

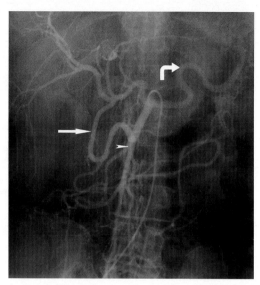

Fig. 2. Selective SMA arteriogram demonstrating gastroduodenal artery (*straight arrow*) serving as a collateral between the CA and SMA (*arrowhead*). Note splenic artery (*curved arrow*).

occurs by way of the gastroduodenal artery, composed by the superior pancreaticoduodenal (a branch of the CA) and the inferior pancreaticoduodenal artery (a branch of the SMA) (Fig. 2). The superior mesenteric and inferior mesenteric systems are joined by the arc of Riolan (Fig. 3)

The IMA originates from the left anterolateral aspect of the infrarenal abdominal aorta, approximately 4 cm proximal to the aortic bifurcation at the level of the L3 vertebral body (see Fig. 1). It quickly divides into an ascending left colic artery and two descending branches: the sigmoid and superior rectal arteries. The IMA thus supplies the descending and rectosigmoid colon [1–4].

The mesenteric arcades and the marginal artery of the colon constitute the intermediate vascular component of the mesenteric circulation. The mesenteric arcades arise from the jejunal and ileal branches of the SMA [5]. The marginal artery originates from distal SMA branches (ileocolic, right colic, and middle colic arteries) and branches of the IMA (left colic and descending branches). Both mesenteric arcades and the marginal artery give rise to small straight arteries (arteriae rectae) that perfuse the serosa of the bowel wall. This vascular arcade provides effective collateral circulation and is generally protective against ischemia.

Additional vascular protection is obtained from direct communication between the three arterial systems. Communication between the celiac system and the superior mesenteric system generally

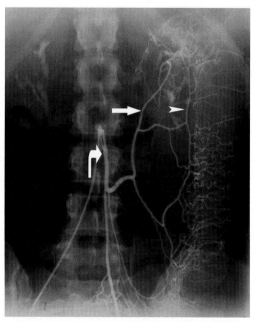

Fig. 3. Selective IMA arteriogram demonstrating IMA (*curved arrow*), Arc of Riolan (*straight arrow*) and marginal artery of Drummond (*arrowhead*).

(formed in the mesentery by anastomoses between adjacent jejunal and ileal arteries), and the marginal artery of Drummond (see Fig. 3) (a portion of the marginal artery of the colon that connects a middle colic artery branch from the SMA to a left colic artery branch from the IMA) [6,7]. In addition, communication also exists between the IMA and branches of the internal iliac arteries by way of the rectum. It is important to recognize that blood flow to the gut can be maintained through these collateral connections even when a major mesenteric artery is completely obstructed. Patients may remain asymptomatic with underlying chronic mesenteric vascular disease. Considerable anatomic variation of these collateral connections exists [8]. In up to 30% of patients, the collateral connections between the superior and inferior mesenteric arteries, including the arc of Riolan and the marginal artery of Drummond, can be weak or nonexistent. The splenic flexure is considered particularly vulnerable to acute ischemia. This region of potentially poor collateral circulation is often referred to as a watershed area [9].

## Mesenteric hemodynamics

Recognition of normal Doppler blood flow patterns is key to successful performance of mesenteric arterial examinations. This section provides a detailed explanation of the dynamics of mesenteric blood flow.

The CA supplies the liver and the spleen, organs with high oxygen demands. To properly function, these organs require continuous forward arterial blood flow during systole and diastole. Like the internal carotid artery, the CA and its branches demonstrate low-resistance arterial flow during Doppler interrogation (Fig. 4). The normal CA flow pattern is not usually affected by fasting or postprandial states, and thus no significant variability in peak systolic velocities is seen [10–13].

In contrast, the SMA and IMA supply the high-resistance vascular beds of the small and large bowel. This allows redirection of blood flow to the vital visceral organs with high oxygen demand during the fasting state and increased perfusion of the bowel only during periods of intestinal digestion. Pulsed Doppler thus reveals high-resistance flow with low diastolic velocities during the fasting state (see Fig. 4C,D) and low-resistance flow with higher diastolic velocities during the postprandial state [10–14]. Physical exercise in humans increases splanchnic vascular resistance with a subsequent reduction in blood flow, predominately because of increased resistance in the CA bed that reduces blood flow to the liver, spleen, and stomach.

Exercise has no effect on SMA resistance during digestion-induced vasodilation [15].

## Natural history of bowel ischemia

Mesenteric ischemia is traditionally classified into four major subcategories based on etiology: acute arterial occlusive disease, nonobstructive mesenteric arterial insufficiency, mesenteric venous occlusion, and chronic mesenteric ischemia.

Acute arterial occlusive disease is most commonly caused by embolus, thrombus, vasculitis, volvulus, or external compression. These patients often present with acute abdominal pain out of proportion to physical findings and rapid development of peritonitis caused by intestinal gangrene. Doppler ultrasonography is generally not useful in this situation because of the rapid time course of the disease and the necessity for emergent medical or surgical intervention.

Nonobstructive mesenteric arterial insufficiency is usually caused by hypotensive shock, blood loss, or sepsis. These are conditions in which blood supply to the bowel is insufficient, and treatment of the underlying condition is the correct management. Although Doppler ultrasonography can be used to exclude the presence of luminal occlusion or narrowing in mesenteric vessels, the clinical history and symptomatology often establish the diagnosis.

Veno-occlusive disease is characterized by the presence of impaired venous drainage and is most often caused by venous thrombus, tumor, volvulus, or adhesions. Doppler ultrasound can be helpful in the evaluation of venous flow anomalies or thrombus, thickened bowel wall, or free intraperitoneal fluid. Slow mesenteric venous flow may be difficult to detect, however, and only the main mesenteric veins and portal vein can be optimally evaluated [16]. Other modalities such as contrast-enhanced CT and magnetic resonance venography are more commonly used to evaluate for mesenteric venous occlusion.

Chronic mesenteric ischemia (CMI) presents a diagnostic dilemma for clinicians, because clinical symptoms are often nonspecific. Doppler ultrasonography can play a major role in screening patients in whom suspicion of CMI is high. CMI is a progressive arterial occlusive process in which bowel blood supply is inadequate to support metabolic and functional demands. It is attributed to atherosclerotic disease in 95% of cases [8]. This uncommon condition occurs in elderly patients who have stenosis or occlusion of at least two of the three principal mesenteric vessels (the CA, SMA, and IMA) [17]. Patients who have CMI usually present with vague symptoms of postprandial abdominal pain, often with accompanying malnutrition

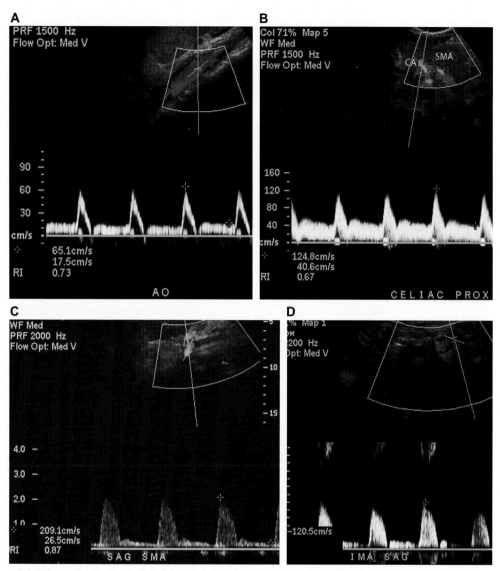

Fig. 4. (A) Color and pulsed Doppler of the abdominal aorta (AO) demonstrating a high-resistance waveform pattern. (B) Color and pulsed Doppler evaluation of the celiac trunk demonstrating a characteristic low-resistance waveform pattern. (C, D) Color and pulsed Doppler evaluation of the SMA and IMA demonstrating high-resistance waveform patterns in the fasting state.

[18]. Until recently visceral angiography was the primary diagnostic modality used in the assessment of patients who have suspected CMI. With recent advances in technology, ultrasound, MR angiography, and CT angiography have proven to be accurate noninvasive alternatives to arteriography for the evaluation of the mesenteric arteries [19–21]. Doppler ultrasonography is useful as a primary screening test for evaluation of CMI [14,22,23]. Advantages of Doppler ultrasonography include direct evaluation of all three mesenteric vessels, assessment of the hemodynamics of blood flow, and determination of the significance of lesions involving the visceral vessels. It is an inexpensive, noninvasive method that requires no contrast material, can be performed portably, and does not have any inherent risks associated with other angiographic studies [14]. Doppler ultrasound also provides adequate visualization of the IMA [24]. It is essential to identify and examine all three mesenteric arteries, because significant two-vessel disease is usually required for the diagnosis of CMI. Doppler ultrasound determines the hemodynamic significance of stenotic lesions by demonstrating pre- and poststenotic waveform changes. These findings can influence the decision to intervene in the

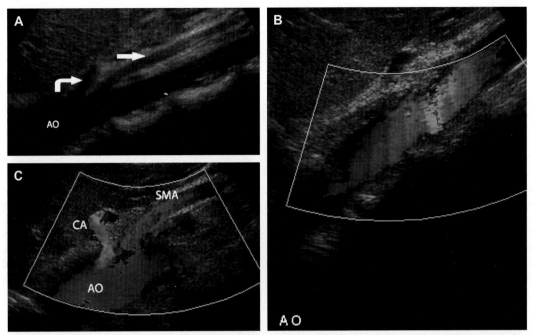

*Fig. 5.* (*A, B*) Sagittal view of the aorta. The aorta (*AO*) is found anterior to the spine and slightly to the left of midline throughout its course. The celiac (*curved arrow*) and SMA (*straight arrow*) arise from the anterior aorta. The aortic wall is easily assessed on the grayscale image. Note the normal color flow patterns in the aorta, on color Doppler. (*C*) On the sagittal color Doppler image, celiac (*CA*) and SMA demonstrate homogeneous anterograde flow.

appropriate clinical setting. In general, CT angiography and MR angiography do not provide hemodynamic information.

## Technique

The Doppler ultrasonographic examination usually includes evaluation of the abdominal aorta and the ostia and proximal portions of the CA, SMA, and IMA. Distal segments of mesenteric arteries cannot be seen with ultrasound because of their small caliber and depth. Because most atherosclerotic plaque occurs at the ostium and proximal segments of vessels, however, visualization of these segments may be sufficient for diagnosis.

The mesenteric arteries should be scanned with the patient in the fasting state to minimize the artifacts caused by overlying bowel gas and to avoid the higher arterial velocities associated with the postprandial state [25]. At the authors' institution, no premedication or water are given to the patient before examination. Given that mesenteric vessels are situated deep in the abdomen, a Doppler scanner with a low-frequency 2- to 5-MHz convex (curvilinear) phased-array transducer is used. This allows for adequate visualization and resolution over a large field of view. Modern ultrasound instruments with high-quality color and power Doppler

imaging and sensitive pulsed Doppler capabilities are preferred for assessment. Most studies are performed at a constant Doppler angle (60° or less) to provide consistency in the Doppler measurements. The angle of insonation used in evaluating the mesenteric arteries should not exceed 60°, because larger Doppler angles skew the obtained velocity to a much higher value.

Patients are examined most often in the supine position by way of an anterior approach. If visualization of the vessels is limited because of overlying bowel gas, patients may be turned to the decubitus or oblique positions for better visualization of the vessels of interest using the liver as an acoustic window. During the study, the patient is asked to breath-hold or breathe quietly to obtain adequate Doppler spectral samples.

The aorta is evaluated by way of an anterior approach by placing the transducer just below the xiphoid process of the sternum. Transverse and sagittal planes are used for visualization. The aorta can be found anterior to the spine and slightly to the left of midline throughout its course (Fig. 5A,B). Quick assessments of aortic diameter (upper limits of normal for aortic diameter are 2.5 cm at the diaphragm, 2.0 cm in the midabdomen, and 1.8 cm at the bifurcation) and integrity of the vascular wall are recommended to ensure absence of aortic aneurysm and significant atherosclerotic changes.

The SMA is best seen on the sagittal view (longitudinal view) arising from the anterior aspect of the aorta (Fig. 5A,C). Because of its distinctive anatomic location, the SMA has served as a landmark for scanning mesenteric vessels in particular and upper abdominal vessels in general. On the transverse view, it can be seen surrounded by a prominent ring of retroperitoneal fat that separates the SMA from the pancreas (see Fig. 6). In patients who have normal bowel rotation, the SMA lies to the right of the superior mesenteric vein. The splenic vein and pancreas lie anterior to the SMA, whereas the left renal vein is situated posteriorly (see Fig. 6). Visualization of these anatomic structures is important in patients who have vascular anomalies or normal variant anatomy. In the most common anatomic variations, one or more of the celiac branches may arise separately from the aorta or from the SMA. This can cause misinterpretation and errors in diagnosis.

Ultrasound visualization of the CA origin is best accomplished in the sagittal (longitudinal) plane, whereas its main branches are best seen in the transverse orientation. The CA arises from the anterior aspect of the aorta just superior to the SMA and bifurcates shortly after its point of origin (see Fig. 5C). Ultrasound visualization of the T-shaped bifurcation (seagull sign) on the transverse view is the characteristic landmark of the CA (Fig. 7A). In older patients, the T-shaped bifurcation may be less apparent because of aortic tortuosity. The IMA can be found by searching for a small branch arising from the left anterolateral aspect of the aorta, just caudally to the renal arteries. This vessel quickly divides into several branches and may occasionally be difficult to detect (Fig. 7B).

Several techniques can be used to optimize assessment of the mesenteric vessels. Harmonic imaging is routinely used to improve resolution and signal-to-noise ratio, especially in obese patients who have significant body wall fat. Optimization of the grayscale and color Doppler parameters assists in the visualization of the vessel wall and detection of atherosclerotic plaque and in the assessment of the residual lumen. Adjustment of color Doppler parameters allows better detection of flow within the vessel. Adjustment of the color Doppler gain, output power, wall filter, color box size, and field of view may improve the detection of blood flow. Adjusting the color/grayscale priority toward color improves the visualization of color in the vessel. Proper selection of pulse repetition frequency (PRF) allows the operator to obtain a homogeneous laminar flow pattern in the normal segments of the aorta and branch vessels. PRF optimization also enables the visualization of high-velocity flow and aliasing to improve the detection of stenosis. A small sample volume (1.5–3.0 mm) is used to ensure the velocity measurements are obtained from the vessel of interest.

Optimized grayscale and Doppler settings allow the examiner to improve the detection of vascular flow abnormalities. Color bruit artifacts, color aliasing, and elevated peak systolic velocities should alert the examiner to the presence of vessel stenosis. Doppler ultrasound can also be used for evaluation of the mesenteric arteries after revascularization and in the initial assessment and follow-up of mesenteric stents.

### Examination protocol

The authors begin assessment with grayscale and color Doppler evaluation of the aorta, looking for the presence of atherosclerotic plaques, luminal narrowing, and aneurysm. We then obtain a baseline velocity measurement with pulsed Doppler in the aorta at the level of the mesenteric arteries, to be compared with mesenteric artery peak systolic velocities. The next step involves identification and color Doppler analysis of the CA and SMA using the characteristic landmarks explained earlier, followed by peak systolic velocity measurements from the origin and proximal segments. The process is repeated for the IMA. The sample volume must be passed slowly from the aorta into the ostium and proximal segments of each vessel, searching for

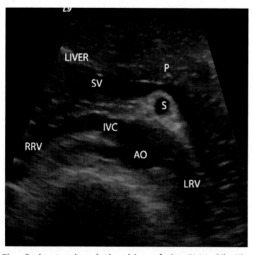

*Fig. 6.* Anatomic relationships of the SMA (*S*). The SMA is surrounded by a layer of echogenic fat. Anterior to the SMA is the pancreas (*P*), posterior to the SMA is the aorta (*AO*), to the left is the left renal vein (*LRV*), and to the right is the right renal vein (*RRV*) and inferior vena cava (*IVC*). Splenic vein (*SV*) is situated between the pancreas and SMA.

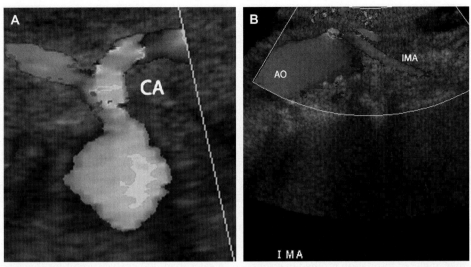

Fig. 7. (A) Transverse color Doppler image reveals a T-shaped bifurcation, the characteristic landmark of the CA. (B) A transverse color Doppler image of the IMA arising from the anterior left lateral aspect of the aorta (AO).

elevated peak systolic velocities, poststenotic turbulence, and bruits.

## Diagnostic criteria

No absolute consensus has been reached on a set of sonographic criteria for the diagnosis of mesenteric arterial stenosis. Multiple conflicting reports advocating different diagnostic parameters exist in the literature. In this section the authors describe the most commonly used set of diagnostic criteria, which was established based on retrospective studies and has since been validated with prospective studies. The diagnostic value of the different diagnostic criteria, including peak systolic velocity (PSV), end-diastolic velocity (EDV), and velocity ratios, is discussed.

The normal blood flow velocity spectrum in the CA is narrow and ranges from 98 to 105 cm/s [26]. In the SMA and IMA the range of flow velocities is wider, running from 97 to 142 and 93 to 189 cm/s, respectively [26].

The most widely accepted criteria for mesenteric stenosis is based on peak systolic velocity measurements. Many investigators, including Moneta and colleagues, Lim and colleagues, and Perko and colleagues, demonstrated that a PSV greater than 275 cm/s in the SMA and 200 cm/s in the CA signified a greater than 50% to 70% stenosis in the affected artery [27–29].

In a retrospective review of mesenteric Doppler examinations in 34 patients, Moneta and colleagues showed that when the aforementioned criteria were met, the sensitivity, specificity, and positive predictive value for a greater than 70% stenosis was 89%, 92%, and 80%, respectively, in the SMA; and 75%, 89%, and 85% in the CA.

Unfortunately IMA values were not assessed in this particular study. These investigators also found that end-diastolic velocities and velocity ratios did not offer any advantage over arterial PSV measurements. In a subsequent prospective study of 100 patients, Moneta and colleagues were able to reproduce their initial preliminary criteria and suggested that duplex evaluation could be used as a screening test for suspected CA and SMA stenosis. In a separate prospective study of 82 patients, Lim and colleagues were able to validate the Moneta criteria for mesenteric artery stenosis, obtaining an overall sensitivity of 100% and specificity 98% in the SMA and 100% and 87% in the CA [30].

In their study of 24 patients, Bowersox and colleagues [31] found that an EDV greater than 45 cm/s or absence of flow was 100% sensitive and 92% specific for the diagnosis of 50% or greater SMA stenosis or occlusion. They also concluded that PSV was less accurate than EDV for the evaluation of mesenteric vessels. A threshold velocity for CA stenosis was not identified in this study; however, they did state that retrograde blood flow in the common hepatic artery was a reliable indicator of severe CA stenosis or occlusion. A similar conclusion regarding the value of EDV in the evaluation of mesenteric ischemia was reached by Zwolak and colleagues and Perko and colleagues [29,32,33]. In their study of 243 patients with 43 correlative angiograms, Zwolak [14] showed EDV to be the most reliable parameter in diagnosing 50% or greater stenosis in the SMA and CA, with a sensitivity of 90%, specificity of 91%, and overall accuracy of 91% for SMA (EDV ≥45 cm/s) and sensitivity of 93%, specificity of 94%, and accuracy of 93% for CA (EDV >55 cm/s). Zwolak later determined that

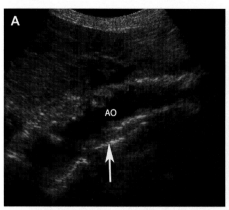
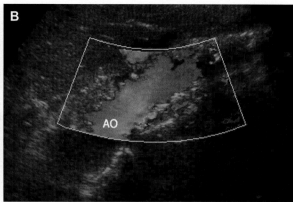

Fig. 8. (A) Sagittal gray-scale image demonstrates marked calcification (*straight arrow*) of the abdominal aorta (*AO*). (B) Color Doppler image of the abdominal aorta demonstrates luminal irregularity.

suboptimal angles of insonation resulted in erroneous PSV measurements. When accurate PSVs were measured, these investigators were able to confirm that the diagnostic criteria based on PSV proposed by Moneta were valid.

Most of the aforementioned studies did not evaluate for IMA stenosis. This is crucial, because the diagnosis of CMI is based on the presence of significant stenosis or occlusion in two of the three mesenteric arteries. Evaluation of the IMA may be essential for establishing this diagnosis. Selective IMA evaluation was performed independently by Mirk and Denys, whose data demonstrated that the IMA was visualized in 88.8% and 92% of cases, respectively [24,34]. Although PSV of the IMA has been shown to range from 93 to 189 cm/s in normal patients, specific criteria for the diagnosis of significant IMA stenosis was never established [6]. Pellerito and colleagues [35] recently reported that a PSV

greater than 200 cm/s is useful for the determination of significant stenosis of the IMA. In another study, Erden and coworkers showed that PSV in the IMA can reach 190 cm/s when the IMA serves as part of a collateral pathway (in the presence of occluded or severely stenotic CA or SMA) [6].

Velocity ratios have also been proposed for the diagnosis of mesenteric artery stenosis [28,33]. A velocity ratio can be calculated by dividing PSV obtained from a mesenteric artery by the PSV at an adjacent site in the abdominal aorta. When the obtained ratio is greater than 3.0 to 3.5, the likelihood of hemodynamically significant stenosis in the mesenteric vessel is high [28]. (The normal value for a velocity ratio is slightly greater than or equal to 1.0.) Moneta and colleagues [28] found no significant advantage for the PSV ratios over absolute PSV measurements obtained from the region of stenosis. In the authors' experience, the use of velocity ratios

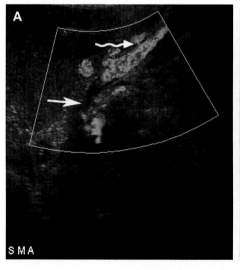
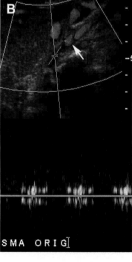

Fig. 9. (A) Color Doppler demonstrates absence of color flow in the origin and proximal SMA consistent with occlusion (*straight arrow*) with reconstitution by collaterals from the CA (*wavy arrow*). (B) Pulsed Doppler evaluation of the occluded segment of the SMA demonstrates thump artifacts and focal retrograde flow in the collateral vessel (*straight arrow*).

**A** **B**

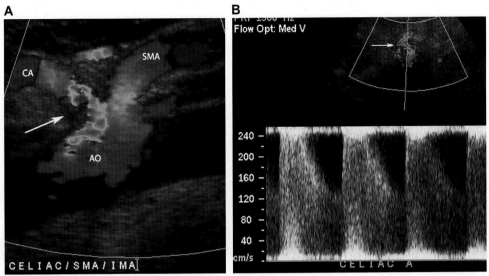

Fig. 10. (A) Color demonstrates aliasing artifact (*arrow*) in the proximal CA consistent with stenosis. Note the normal color flow pattern in the aorta (*AO*) and SMA. (B) Pulsed Doppler reveals high velocity flow (>200 cm/s) in the CA stenosis.

proved to be most useful in patients who have abnormally low systolic flow velocities (secondary to cardiac dysfunction, blood loss, or other low flow states) and in patients who have high peak systolic flow velocities (young adults, patients with metabolic/hormonal abnormalities, or patients who have right-to-left shunts). An elevated velocity ratio greater than 3.0 in these groups is suspicious for underlying mesenteric stenosis. The authors recently performed a comparative study of multiple diagnostic criteria that demonstrated that absolute PSV measurements are the most accurate criteria in diagnosis of mesenteric stenosis [36]. The use of resistive index, pulsatility, and mean velocity were also not shown to be as reliable as PSV criteria for the diagnosis of mesenteric artery stenosis.

### Key points to successful evaluation

The authors generally assign an experienced examiner to perform mesenteric evaluation. A junior sonographer or trainee is supervised by a more experienced staff member during the training of abdominal Doppler studies. Before starting the examination, we confirm that the patient is adequately prepared for the study (the patient must have fasted for at least 12 hours before evaluation is performed, otherwise the obtained findings may not be reliable). We review images and reports from prior studies and correlative studies when available. Our most sensitive Doppler machines are used in the evaluation.

The authors begin with an examination of the abdominal aorta and branch vessels using grayscale and color Doppler. Grayscale evaluation allows

identification of intraluminal echoes, such as those associated with plaque or thrombus. Wall thickness abnormalities, which can be related to the presence of atherosclerotic plaques, can also be readily detected by grayscale imaging (Fig. 8). Irregularity of the vascular wall or the presence of a beading pattern can be suggestive of vasculitis or fibromuscular dysplasia. The presence of normal vessels, free of atherosclerotic changes, reduces the risk for CMI.

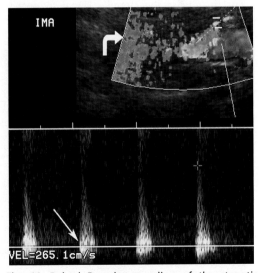

Fig. 11. Pulsed Doppler sampling of the stenotic region in the IMA demonstrates elevated PSVs and Doppler bruit artifact (*straight arrow*) consistent with hemodynamically significant stenosis. Note color bruit on color Doppler image (*curved arrow*).

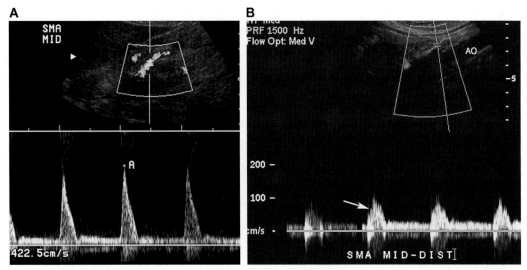

*Fig. 12.* (*A*) Severe stenosis of the SMA with high-velocity flow. (*B*) Pulsed Doppler evaluation of the mid-distal SMA in a patient who had SMA-origin stenosis demonstrates low-velocity rounded (tardus-parvus) waveforms (*arrow*) in the poststenotic zone.

Color Doppler is a powerful tool for the assessment of vascular stenosis or occlusion and provides several useful signs of vascular disease. Nonvisualization of color flow in a vessel is suspicious for arterial occlusion (Fig. 9A). This finding should be confirmed by the absence of arterial signals during pulsed Doppler interrogation (Fig. 9B). Color aliasing may be present in the setting of significant arterial stenosis (Fig. 10A). Aliasing typically manifests as an apparent reversal of flow direction on color Doppler, occurring when the sampling rate is lower than the Nyquist limit, that is, when the PRF is less than twice the Doppler signal frequency. This artifact occurs in areas of increased velocity or

stenosis, when actual velocities exceed the velocity scale settings of the machine and are mistakenly assigned a much lower value. In severe arterial stenosis, color Doppler may show the presence of extensive collateral circulation. Another sign that increases the detection of arterial stenosis is the presence of a color bruit artifact. A mixture of colors is seen within the soft tissues adjacent to the stenotic blood vessel as a result of turbulent vibration in the vessel wall and surrounding soft tissues (Fig. 10B). This phenomenon may also be seen in arteriovenous fistulas and pseudoaneurysms.

Reversal of flow is another useful sign of vascular occlusion, caused by redirection of blood into

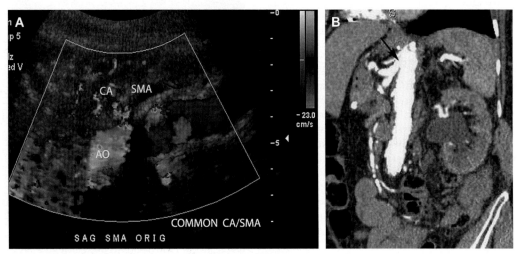

*Fig. 13.* (*A*) Normal variant anatomy of the mesenteric vessels: common origin of the CA and SMA. Color Doppler evaluation of a patient who had common celiac and SMA origin. (*B*) Sagittal MRA of the abdominal aorta demonstrates common origin of the CA and SMA (*arrow*).

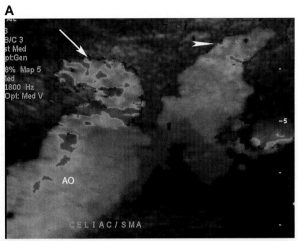

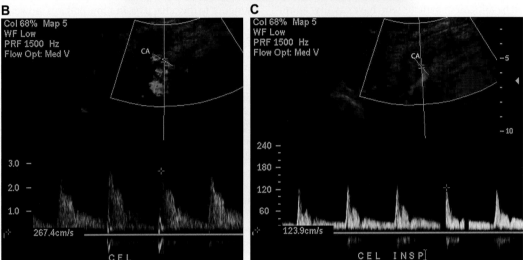

*Fig. 14.* Median arcuate ligament syndrome. (*A*) Color Doppler image reveals a "fishhook" appearance (*straight arrow*) of the CA in expiration. SMA is seen (*arrowhead*). (*B*) Pulsed Doppler sample of the CA in expiration reveals elevated velocities (267 cm/s) caused by compression by the median arcuate ligament. (*C*) There is a marked decrease of PSV in the CA on inspiration.

collateral pathways. For example, reversal of flow in the gastroduodenal artery and hepatic artery occurs when the celiac ostium is occluded.

Finally, pulsed Doppler evaluation is crucial in the assessment of stenosis and occlusion. Doppler examination determines the hemodynamic significance of a stenotic segment by showing elevated peak systolic velocities and the presence of poststenotic turbulence (Fig. 11). The detection of poststenotic turbulence confirms the presence of a significant stenosis. Blood flow in the immediate poststenotic region is no longer laminar but turbulent with decreased flow velocities and altered Doppler waveform pattern. Low-velocity, monophasic waveforms (tardus-parvus waveforms) indicate significant proximal disease and are characterized by prolonged acceleration and a rounded systolic peak (Fig. 12*A*, *B*)

[37–40]. Mesenteric/aortic velocity ratios should also obtained for confirmation of stenosis or in low- or high-flow states as described.

The secret to successful evaluation of mesenteric arterial disease lies in the detection of these specific diagnostic features that, when analyzed together, cinch the diagnosis. Discordant sonographic findings should be further investigated by other modalities such as CT angiography, MR angiography, or conventional angiography.

## Pitfalls

Several pitfalls must be considered in evaluation of the mesenteric arteries to avoid misinterpretation of the obtained results.

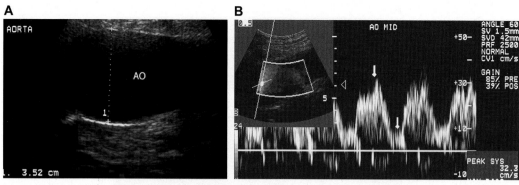

**Fig. 15.** (*A*) Grayscale image demonstrates an abdominal aortic aneurysm measuring 3.5 cm. (*B*) Color and pulsed Doppler evaluation of the aneurysm reveals low-velocity flow, with PSV measuring 32 cm/s.

Locating the main mesenteric arterial branches can be difficult in patients who have vascular anomalies or normal anatomic variants. The most frequent anomaly is the replaced right hepatic artery, wherein the right hepatic artery originates from the SMA rather than the CA (by way of the common hepatic). Other, less frequent variants include anomalous origin of the common hepatic artery (from the SMA or directly from the aorta) and a common origin of the celiac–mesenteric trunk from the aorta (Fig. 13 *A,B*) [14]. An examiner not familiar with the presence of these variants may misinterpret increased EDV associated with an anomalous hepatic artery waveform as a potential SMA stenosis. This possible pitfall can be avoided by following the course of arterial branches.

A potential pitfall for CA stenosis is the median arcuate ligament syndrome (MALS). The median arcuate ligament (MAL) is a fibrous arch that unites the diaphragmatic crura on either side of the aortic hiatus. In a healthy individual, the MAL passes just superior to the celiac axis. In some patients, however, the MAL passes anteriorly to the CA and may compress it during expiration, because of upward motion of the diaphragm that displaces the CA cephalad. With pulsed Doppler, mechanical compression of the CA by the MAL is detected as an increased PSV during expiration. On inspiration, however, the CA is in its uncompressed caudad position and a normal PSV is observed. When MALS is suspected, inspiratory and expiratory velocity measurements therefore should be obtained (Fig. 14*A–C*).

As stated, it is crucial that the sample volume be passed slowly from the aorta into the ostium and proximal segments of each vessel when evaluating for stenosis or occlusion. Proximal occluded segments can be missed, because occlusions can be reconstituted distally by way of collateral

**Fig. 16.** Pulsed Doppler evaluation of the IMA demonstrates variable PSV caused by cardiac arrhythmia with maximal PSV reaching 220 cm/s and minimal 150 cm/s in the IMA. No secondary signs of stenosis are identified.

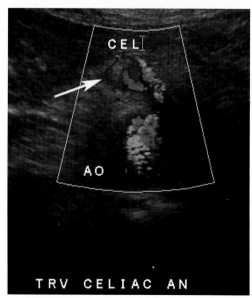

**Fig. 17.** CA aneurysm. The lumen of the CA is dilated (*arrow*) and demonstrates disturbed flow on the color Doppler image.

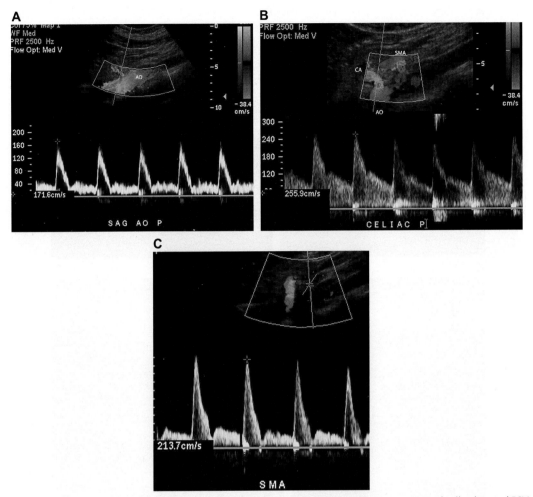

**Fig. 18.** Hyperemia caused by pregnancy. (*A, B*) Pulsed Doppler evaluation demonstrates markedly elevated PSVs in the aorta (*AO*) (PSV = 172 cm/s) and CA (PSV = 256 cm/s). The color Doppler evaluation of the CA demonstrates a normal flow pattern without color aliasing, bruit, and poststenotic turbulence. (*C*) Pulsed Doppler evaluation of the SMA demonstrates high-velocity, high-resistance flow.

pathways and normal distal flow velocities may be observed (see Fig. 9 *A, B*).

It may be difficult to obtain optimal angles of insonation in tortuous vessels or in obese patients who have deeply situated mesenteric arteries, and as a result velocities may be incorrectly calculated. If the angle is too large or greater than 60°, it provides falsely elevated velocity measurements [41].

Assessment of the aorta for the presence of aneurysms is essential. Elevated aortic velocities may be detected with aortic stenosis, and decreased velocities can be seen with aortic dilatation and aneurysm (Fig. 15A, *B*). Variable flow velocities may be seen in patients who have cardiac arrhythmias, caused by disproportionate cardiac output during ectopic heart beats (Fig. 16). Color and pulsed Doppler imaging can also detect aneurysmal dilatation of the aortic branches (Fig. 17).

In the presence of significant stenotic disease in one of the mesenteric vessels, an increase in flow velocity in another mesenteric vessel may be seen, caused by compensatory blood flow to the intestines [33]. It is believed that the compensatory increase in blood flow allows perfusion of collaterals (pancreaticoduodenal) that exist between the celiac and SMA and may prevent ischemia. This increase in flow in the normal vessel should not be misinterpreted as stenotic disease, and there is a conspicuous absence of other secondary signs of stenosis in the hyperemic vessel, including poststenotic turbulence, bruit artifacts, or tardus-parvus waveforms.

In elderly patients, underlying processes, such as cardiac hypotension, septic shock, or blood loss, may result in low-flow velocities, and strict criteria for stenosis based on normotensive individuals may not be met [42]. Conversely in patients who

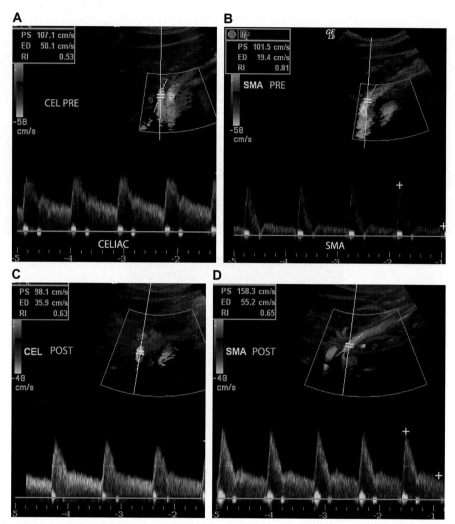

*Fig. 19.* (*A, B*) Normal waveforms obtained from the CA and SMA in the fasting state. (*C, D*) After a meal no significant change in blood flow is noted in the CA. Increased systolic and diastolic flow with a decrease in resistance is noted in the SMA following a meal.

have high cardiac output or in young individuals, PSVs may be high without clinical evidence of disease (Fig. 18). The aortic-mesenteric PSV ratio can improve diagnostic accuracy in these situations.

It is a well known phenomenon that intestinal blood flow increases after a meal because of a reduction in the bowel's peripheral vascular resistance and a compensatory increase in diastolic blood flow. Postprandial hyperemia may therefore lead to spuriously high velocity measurements, thus emphasizing the importance of patient fasting before examination (Fig. 19) [25,43].

the authors' experience, color and pulsed Doppler ultrasound is an excellent screening test for patients undergoing evaluation for chronic mesenteric ischemia. Specific ultrasound findings allow the determination of vascular stenosis and the hemodynamic significance of the lesion. The technique can also be used to assess response to revascularization of the mesenteric arteries. It can provide additional information and in many situations, is complimentary to other modalities such as CTA, MRA, and conventional angiography.

## Summary

An understanding of basic anatomy, normal flow dynamics, and Doppler principles is essential for the evaluation of the mesenteric circulation. In

## Acknowledgments

The authors would like to thank Nanaz Maghool for her sonographic expertise and Dr. James Naidich for his insights and humor.

## References

[1] Ruzika FF Jr, Rossi P. Normal vascular anatomy of the abdominal viscera. Radiol Clin North Am 1970;8:3–29.

[2] Michels NA. Blood supply and anatomy of the upper abdominal organs. Philadelphia: HB Lippincott; 1955.

[3] Kornblith PL, Boley SJ, Whitehouse BS. Anatomy of the splanchnic circulation. Surg Clin North Am 1992;72:1–30.

[4] Lin PH, Chaikof EL. Embryology, anatomy and surgical exposure of the great abdominal vessels. Surg Clin North Am 2000;80:417–33.

[5] Chow LC, Chan FP, Li KC. A comprehensive approach to MR imaging of mesenteric ischemia [Review]. Abdom Imaging 2002;27(5):507–16.

[6] Erden A, Yurdakul M, Cumhur T. Doppler waveforms of the normal and collateralized inferior mesenteric artery. AJR Am J Roentgenol 1998;171(3):619–27.

[7] Horton Karen M, Fishman Elliot K. Volume-rendered 3D CT of the mesenteric vasculature: normal anatomy, anatomic anatomy, anatomic variants, and pathologic conditions. Radiographics 2002;22:161–72.

[8] Cunningham CG, Reilly LM, Stoney R. Chronic visceral ischemia. Surg Clin North Am 1992;72:231–44.

[9] Fisher DF, Fry WJ. Collateral mesenteric circulation. Surg Gynecol Obstet 1959;108:641–50.

[10] Van Bel F, Van Zwielen PHT, Guit GL, et al. Superior mesenteric artery blood flow velocity and estimated volume flow: duplex Doppler US study of preterm and term neonates. Radiology 1990;174:165–9.

[11] Perry MA, Ardell JL, Barrowman JA, et al. Physiology of splanchnic circulation. In: Kveitys PR, Barrowman JA, Granger DN, editors, Pathophysiology of the splanchnic circulation, vol 1. Boca Raton: Fla: CRC; 1987. p. 1–56.

[12] Granger DN, Richardson PDI, Kveitys PR, et al. Intestinal blood flow. Gastroenterology 1980;78:837–63.

[13] Lewis BD, James EM. Current applications of duplex and color Doppler ultrasound imaging: abdomen. Mayo Clin Proc 1989;64:1158–69.

[14] Zwolak RM. Can duplex ultrasound replace arteriography in screening for mesenteric ischemia? Semin Vasc Surg 1999;12:252–60.

[15] Perko MJ, Nielsen HB, Skak C, et al. Mesenteric, coeliac and splanchnic blood flow in humans during exercise. J Physiol 1998;513:907.

[16] Bradbury MS, Kavanagh PV, Betchtold RE, et al. Mesenteric venous thrombosis: diagnosis and noninvasive imaging. Radiographics 2002;22:527–41.

[17] Baxter BT, Pearce H. Diagnosis and surgical management of chronic mesenteric ischemia. In: Strandness DE, Van Brida A, editors. Vascular diseases surgical and interventional therapy. 1st edition. New York: Churchill Livingstone Publishers; 1994. p. 795–802.

[18] Moawad J, Gewertz BL. Chronic mesenteric ischemia. Clinical presentation and diagnosis. Surg Clin North Am 1997;77:357–69.

[19] Meany JF, Prince MR, Nostrand TT. Gadolinium-enhanced magnetic resonance angiography in patients with suspected chronic mesenteric ischaemia. J Magn Reson Imaging 1997;7:171–6.

[20] Carlos RC, Stanley JC, Stafford-Johnson D, et al. Interobserver variability in the evaluation of chronic mesenteric ischemia with gadolinium enhanced MR angiography. Acad Radiol 2001; 8(9):879–87.

[21] Savastano S, Teso S, Corra S, et al. Multislice CT angiography of the celiac and superior mesenteric arteries: comparison with arteriographic findings. Radiol Med (Torino) 2002;103(5–6):456–63.

[22] Harward TR, Smith S, Seeger JM. Detection of celiac axis and superior mesenteric artery occlusive disease with use of abdominal duplex scanning. J Vasc Surg 1993;17(4):738–45.

[23] Moneta GL. Screening for mesenteric vascular insufficiency and follow-up of mesenteric artery bypass procedures. Semin Vasc Surg 2001;14(3):186–92.

[24] Denys AL, Lafortune M, Aubin B, et al. Doppler sonography of the inferior mesenteric artery: a preliminary study. J Ultrasound Med 1995;14(6):435–9.

[25] Gentile AT, Moneta GL, Lee RW, et al. Usefulness of fasting and postprandial duplex ultrasound examination for predicting high grade superior mesenteric artery stenosis. Am J Surg 1995;169:476–9.

[26] Jager K, Bollinger A, Valli C, et al. Measurement of mesenteric blood flow by duplex scan. J Vasc Surg 1986;3:462–9.

[27] Lim HK, Lee WJ, Kim SH, et al. Splanchnic arterial stenosis or occlusion: diagnosis at Doppler ultrasound. Radiology 1999;211:405–10.

[28] Moneta GL, Yeager RA, Dalman R, et al. Duplex ultrasound criteria for diagnosis of splanchnic artery stenosis or occlusion. J Vasc Surg 1991;14:511–20.

[29] Perko MJ, Just S, Schroeder TV. Importance of diastolic velocities in the detection of celiac and mesenteric artery disease by duplex ultrasound. J Vasc Surg 1997;26:288–93.

[30] Moneta GL, Lee WL, Yeager RA, et al. Mesenteric duplex scanning: a blinded prospective study. J Vasc Surg 1993;17:79–86.

[31] Bowersox JC, Zwolak RM, Walsh DB, et al. Duplex ultrasonography in the diagnosis of celiac and mesenteric artery occlusive disease. J Vasc Surg 1991;14(6):780–6.

[32] Zwolak RM, Fillinger MF, Walsh DB, et al. Mesenteric and celiac duplex scanning: a validation study. J Vasc Surg 1998;27:1078–88.

[33] Healy DA, Marsha M, Neumyer BS, et al. Evaluation of celiac and mesenteric vascular disease

with duplex ultrasonography. J Ultrasound Med 1992;11:481–5.

[34] Mirk P, Palazzoni G, Cotroneo AR, et al. Sonographic and Doppler assessment of the inferior mesenteric artery: normal morphologic and hemodynamic features. Abdom Imaging 1998;23:364–9.

[35] Pellerito JS, Revzin MV, Axelrod DJ, et al. Comparative analysis of Doppler criteria for the diagnosis of mesenteric stenosis. Presented at the 92nd Scientific Assembly and Annual Meeting Radiological Society of North America, Chicago, Illinois, November 26-December 12006.

[36] Pellerito JS, Revzin MV, Axelrod DJ, et al. Duplex and color Doppler ultrasound evaluation of chronic mesenteric ischemia. Presented at the 92nd Scientific Assembly and Annual Meeting Radiological Society of North America, Chicago, Illinois, November 26-December 1, 2006.

[37] Baker D. Application of pulsed Doppler techniques. Radiol Clin North Am 1980;18:79–103.

[38] Douville Y, Johnston KW, Kassam M. Determination of the hemodynamic factors which influence the carotid Doppler spectral broadening. Ultrasound Med Biol 1985;11:417–23.

[39] Kotval PS. Doppler waveform parvus and tardus. J Ultrasound Med 1989;8:435–40.

[40] Nicholls SC, Kohler TR, Martin RL, et al. Use of hemodynamic parameters in the diagnosis of mesenteric insufficiency. J Vasc Surg 1986;3:507–10.

[41] Rizzo RJ, Sandager G, Astleford P, et al. Mesenteric flow velocity variations as a function of angle of insonation. J Vasc Surg 1990;11:688–94.

[42] Perko MJ, Perko G, Just S, et al. Changes in superior mesenteric artery Doppler waveform during reduction of cardiac stroke volume and hypotension. Ultrasound Med Biol 1996;22(1):11–8.

[43] Moneta GL, Taylor DC, Helton WS, et al. Duplex ultrasound measurement of postprandial intestinal blood flow: effect of meal composition. Gastroenterology 1988;95:1294–301.

ELSEVIER
SAUNDERS

ULTRASOUND
CLINICS

Ultrasound Clin 2 (2007) 493–523

# Ultrasound Evaluation of the Acute Abdomen

Leslie M. Scoutt, MD[a],*, Steven R. Sawyers, MD[a],
Jamal Bokhari, MD[a], Ulrike M. Hamper, MD, MBA[b]

The acute abdomen is a medical term used to describe a patient who presents with sudden onset of severe abdominal pain sometimes accompanied by nausea, vomiting, diarrhea, abdominal distension, and even hypotension or shock. As there are numerous etiologies that can result in the acute abdomen, prompt, accurate diagnosis is necessary to ensure proper patient management. Although helical and/or multidetector CT generally is considered the diagnostic imaging gold standard for evaluating patients who have acute abdominal pain, ultrasound may, nonetheless, be the first imaging test performed, particularly in unstable patients and in patients suspected of having gallbladder or biliary tract disease. In addition, ultrasound may be performed first in children and pregnant women because of the perceived risk of ionizing radiation from CT.

Ultrasound is a well-established imaging modality for evaluating the abdomen, as it is noninvasive, portable, readily obtainable, relatively inexpensive,

and without the risks of ionizing radiation or iodinated intravenous contrast. In addition, ultrasound has extremely high diagnostic accuracy in many clinical scenarios equivalent or even superior to CT [1]. A recent study reported that abdominal ultrasound performed in patients with acute abdominal pain confirmed the preultrasound diagnosis in 29% of cases, rejected the leading pretest diagnosis in 43% of patients, established a diagnosis in 10% of patients in whom there was no leading pretest diagnosis, provided significant increase in clinical diagnostic confidence, and changed patient management in nearly 25% of patients [1]. In addition, high-resolution ultrasound provides better spatial and soft tissue resolution of some structures such as the gallbladder, ovaries, uterus, and appendix than CT, at least in thin patients [2]. Furthermore, the dynamic, real-time capability of ultrasound and the interactive nature of the ultrasound examination are unique and allow the sonographer to correlate the ultrasound findings

[a] Department of Diagnostic Radiology, Yale University School of Medicine, 20 York Street, 2-272 WP, New Haven, CT 06504, USA
[b] Department of Radiology, Johns Hopkins University School of Medicine, 600 North Wolfe Street, Baltimore, Maryland 21287, USA
* Corresponding author. Department of Diagnostic Radiology, Yale University School of Medicine, 333 Cedar Street, New Haven, CT 06520.
E-mail address: leslie.scoutt@yale.edu (L.M. Scoutt).

1556-858X/07/$ – see front matter © 2007 Elsevier Inc. All rights reserved.
ultrasound.theclinics.com

doi:10.1016/j.cult.2007.07.002

with the physical examination and to identify and focus on the precise location of the patient's point of maximum tenderness [2].

This article reviews the role of high-resolution ultrasound in the evaluation of various nontraumatic conditions involving the biliary tree, liver, pancreas, kidney, and gastrointestinal tract that can cause acute abdominal pain. In addition, the ultrasound imaging findings of conditions resulting in acute intra-abdominal hemorrhage and select gynecological conditions that also can present with acute abdominal pain and mimic upper abdominal disease are discussed.

## The biliary tract

The most common cause of acute right upper quadrant (RUQ) pain in adults is acute cholecystitis. Ultrasound largely has replaced scintigraphy (HIDA scan) as the initial imaging modality of choice for evaluating patients with clinical suspicion of acute cholecystitis, as ultrasound is as accurate as scintigraphy in diagnosing acute cholecystitis, but less time-consuming. Furthermore, ultrasound has the additional advantages of being able to demonstrate potential complications of acute cholecystitis, such as perforation and gangrene, and the potential to identify nonbiliary causes of RUQ pain. Hence, currently in most departments, scintigraphy is performed to assess patients for acute cholecystitis only when clinical suspicion is high, and ultrasound examination is negative or equivocal.

The two most important diagnostic criteria for the diagnosis of acute cholecystitis on ultrasound examination are the presence of gallstones and a positive sonographic Murphy's sign. In combination, these two findings have been shown by Ralls and colleagues [3] to have a positive predictive value of 92% for the diagnosis of acute cholecystitis (Fig. 1). As acute cholecystitis is an obstructive process, the gallbladder also typically is distended. Hence, a careful search should be made for an obstructing stone in either the cystic duct or the neck of the gallbladder [4]. Thickening of the gallbladder wall and the presence of pericholecystic fluid are secondary findings of acute cholecystitis on ultrasound examination, but are neither sensitive nor specific (Fig. 2). Ultrasound examination also can be helpful in patients who have persistent pain and fever following cholecystectomy to evaluate for retained stones, bile leaks, or abscess/hematoma in the gallbladder fossa (Fig. 3).

Patients who have biliary colic most commonly complain of acute, spasmodic RUQ pain that may mimic acute cholecystitis but typically is not associated with fever or elevation of the white blood cell count (WBC). Patients who have choledocholithiasis also may present with jaundice and abnormal liver function tests, and choledocholithiasis is known to be a common precipitating cause of acute pancreatitis. Biliary colic should be suspected in patients with acute RUQ pain who are found to have small-to-tiny gallstones in a nondistended gallbladder but no sonographic Murphy's sign, gallbladder wall thickening, or peri-cholecystic fluid (Fig. 4). The presence of an echogenic, shadowing focus (choledocholithiasis) in the common bile duct (CBD) and/or biliary ductal dilatation will help to confirm the diagnosis. The biliary tree may be dilated secondary to retained stones, spasm, or edema. In some cases, however, neither

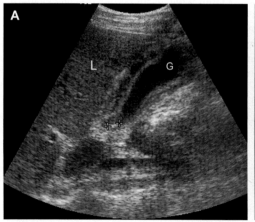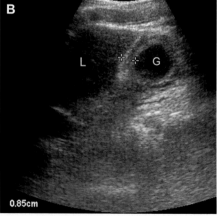

Fig. 1. Acute cholecystitis. Sagittal *(A)* and transverse *(B)* views of gallbladder in a 68-year-old man presenting with acute right upper quadrant pain and fever demonstrate a thick, edematous gallbladder wall (8.5 mm in B) with a stone impacted in the neck of the gallbladder (calipers in A). The patient had a positive sonographic Murphy's sign. *Abbreviations:* G, gallbladder; L, liver.

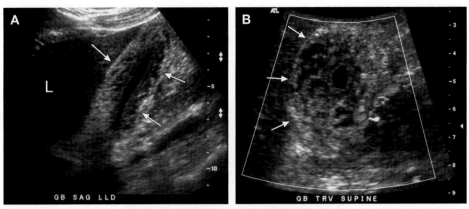

Fig. 2. HIV cholangiopathy. On both sagittal *(A)* and transverse *(B)* views of the gallbladder, the wall *(arrows)* is thickened markedly and heterogeneous in echotexture with numerous linear hypoechoic to anechoic striations. The gallbladder is not distended, however, and the lumen is slit-like. This HIV-positive patient was asymptomatic. If the gallbladder lumen is not distended, one should question a diagnosis of acute cholecystitis. *Abbreviation:* L, Liver.

intra- nor extrahepatic biliary ductal dilatation will be observed. The sensitivity of ultrasound in detecting stones in the CBD is directly related to experience and effort. The sensitivity of ultrasound in detecting choledocholithiasis has been reported to range from 70% to 89% in experienced hands [4,5]. Images should be obtained in supine, semierect, left posterior oblique (LPO) and right posterior oblique (RPO) positions using multiple scanning planes (Fig. 5) [5,6]. Stones in the proximal CBD are easier to identify than stones in the distal CBD. Magnetic resonance cholangiopancreatography (MRCP) and endoscopic retrograde cholangiopancreatography (ERCP) are more sensitive than ultrasound for the detection of ductal stones, with the later modality having the additional advantage of being also therapeutic. Choledocholithiasis may not always be demonstrable in

patients who have biliary colic, as the stones may have passed before the examination was performed or because the CBD often is partially obscured by overlying bowel gas.

## Liver

Patients who have hepatic abscesses most commonly present with acute onset of RUQ pain associated with fever and elevated WBC, although some patients may present with more chronic and milder symptoms of fever, malaise, fatigue, weight loss, and abdominal discomfort. Pyogenic hepatic abscesses may occur secondary to hematogenous dissemination, superinfection of necrotic tissue, or direct extension into the liver parenchyma from ascending cholangitis or an infected gallbladder. Most hepatic abscesses are

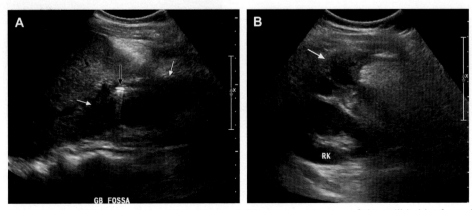

Fig. 3. Abscess in the gallbladder fossa. *(A)* Sagittal and *(B)* transverse images of the gallbladder fossa demonstrate an irregular, ill-defined hypoechoic collection *(white arrows)* in a patient with persistent pain and fever s/p cholecystectomy. Note linear echogenic focus with ring down artifact *(black arrow)* in *(A)* consistent with postsurgical clips. A postoperative hematoma could have a similar appearance. *Abbreviation:* RK, right kidney.

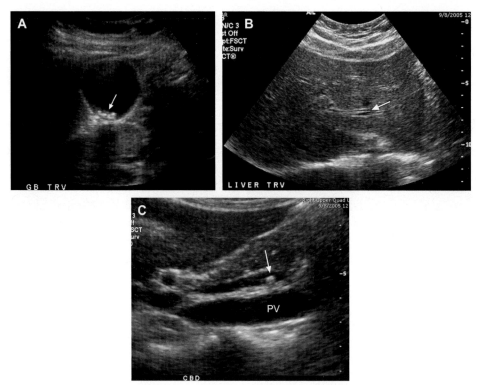

*Fig. 4.* Biliary colic. *(A)* There are numerous small gallstones *(arrow)* on this transverse view of the gallbladder in a patient with right upper quadrant pain. *(B)* Note mild intrahepatic ductal dilatation *(arrow)*. *(C)* View of the common bile duct reveals a nonobstructing stone *(arrow)*. *Abbreviation:* PV, portal vein.

polymicrobial, although *Escherichia coli* and anaerobes are the most common pathogens. With early diagnosis and percutaneous aspiration, mortality rates and the need for surgical intervention have decreased dramatically [7,8]. On ultrasound, a liver abscess most commonly appears as a complex cystic mass with an irregular, shaggy border that

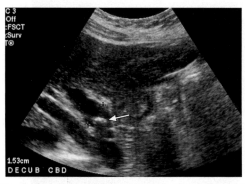

*Fig. 5.* Choledocholithiasis. Decubitus or right posterior oblique views can be very helpful in evaluating the distal common bile duct. Note obstructing echogenic stone *(arrow)* in the dilated (1.5 cm) distal common bile duct (calipers).

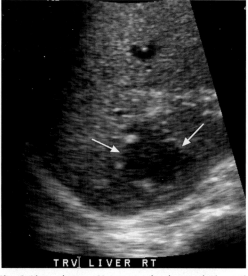

*Fig. 6.* Liver abscess. Note complex hypoechoic cystic mass *(arrows)* with an ill-defined irregular shaggy border and low-level internal echoes in the right lobe of the liver. This patient presented with right upper quadrant pain, fever, and bacteremia.

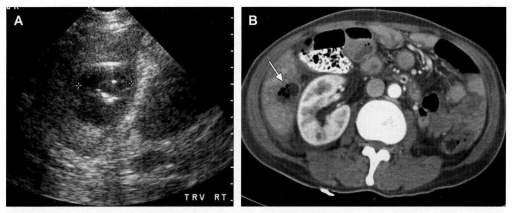

*Fig. 7.* Liver abscess. *(A)* Gray scale image demonstrating a complex hypoechoic cystic lesion in the liver (calipers). Echogenic material with dirty distal shadowing represents air in the abscess. *(B)* Corresponding CT scan demonstrating air in the hepatic abscess *(arrow)*.

demonstrates increased through transmission (Fig. 6). The ultrasound appearance, however, can be quite variable, and a liver abscess can appear completely anechoic or even echogenic because of the presence of internal debris or hemorrhage. Septations, stranding, or brightly echogenic foci of gas with distal shadowing may be noted (Fig. 7), and sometimes liver abscesses may appear to be solid. Ultrasound has been reported to have a 90% sensitivity in detecting liver abscesses [9]. Clinical correlation, however, is extremely important when evaluating focal liver lesions, as the ultrasound appearance is often nonspecific. A miliary pattern of microabscesses can be observed in patients who have hepatic fungal infections, in immunosuppressed patients, or in patients who have staphylococcal septicemia. Hepatic abscess is also the most common extraintestinal complication of amebiasis. Patients are

often extremely ill, even toxic, at presentation with severe RUQ pain and fever. The specific diagnosis is made when there is strong clinical suspicion and positive serologies. Percutaneous drainage is usually not necessary, as oral metronidazole is highly effective. On ultrasound, amebic abscesses usually appear cystic, demonstrating increased through transmission and containing low-level, occasionally layering, internal echoes, representing the so-called anchovy paste which is found characteristically in amebic abscesses. Hepatic amebic abscesses are most commonly peripheral in location. Extrahepatic extension is the most common complication.

Occasionally patients who have metastatic liver disease may present with acute RUQ pain. In some patients, this may be the initial presentation of their malignancy. In patients who have diffuse metastatic disease, the pain likely is caused by

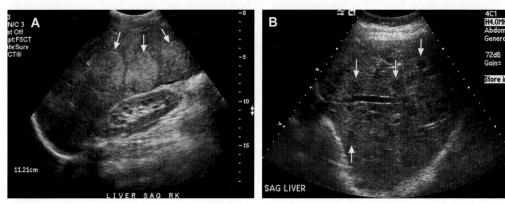

*Fig. 8.* Metastatic liver disease. *(A)* This 58-year-old man presented with acute right upper quadrant (RUQ) pain. He was not known to have an underlying malignancy. The liver is markedly enlarged. Note multiple echogenic liver masses *(arrows)*. *(B)* This 62-year-old women presented with acute onset RUQ pain caused by unsuspected liver metastases from breast cancer. Note multiple small hypoechoic liver masses *(arrows)*.

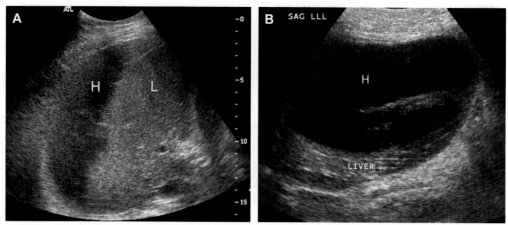

*Fig. 9.* Subcapsular hematomas. (*A*) The large hypoechoic subcapsular hematomas (H) deforms the surface contour of the liver in a patient presenting with acute right upper quadrant pain. (*B*) This patient has a more hypoechoic nearly anechoic subcapsular hematoma (H) that is so large it compresses the liver, which has a concave border. An abscess or superinfection could have a similar appearance. Subcapsular liver hematomas can occur spontaneously but also may be seen secondary to trauma, coagulopathies, or rupture of underlying hepatic masses or arteriovenous malformations. *Abbreviation:* L, liver.

swelling of the liver and stretching of the liver capsule (Fig. 8). Hemorrhage into a liver mass or metastasis, however, also may cause acute RUQ pain. Subcapsular hematomas or free intraperitoneal hemorrhage also may occur following rupture a liver mass. If bleeding is extensive, patients may become hypotensive. Hepatic adenomas, hepatocellular carcinomas (HCCs), and vascular metastases are the liver masses most prone to hemorrhage. Hepatic adenomas occur most commonly in women taking oral contraceptives, patients taking anabolic steroids, or in patients who have type I glycogen storage disease. The risk of rupture is related to size and location, with larger size and subcapsular location being significant risk factors. On ultrasound, a subcapsular hematoma will appear as a crescentic-shaped area compressing the liver parenchyma and deforming the surface contour of the liver (Fig. 9). The mass is typically heterogenous in echotexture, with both anechoic and echogenic areas caused by acute and subacute hemorrhage [10]. Spontaneous hemorrhage or rupture has been estimated to occur in up to 10% of HCCs [11], and intraperitoneal rupture has grave prognostic implications. An echogenic rind surrounding the liver has been described as a common finding in this clinical scenario, representing either acute hemoperitoneum or subcapsular hematoma (Fig. 10)

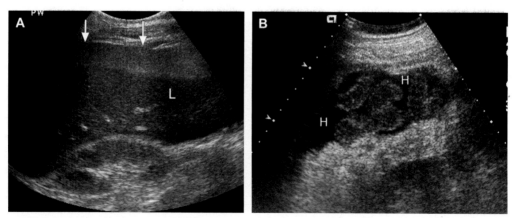

*Fig. 10.* Acute hemorrhage from hepatocellular carcinoma. (*A*) Note echogenic rind *(arrows)* around the liver in this patient who bled from a hepatocellular carcinomas (HCC). (*B*) Ultrasound of the midabdomen in another patient with intraperitoneal hemorrhage (H) following a bleed from an HCC demonstrates echogenic clot within more anechoic intraperitoneal fluid. *Abbreviation:* L, liver.

[4]. Giant cavernous hemangiomas have been reported to rupture in the setting of trauma and pregnancy [12,13].

## The pancreas

Acute pancreatitis is a common cause of midepigastric pain, which may be accompanied by nausea, vomiting, and fever. The diagnosis is confirmed by elevation of the serum amylase and lipase levels. Alcohol abuse and gallstones are the two most common precipitating causes in the United States [14]. Toxins (including drugs), trauma, vasculitis, and viral or parasitic infections are less common causes. CT is considered the imaging modality of choice for staging pancreatitis and for evaluation of potential complications such as pancreatic necrosis, hemorrhage, pseudocysts, pseudoaneurysms, thrombophlebitis, and abscess formation. Patients who have acute pancreatitis often develop an ileus, and the pancreas is, therefore, commonly surrounded by dilated, air-filled loops of bowel. Thus, ultrasound is typically quite limited in the initial evaluation of patients who have pancreatitis, as visualization of the pancreas often is obscured by artifact from bowel gas. Additionally, the pancreas may have an entirely normal sonographic appearance acutely. Thus, in patients clinically suspected of having acute pancreatitis, the primary role of ultrasound is to assess for gallstones and biliary obstruction, as the identification of choledocholithiasis and/or biliary ductal dilatation will result in emergent triage to ERCP for decompression [14–16]. The ultrasonographer should be aware of the ultrasound findings of acute pancreatitis, however, because many patients who have nonspecific acute abdominal pain may be evaluated initially by ultrasound, and ultrasound examination may reveal clinically unsuspected pancreatic abnormalities suggesting the diagnosis of pancreatitis.

Although the pancreas may be initially completely normal sonographically in patients with acute pancreatitis, ultimately, the inflamed pancreas will become enlarged and hypoechoic (Fig. 11). Focal pancreatitis will result in a localized hypoechoic area that may be indistinguishable from a pancreatic adenocarcinoma. The margins of the gland will become ill-defined and distorted because of inflammation and edema in the surrounding peri-pancreatic fat (Fig. 12). Hypoechoic streaking or thickening of tissue planes surrounding the pancreas, adjacent vessels, and the peri-renal and anterior and posterior para-renal spaces may be observed (Fig. 13) [17]. Such hypoechoic inflammatory changes may be difficult to differentiate from fluid, which also is observed commonly

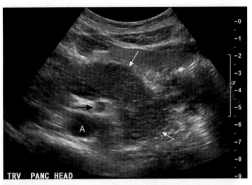

Fig. 11. Acute Pancreatitis. On this transverse view of the midabdomen, the tail of the pancreas (white arrows) is enlarged and hypoechoic. Abbreviations: A, aorta; SMA, superior mesenteric artery (black arrow).

surrounding the pancreas, within the lesser sac, and/or anterior para-renal space (Fig. 14). The walls of the adjacent bowel and/or blood vessels may be thickened. Thrombosis of the portal, splenic, or superior mesenteric veins, pseudoaneurysms, pseudocysts, ascites and pleural effusions may develop (Fig. 15) [17,18]. If the pancreatic duct is dilated, a careful search for an obstructing stone or lesion should be made.

It may be difficult to visualize the pancreas in the setting of acute pancreatitis because of shadowing from overlying bowel gas and guarding on examination. In addition, such patients are typically NPO, and therefore, the stomach cannot be filled with fluid to provide an improved acoustic window. Placing the patient in the RPO or right decubitus position often will improve visualization of the

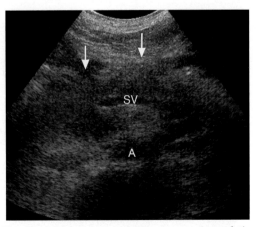

Fig. 12. Acute pancreatitis. Transverse view of the midabdomen reveals an enlarged, hypoechoic pancreas (arrows). The margins of the gland are indistinct. Abbreviations: A, aorta; SV, splenic vein.

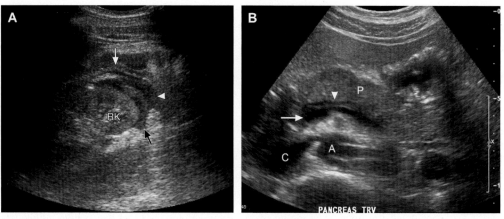

Fig. 13. Acute pancreatitis. (A) Oblique view through the right flank in a patient with upper abdominal pain reveals fluid in the peri-renal space *(black arrow)* and para-renal space *(arrowhead)*. Note hypoechoic, thickened para-renal fat *(white arrow)*. (B) Note linear, hypoechoic plane *(arrowhead)* between the pancreas (P) and splenic vein/portal confluence *(arrow)* in a patient with acute right upper quadrant pain and elevated serum amylase and lipase. *Abbreviations:* A, aorta; C, inferior vena cava; RK, right kidney.

pancreas, as air in the duodenum and antrum of the stomach will rise to the fundus on the left, and the antrum and duodenum will fill with fluid, providing a better acoustic window.

## The kidney

Patients who have renal colic typically present with acute, severe spasmodic abdominal pain radiating to the flank. Acute obstruction of the urinary tract most commonly is caused by ureteral calculi, but also may be caused by blood clots, fungal balls, or neoplasms. Hematuria is present in only approximately 50% of cases. Although noncontrast helical CT is the current gold standard for diagnosing ureteral calculi, the radiation dose is very high;

therefore, ultrasound should be considered in patients who are young, pregnant, or who present with recurrent symptoms. Complete ultrasound evaluation for renal colic requires gray scale imaging of the kidney, ureters, and bladder to assess for hydronephrosis and ureteral calculi; pulse Doppler interrogation to assess for elevation of the intraparenchymal renal artery resistive index (RI); and color Doppler imaging to search for ureteric jets within the bladder. Gray scale imaging is quite sensitive for diagnosing dilation of the intrarenal collecting system (Fig. 16), but less specific in differentiating obstructive hydronephrosis from nonobstructive causes of dilation such as reflux, congenital megacalyces, diabetes insipidus, or pregnancy. Para-pelvic cysts may result in

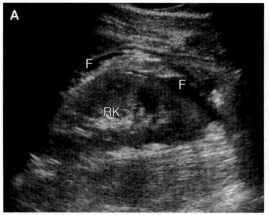
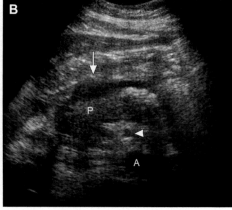

Fig. 14. Acute pancreatitis. (A) Sagittal image of the right kidney (RK) reveals fluid (F) in the peri- and para-renal spaces. (B) Transverse midabdominal imaging plane reveals hypoechoic fluid *(arrow)* anterior to the pancreas (P). Abbreviations: A, aorta; SMA, arrowhead.

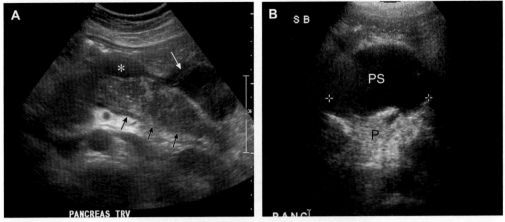

*Fig. 15.* Pseudocyst. *(A)* The pancreatic parenchyma *(black arrows)* is markedly heterogeneous and hypoechoic in this patient with acute pancreatitis. Note fluid (*) anterior to the body of the pancreas and a pseudocyst *(white arrow)* containing debris (internal echoes) anteriolateral to the tail of the pancreas. Hemorrhage or superinfection cannot be excluded. *(B)* In another patient, note large anechoic pseudocyst (PS) anterior to the tail of the pancreas (P). The pancreatic parenchyma is echogenic, indicating that the pseudocyst is likely chronic.

a false-positive diagnosis of hydronephrosis. Elevation of the RI (greater than .7 or 0.1 greater than the RI in the contralateral kidney) has been reported to help differentiate obstructed from nonobstructed dilation of the intrarenal collecting system [19,20]. If hydronephrosis is noted, the ureter should be followed as distally as possible toward the bladder to identify the level of obstruction with special attention to the ureteropelvic junction (UPJ) and ureterovesicular junction (UVJ) (Fig. 17). Filling the bladder aids in evaluation of the UVJ and distal ureter by providing an improved sonographic window. The UVJ sometimes can be

visualized best on endovaginal ultrasound (EVUS) examination, particularly in pregnant women who may not be able to adequately distend their bladder (Fig. 18). The presence of echogenic material within the collecting system suggests pyonephrosis (Fig. 19). Pyonephrosis is considered a urologic emergency requiring immediate decompression. On ultrasound, renal/ureteral calculi are brightly echogenic foci with distal shadowing. Sensitivity for detection of renal calculi may be increased by using color Doppler imaging, which will produce a twinkle artifact posterior to the calculus (Fig. 20) [21]. Ultrasound, however, is less sensitive

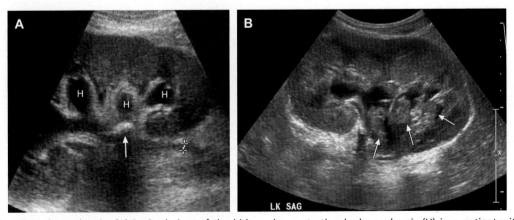

*Fig. 16.* Hydronephrosis. *(A)* Sagittal view of the kidney demonstrating hydronephrosis (H) in a patient with acute flank pain. Note echogenic, shadowing calculus *(arrow)* obstructing the collecting system at the level of the ureteropelvic junction. The proximal ureter (calipers) is normal in caliber. *(B)* In another patient with acute flank pain, blood clot (lobular, medium echogenicity, and without evidence of distal acoustic shadowing) *(arrows)* in the collecting system is causing obstruction and hydronephrosis.

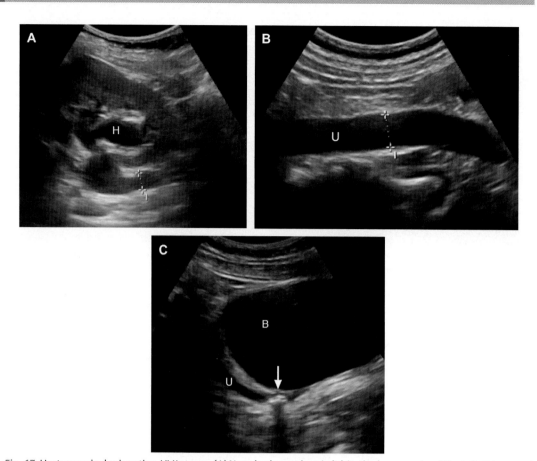

*Fig. 17.* Ureterovesicular junction UVJ stone. *(A)* Note hydronephrosis (H) in the lower pole of the left kidney and dilatation of the proximal ureter (calipers). *(B)* The midureter (U) also is dilated. *(C)* Images of the bladder (B) reveal a dilated distal ureter (U) and an echogenic, shadowing stone *(arrow)* obstructing the UVJ.

than CT for visualizing renal calculi (especially small stones), with the exception of indinavir stones, which are radiolucent on CT. Furthermore, the ureter will be visualized incompletely in the midabdomen and upper pelvis in most patients on ultrasound because of overlying bowel gas.

Normally, the passage of urine from the distal ureter into the bladder will cause a linear flash of color on color Doppler interrogation of the bladder trigone. Absence of the ureteral jet

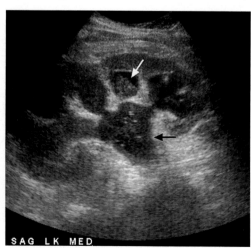

*Fig. 19.* Pyonephrosis. Note echogenic debris *(black arrow)* that layers *(white arrow)* in a midpole calyx in the dilated collecting system.

*Fig. 18.* Ureterovesicular junction (UVJ) stone. Endo-vaginal ultrasound reveals an echogenic shadowing calculus *(arrow)* at the right UVJ in this pregnant patient with acute right flank pain. *Abbreviations:* B, bladder; A, amniotic fluid.

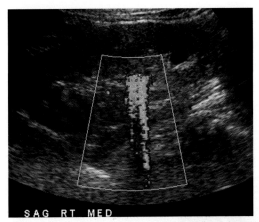

Fig. 20. Twinkle artifact. Sagittal color Doppler image of the right kidney demonstrates a cascade of color from the renal sinus. This is the so-called twinkle color Doppler artifact from an underlying renal calculus that was not well-seen on the gray scale image.

indicates complete obstruction of the ureter (Fig. 21) [22].

Patients who have pyelonephritis present with symptoms of cystitis, flank pain, elevated WBC, and fever. On ultrasound, the kidney typically is enlarged and hypoechoic with poor cortico–medullary differentiation. Pyelonephritis may be diffuse or focal. Hemorrhagic areas will be echogenic (Fig. 22). Hence, the renal cortex also may have a striated, heterogenous appearance. Ultrasound primarily is used in the work up of patients suspected of having pyelonephritis, urinary sepsis, or a urinary tract infection nonresponsive to

standard therapy to exclude obstruction of the collecting system and/or pyonephrosis and complications of infection such as a renal or perinephric abscess. An intraparenchymal renal abscess will appear on ultrasound as a complex fluid collection or cystic mass in the renal cortex demonstrating peripheral vascularity and increased through transmission (see Figs. 22A and 23). A perinephric abscess will result in a heterogeneous crescent-shaped fluid collection surrounding the kidney that may deform the renal cortex (Fig. 24). Emphysematous pyelonephritis is an uncommon, but life-threatening, infection of the renal parenchyma characterized by gas formation [23]. Most patients are female with a female-to-male ratio of 2:1, and 90% of patients are diabetic. *E coli* is the most common causative agent. Patients are typically extremely ill, often toxic, presenting with fever, flank pain, acidosis, hyperglycemia, dehydration, and electrolyte imbalance [24]. The presence of gas, which produces confluent echogenic foci with dirty acoustic shadowing within the renal parenchyma, is diagnostic. Shadowing from intraparenchymal gas may limit evaluation of underlying deeper structures, however (Fig. 25).

Renal emboli/infarcts are rare causes of acute flank pain. In patients who have a segmental renal infarct, color or power Doppler ultrasound will reveal a wedge-shaped avascular area in the renal cortex (Fig. 26). Emboli or thrombosis of the main renal artery will result in absence of blood flow to the entire kidney.

Hemorrhage into a renal cell carcinoma or angiomyolipoma is a rare cause of acute abdominal pain (Fig. 27). Peri-renal hemorrhage also may occur in

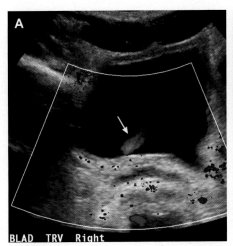

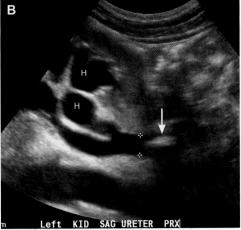

Fig. 21. Absence of ureteral jet. (A) Transverse color Doppler image of the bladder reveals a right ureteral jet (j) but no left jet in a child with acute left-sided flank pain. (B) Oblique sagittal view of the patient's left kidney demonstrates hydronephrosis (H), a dilated proximal ureter (calipers), and an obstructing echogenic calculus *(arrow)* in the upper ureter. Absence of the ureteral jet is consistent with complete obstruction of the upper ureter.

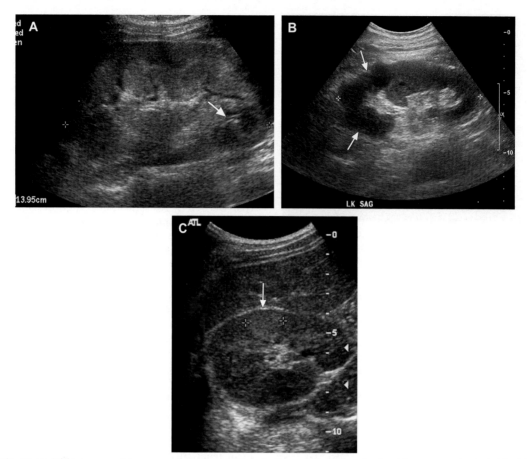

Fig. 22. Variable sonographic appearance of the kidney in three different patients with acute pyelonephritis. *(A)* Diffuse swelling of the left kidney (calipers) with loss of corticomedullary differentiation. The kidney measures 13.95 cm in length. Note small cystic mass at the lower pole *(arrow)* with internal echoes consistent with a renal abscess. *(B)* The cortex of the upper pole of the kidney *(arrows)* is hypoechoic consistent with focal pyelonephritis. *(C)* Note focal area of increased echogenicity *(arrow)* consistent with focal hemorrhage pyelonephritis.

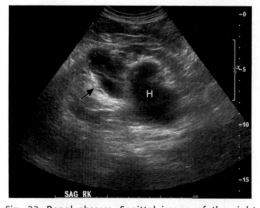

Fig. 23. Renal abscess. Sagittal image of the right kidney reveals a complex cystic mass *(arrow)* separate from the dilated collecting system (H) consistent with renal abscess in a patient with flank pain and persistent bacteremia.

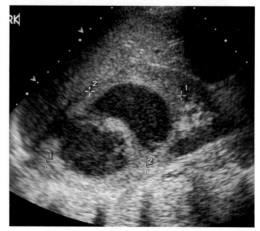

Fig. 24. Perinephric abscess. Note complex fluid collection (calipers) with an echogenic rim compressing the renal cortex.

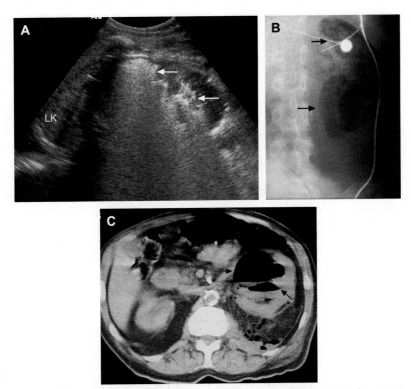

Fig. 25. Emphysematous pyelonephritis. *(A)* Note echogenic area with distal acoustic dirty shadowing *(arrows)* obscuring visualization of most of the mid- and lower poles of the left kidney (LK) in this diabetic male with flank pain, fever, and urinary tract infection. *(B)* Plain abdominal radiograph demonstrates reniform collection of air *(arrows)* in left flank. *(C)* CT confirms the presence of intraparenchymal renal air *(arrows)* and retroperitoneal air posterior to the kidney.

the setting of coagulopathies, anticoagulation therapy, renal artery aneurysms, arteriovenous fistulae, or trauma. Ultrasound examination will demonstrate heterogeneous complex material surrounding the kidney (Fig. 28). If the hemorrhage is subcapsular, the renal cortex will be deformed and compressed.

In adults, acute adrenal hemorrhage occurs most often in the setting of trauma, coagulopathies, anticoagulation therapy, or sepsis. Patients may present with abdominal or flank pain, but are often asymptomatic. Ultrasound will demonstrate a heterogeneous suprarenal avascular mass (Fig. 29).

### The spleen

Spontaneous, nontraumatic splenic rupture occurs most commonly in the setting of splenomegaly in patients who have an underlying hematologic disorder, lymphoproliferative malignancy, or viral infection. Patients typically present with acute left upper quadrant (LUQ) pain. The echotexture of intraparenchymal splenic hemorrhage may range from echogenic to anechoic depending upon the time of hemorrhage. Acute hemorrhage is typically

anechoic or demonstrates low-level internal echoes, becoming more echogenic 24 to 48 hours after bleeding and then becoming anechoic again as clots develop (Fig. 30). Perisplenic clot or free intraperitoneal hemorrhage may be observed.

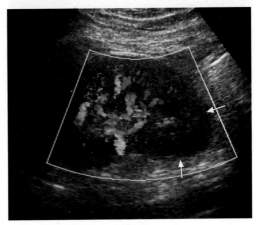

Fig. 26. Renal infarct. Sagittal color Doppler image of the left kidney in a patient with acute onset of left flank pain reveals a focal avascular area at the lower pole *(arrows)* consistent with a segmental renal infarct.

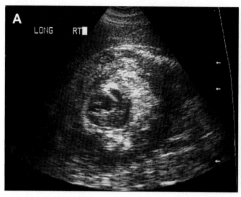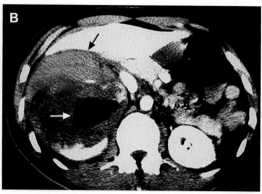

Fig. 27. Hemorrhage into renal angiomyolipoma (AML). *(A)* Note complex echogenic (fat-containing) mass in the right kidney. Hypoechoic central area and surrounding hypoechoic rind represent acute hemorrhage. This woman presented with acute-onset of right flank pain. *(B)* Corresponding CT scan demonstrating large complex fat containing mass *(white arrow)* with central and surrounding hemorrhage *(black arrow)* replacing most of the upper pole of the right kidney.

Splenic infarcts also may cause acute LUQ pain and occur most commonly either secondary to emboli, splenic vein thrombosis, or as complications of leukemia or sickle cell disease. Ultrasound examination will reveal avascular wedge-shaped or rounded defects extending to the splenic capsule (Fig. 31). The echotexture and shape will evolve over time. Healed infarcts are typically echogenic and wedge-shaped [25], while acute infarcts may be hyperechoic, heterogenous, and more rounded. Rupture or superinfection of splenic cysts rarely may cause pain and/or hemoperitoneum. Thick walls and internal debris suggest infection but are nonspecific findings that can be seen in splenic hematomas, complex cysts, or necrotic tumor [26,27].

Gas within a splenic mass or cyst is a more diagnostic finding of infection and is evidenced on ultrasound by echogenic ill-defined foci with dirty shadowing or comet tail artifact (Fig. 32).

## The aorta

Rupture of an abdominal aortic aneurysm (AAA) is a catastrophic cause of acute abdominal pain and a true surgical emergency. Rupture of an AAA should be suspected in the elderly patient presenting with severe acute abdominal or back pain and hypotension. Although ultrasound is highly

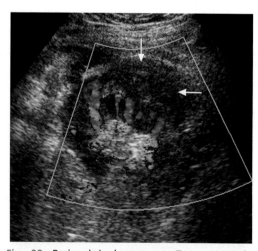

Fig. 28. Perinephric hematoma. Transverse color Doppler image of the left kidney demonstrates a subcapsular hypoechoic avascular collection *(arrows)* that deforms the underlying renal cortex in this patient with acute left flank pain.

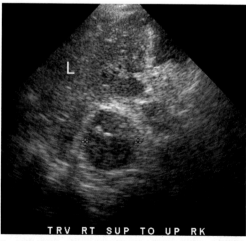

Fig. 29. Adrenal hemorrhage. Note right complex suprarenal mass (calipers) representing adrenal hemorrhage in this coagulopathic young man s/p trauma. Color Doppler imaging (not shown) revealed no flow, which argues against an underlying neoplasm. The mass resolved on follow up imaging. *Abbreviation:* L, liver.

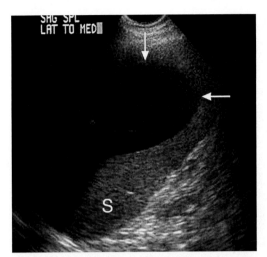

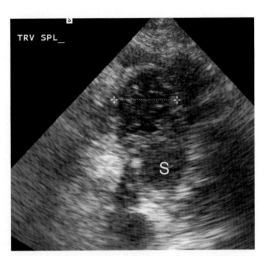

*Fig. 30.* Acute spontaneous subcapsular splenic hemorrhage. Note anechoic fluid collection *(arrows)* around the spleen (S), which deforms the contour of the splenic parenchyma. There was no underlying mass or trauma in this elderly man who presented with acute left upper quadrant pain. The subcapsular hemorrhage resolved on follow-up imaging.

*Fig. 32.* Splenic abscess. Note hypoechoic area (calipers) containing punctate echogenic foci consistent with air within a splenic abscess in this patient with left upper quadrant pain and fever. *Abbreviation:* S, spleen.

accurate and sensitive in identifying AAAs, it is much less sensitive (approximately 4%) in detecting peri-aortic hemorrhage [28], which is much more accurately detected by CT. Identification of an AAA in the setting of acute onset of abdominal/back pain and hypotension, however, correlates strongly with aortic rupture and should prompt emergent surgery (Fig. 33). Findings on ultrasound

that suggest rupture of an AAA include deformation of the wall of the aneurysm, a hypoechoic break in the wall, interruption of intraluminal thrombus, floating thrombus, a para-aortic hypoechoic mass, retroperitoneal/psoas hematoma, and hemoperitoneum (see Fig. 33) [29]. On ultrasound, retroperitoneal bleeds will appear as echogenic, ill-defined infiltrative masses or asymmetric enlargement of the psoas muscle. Subacutely, retroperitoneal hematomas will liquefy, becoming more hypo or anechoic, and they may be difficult to distinguish from fluid collections or abscess. Evaluation with CT and/or needle aspiration may be required.

Dissection of the abdominal aorta also may cause acute-onset of severe abdominal or back pain. Ultrasound will reveal an echogenic flap present within the aortic lumen (Fig. 34). If the false lumen is patent, Doppler interrogation will reveal flow on either side. When evaluating a patient with an aortic dissection, it is important to determine if the dissection extends into the origins of the major intra-abdominal branches of the aorta and whether these vessels arise from the true or false lumen.

## Gastrointestinal tract

Appendicitis is one of the most common causes of acute abdominal pain in the United States. Prompt diagnosis and surgical intervention are imperative to minimize the rate of appendiceal perforation. In adults, CT is considered the imaging modality of choice and has been shown to substantially reduce the false-negative (FN) appendectomy rate to 4% to 6% from a previously observed FN rate

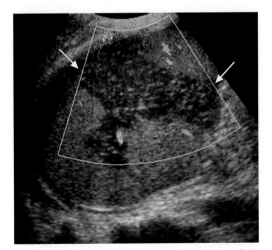

*Fig. 31.* Splenic Infarct. Color Doppler image of the spleen demonstrates a hypoechoic area *(arrows)* in the spleen. Straight margins and wedged-shaped contour with the apex pointing toward the splenic hilum suggest the vascular nature of the mass.

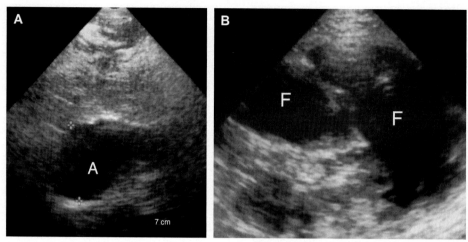

**Fig. 33.** Ruptured abdominal aortic aneurysm. *(A)* Sagittal image of the proximal abdominal aorta obtained in a patient being resuscitated following cardiac arrest demonstrates a 7 cm abdominal aortic aneurysm (calipers). *(B)* Image of the right lower quadrant demonstrates anechoic free fluid (F) from acute hemoperitoneum. The patient died during emergent surgery for aortic repair.

of 15% to 20% when only clinical criteria were used for diagnosis [30–32]. Ultrasound, however, should be recommended as the initial imaging technique in children and in young or pregnant women to avoid exposure to ionizing radiation. Furthermore, ultrasound is more sensitive and specific than CT in diagnosing gynecologic causes of acute abdominal or pelvic pain, which are the most common clinical mimics of appendicitis in young women.

Ultrasound evaluation of the appendix is particularly operator-dependent, and there is a relatively long learning curve. Ultrasound examination of the appendix also is limited in the obese patient. The examination is performed using the technique of graded compression with a high-resolution 5 to 12 MHz linear array transducer, depending upon body habitus, although graded compression can be applied with a curved array transducer if a lower frequency transducer is required for deeper penetration in the obese patient. Slowly progressive, continuous compression improves resolution by decreasing depth and by displacing and/or compressing normal gas-filled loops of bowel. Rebound tenderness and patient discomfort caused by movement of the transducer also are avoided. Most importantly, the technique of graded compression serves to localize the point of maximal tenderness (ie, pathology).

One begins searching for the appendix by asking the patient to point to the area of maximum discomfort or by scanning transversely down the ascending colon from the right lobe of the liver into the pelvis. The appendix will be found arising from the posterior medial wall of the cecum

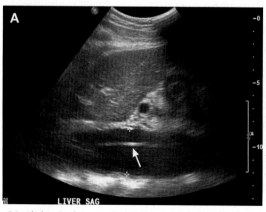
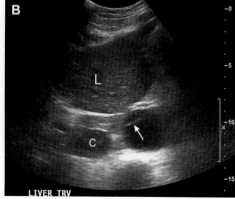

**Fig. 34.** Abdominal aortic dissection. *(A)* Sagittal and *(B)* transverse views of the abdominal aorta demonstrating an echogenic intraluminal intimal flap *(arrow)*. *Abbreviations:* C, inferior vena cava; L, liver.

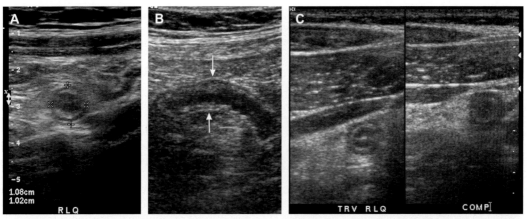

*Fig. 35.* Acute appendicitis. *(A)* The appendix measures more than 1 cm on this transverse image consistent with appendicitis. *(B)* Sagittal image of a different patient with appendicitis reveals a distended fluid-filled appendix *(arrows)* that does not compress on *(C)* transverse view.

approximately 3 cm below the ileocecal valve/ terminal ileum. It is visualized on ultrasound as a blind ending, tubular structure with the characteristic gut wall signature, namely alternating hypoechoic and echogenic rings best visualized on transverse images. The diagnostic ultrasound criteria for appendicitis include noncompressibility and distension with a diameter greater than 6 mm from outer wall to outer wall (Fig. 35) [33,34]. A cutoff diameter of greater than 7 to 8 mm has been reported to increase specificity in adults [35]. Identification of an echogenic, shadowing appendicolith (Fig. 36) also is considered diagnostic of appendicitis regardless of the diameter of the appendix. Increased vascularity in the wall of the appendix (Fig. 37), a large amount of intraluminal fluid, and echogenic noncompressible, vascular peri-appendiceal fat also may be noted [36]. Although peri-appendiceal fluid is a nonspecific finding, focal loss of the laminated appearance of the appendiceal wall suggests impending perforation and/or gangrene [37]. Perforation may result in an ill defined hypoechoic peri-appendiceal mass or fluid collection, which may contain air (Fig. 38) [30,37]. Inflamed peri-appendiceal fat is more common in patients who have perforation. To exclude appendicitis by ultrasound examination, the entire appendix, including the tip, must be visualized; the appendix must be fully compressible and measure less than 6 mm in diameter.

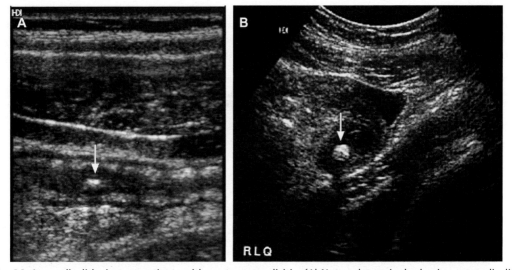

*Fig. 36.* Appendicoliths in two patients with acute appendicitis. *(A)* Note echogenic shadowing appendicolith *(arrow)* on a sagittal view of an inflamed appendix. *(B)* In this pregnant patient presenting with acute right lower quadrant pain, an appendicolith *(arrow)* is visualized on a transverse image of a distended appendix.

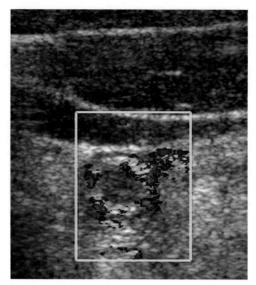

*Fig. 37.* Acute appendicitis. Transverse color Doppler image of the appendix demonstrates increased vascularity in the wall of the inflamed appendix.

Ultrasound has been reported to have an accuracy of 71% to 97%, a sensitivity of 75% to 90%, and a specificity of 86% to 100% for diagnosing acute appendicitis [34,38–43]. Inconclusive examinations, however, are common, the most common cause being nonvisualization of the appendix, as the normal appendix is especially difficult to identify. Ultrasound examination is limited in the obese patient and in patients with severe pain, ascites or markedly distended loops of bowel. Furthermore, it may be difficult to visualize even the abnormal appendix in a retrocecal or deep pelvic location and in pregnant patients in whom the appendix may be displaced quite posteriorly and superiorly by the gravid uterus. EVUS may be helpful for visualizing the deep pelvic appendix in women

(Fig. 39). An inflamed appendix distended with gas also may be difficult to appreciate [35,44]. Other pitfalls that may cause FN examinations include a markedly enlarged appendix that may be misinterpreted as small bowel and lack of visualization of the entire length of the appendix, thereby missing a distal tip appendicitis. In addition, the appendix may deflate following perforation, resulting in FN examination. False-positive ultrasound examinations have been reported in patients with thickening of the appendiceal wall caused by cecal carcinoma, diverticulitis, or inflammatory bowel disease. A thick terminal ileum caused by infectious or inflammatory bowel disease also may be mistaken for an abnormal appendix. Occasionally, a truly inflamed appendix may resolve without surgery because of spontaneous decompression of a soft fecalith or resolution of lymphoid hyperplasia. This, however, should not be considered a true false positive examination.

The presence of multiple (more than five) enlarged round hypoechoic hypervascular mesenteric lymph nodes in a child or young adult without an abnormal appendix suggests the diagnosis of mesenteric adenitis. The wall of the terminal ileum also may be minimally thickened. Mesenteric adenitis is believed to be a consequence of a viral infection and is a self-limited disease process not requiring intervention. In older patients, however, visualization of multiple enlarged pelvic or mesenteric lymph nodes should prompt consideration of appendicitis or malignancy. Isolated mesenteric lymph nodes are usually of no clinical significance.

Primary epiploic appendagitis often is clinically mistaken for appendicitis. In this condition, torsion, ischemia, or inflammation of the epiploic appendices, which arise from the serosal surface of the colon, can cause severe, localized abdominal pain. Although ultrasound has limited sensitivity in making this diagnosis, and CT is considered the

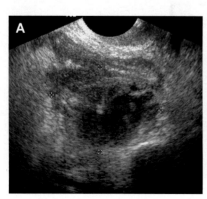

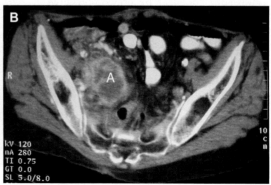

*Fig. 38.* Perforated appendix. *(A)* Complex fluid collection (calipers) in the right lower quadrant (RLQ) represents an abscess secondary to a perforated appendix. *(B)* Corresponding CT scan demonstrating RLQ abscess (A).

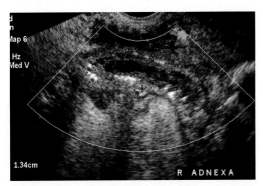

Fig. 39. Acute appendicitis. This dilated appendix (calipers), measuring .79 cm in diameter, was seen best on endovaginal ultrasound because of the deep pelvic location of the appendix in this woman with acute right lower quadrant pain.

gold standard, the presence of small oval noncompressible echogenic masses located anteromedially to the colon underneath the anterior abdominal wall at the site of maximum tenderness suggests the diagnosis [45].

Sigmoid diverticulitis is one of the most common causes of left lower quadrant pain. Upper abdominal pain, however, can be caused by diverticulitis involving the transverse colon or colonic flexures. Although much less common, right-sided diverticulitis tends to occur in younger female patients and may mimic the clinical presentation of appendicitis. Diverticula can be recognized on ultrasound as fluid- or gas-filled small rounded structures adjacent to the outer wall of the colon. If the diverticulum contains a fecalith, it will be brightly echogenic and cast a sharp distal acoustic shadow. Because the wall of a diverticulum is comprised solely of colonic mucosa, it is too thin to be normally visible on ultrasound. When inflammation occurs, the wall of the adjacent colon becomes thickened and hypoechoic with loss of the normal striated pattern of alternating hypoechoic and echogenic rings (Fig. 40). The diverticulum may be surrounded by a hypoechoic rim and later by noncompressible hyperemic echogenic tissue representing inflamed omental fat and mesentery [46–48]. Peri-colonic abscesses or fluid may be observed (see Fig. 40). The sensitivity of ultrasound for diagnosing diverticulitis has been reported to be as high as 84% to 100% [47,49,50]. FN results may occur because of limited visualization in obese patients and when inflammation is minimal. In addition, sensitivity is limited by air in the colon, which may preclude evaluation of the entire colonic wall, or by redundancy of the colon, which may make it difficult to evaluate the entire colon, especially posterior loops. In women, EVUS can be helpful in identifying deep pelvic diverticulitis.

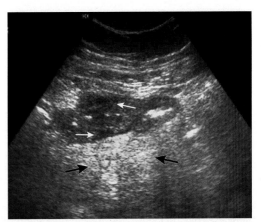

Fig. 40. Acute diverticulitis. Note thickened wall of the left colon with loss of the normal striated gut signature. Echogenic air is noted in the minimally distended lumen. Increased echogenicity of the adjacent fat (black arrows) suggests inflammation. There is a small amount of peri-colonic fluid (white arrows), indicative of perforation. Although no diverticulum is seen, acute diverticulitis is the most likely diagnosis in a 55-year-old woman presenting with acute left lower quadrant pain and an inflamed left colon.

Diffuse thickening of the bowel wall on ultrasound is indicative of colitis, the specific type usually inferred by pattern, distribution, and clinical presentation. Patients who have Crohn's disease typically demonstrate wall thickening of the terminal ileum and cecum. Skip lesions are common, and the bowel will demonstrate diminished peristalsis, lack of compressibility, hyperemia, and stricture. Gut wall involvement may be asymmetric, with less thickening of the antimesenteric bowel

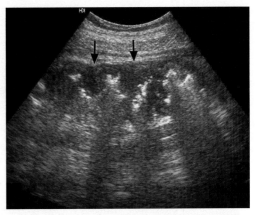

Fig. 41. Ascending colitis from typhlitis. Note diffuse thickening of the wall of the right colon (arrows) with loss of the normal striated gut signature. Only the antimesenteric wall of the colon can be seen, as the distal wall is obscured by artifact from air within the colon.

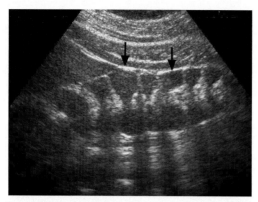

Fig. 42. Pseudomembranous colitis. Image of the transverse colon demonstrates marked thickening of the haustra *(arrows)* in this patient with diarrhea on antibiotics for pneumonia.

wall, which may result in sacculation. Inflammation of the surrounding fat and mesentery results in hyperemic, noncompressible echogenic tissue, so-called creeping fat, adjacent to the bowel. Hypoechoic streaks within this tissue are postulated to represent liponecrotic tracts [44,51,52]. Creeping fat is observed most often near the terminal ileum or cecum [51]. Small echolucencies within the submucosa are the earliest reported finding [52]. Eventually all layers of the bowel wall become thickened, and the normal striated gut wall signature is lost. Echogenic foci within the hypoechoic muscularis layer may represent ulceration or fissures. Echogenic intraluminal mural nodules, representing inflammatory pseudopolyps, may be seen in some patients, and are particularly easy to

see if the bowel is dilated with fluid [51]. Abscesses, phlegmons, and fistulae may develop and present sonographically as complex fluid collections, or less commonly as more solid-appearing masses containing air.

The rectum is the first part of the bowel to become involved in patients who have ulcerative colitis. Thickening of the bowel wall progresses proximally. In patients who have infectious ileitis, the mucosa and submucosa are affected primarily. Lymphadenopathy is noted frequently. The surrounding omentum and mesentery, however, remain normal. Typhilitis occurs primarily in neutropenic patients and is most often secondary to infection with cytomegalovirus (CMV) or *Mycobacterium tuberculosis*. Wall thickening occurs predominately in the cecum and ascending colon (Fig. 41). Patients treated with antibiotics may develop pseudomembranous colitis, due to *Clostridium difficile* infection. In severe cases, pseudomembranous colitis causes edema and diffuse wall thickening of the entire colon (Fig. 42). In patients who have ischemic colitis, wall thickening primarily affects the splenic flexure and descending colon, the so-called watershed areas. If the bowel lumen is distended with fluid, thumbprinting may be identified. In patients who have shock bowel, the bowel wall will be thickened, and the mucosa will be brightly echogenic. This is observed most often in the small bowel (Fig. 43).

Although ultrasound is not considered a first-line imaging modality for clinically suspected bowel obstruction or perforation, the diagnosis occasionally can be made on ultrasound. Dilated fluid-filled loops of bowel can be identified easily on

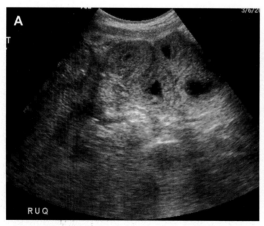

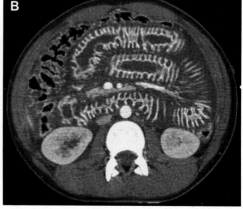

Fig. 43. Shock bowel. *(A)* Note multiple thickened loops of small bowel in this patient with hypotension and acute abdominal pain. The mucosa is slightly more echogenic than the rest of the thickened bowel wall. Rounded hypoechoic areas within the thickened bowel wall likely represent edema or necrosis. There is trace ascites containing debris. *(B)* CT scan demonstrating multiple dilated loops of small bowel with mucosal enhancement and ascites.

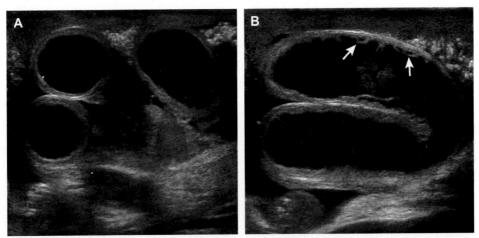

*Fig. 44.* Small bowel obstruction. Transverse *(A)* and longitudinal *(B)* views of multiple dilated loops of small bowel in a patient with a distal small bowel obstruction. There is a small amount of adjacent ascites. Curvilinear echogenic lines *(arrows on B)* within the lumen of the bowel adjacent to the wall represent sloughed mucosa caused by ischemia and/or necrosis of the bowel wall. *(Courtesy of Dr. Rob Goodman.)*

ultrasound, and the small bowel can be distinguished from the colon by the presence of the thin valvulae conniventes in the small bowel versus the thicker haustral markings of the colon (Fig. 44). If the dilated bowel can be followed distally, the cause of the obstruction may be observed. Otherwise, further evaluation with CT and/or plain films is warranted.

Intussusception is a common cause of bowel obstruction in children, although it is much less common in adults. Patients present with abdominal pain, which may be intermittent and crampy, nausea, vomiting, a palpable abdominal mass, and currant jelly stool. On ultrasound examination, one will observe a hypoechoic oval mass with bright central echoes described as either a doughnut

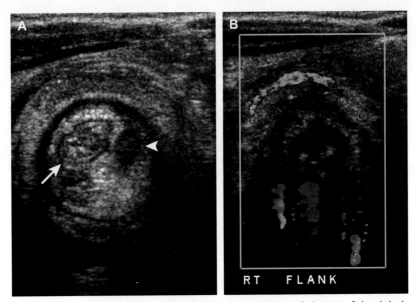

*Fig. 45.* Ileocolic intussusception in a 3-year-old boy. *(A)* Transverse gray-scale image of the right lower quadrant demonstrates the typical doughnut appearance. Echogenic mesenteric fat is noted adjacent to the bowel *(white arrow)* within the intussusceptum. A hypoechoic lymph node *(arrowhead)* is likely the lead point. *(B)* Transverse color Doppler ultrasound shows normal blood flow to the intussuscepted bowel indicating viability. Air enema reduction was initially successful. Repeat reduction with water-soluble contrast agent was necessary, however, as the intussusception recurred.

or target sign on transverse views or as the pseudo kidney sign on longitudinal imaging [53]. Concentric rings of bowel within bowel will be observed (Fig. 45), the intussuscipiens represented by a hypoechoic ring caused by edema of the bowel wall, and the intussusciptum represented by a central echogenic heterogeneous area formed by the echogenic mesenteric fat, bowel, and lead points (often lipomas or lymph nodes) surrounded by hypoechoic fluid. The invaginating echogenic mesenteric fat is usually slightly eccentric within the intussusceptum. The presence of blood flow on color Doppler imaging within the wall of the intussusceptum has been reported to indicate decreased potential risk of perforation from ischemic bowel during reduction maneuvers (see Fig. 45B) [54,55].

Free air, suggesting bowel perforation, also can be detected on ultrasound by the identification of linear echogenic foci with ill-defined shadowing and/or comet-tail artifact between the liver and the diaphragm, between the right lobe of the liver and the kidney (Fig. 46), under the left lobe of the liver, in Morrison's pouch, or by the anterior peritoneal interface. Placing the patient in the left lateral decubitus position may be helpful, as free air will rise under the diaphragm. Asymmetric thickening of the duodenum may suggest peptic ulcer disease. Occasionally, the ulcer crater itself may be identified. Air in the bowel wall may be identified in infants who have necrotizing enterocolitis or in adults who have pneumatosis. In a patient who has thickened loops of dilated bowel, the identification of air in the portal vein is strongly

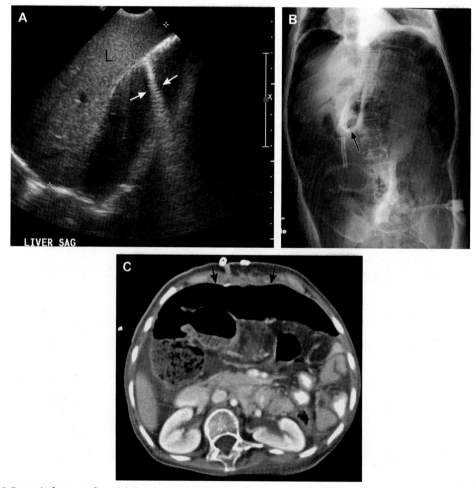

*Fig. 46.* Free air from perforated duodenal ulcer. This patient presented with an acute abdomen and rebound tenderness. *(A)* Note brightly echogenic linear arc with ring down artifact *(arrows)* underneath the right lobe of the liver (L). This represents free intraperitoneal air, which was confirmed on *(B)* plain abdominal radiograph. Note falciform ligament *(arrow)* outlined by air, the so-called Rigler's sign and *(C)* CT scan *(arrows).*

suggestive of ischemic bowel. On ultrasound, air in the portal vein can be identified by direct visualization of echogenic bubbles of gas in the portal veins, which move peripherally into the liver, or by the presence of a classic spike-like artifact caused by the intravenous air bubbles on pulse Doppler tracings of the portal vein.

## Gynecological etiology

Occasionally, acute gynecological pathology may cause acute abdomen pain, either because of referred pain from the pelvis, or from irritation of the diaphragm and peritoneal surfaces secondary to hemoperitoneum or peritonitis. Hence, the radiologist should consider such diagnoses as ectopic pregnancy (EP), hemorrhagic cysts, pelvic inflammatory disease (PID), or ovarian torsion in women of child-bearing age who present with acute abdominal pain.

Women harboring EPs most often come to medical attention because of pelvic pain, adnexal tenderness, and/or vaginal bleeding. Patients, however, occasionally present with acute abdominal pain either because of an intra-abdominal location of the EP or irritation of the peritoneum by intra-abdominal hemorrhage. Risk factors for EP include PID, prior EP, intrauterine devices (IUD), ovulation induction, or other assisted reproductive techniques and prior tubal surgery. Risk factors are additive [56].

The diagnosis of ultrasound for the diagnosing EP is estimated to be approximately 84% [57]. Identification of an extrauterine gestational sac containing a yolk sac and/or embryo is the most specific finding and has a 100% positive predictive value (PPV) (Fig. 47) [57]. In patients who have a B-hCG level above 2,000 mIU/mL (IRP) and no evidence of an intrauterine pregnancy on EVUS, however, identification of an echogenic tubal ring

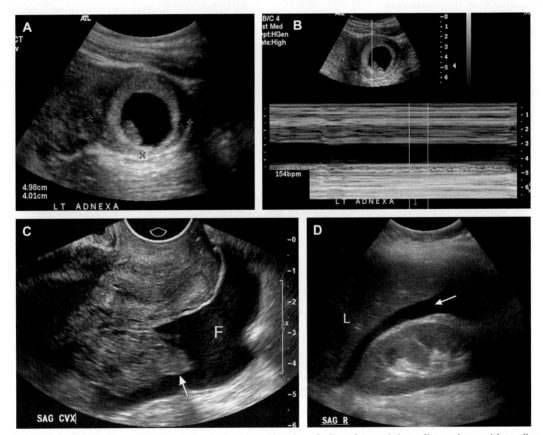

**Fig. 47.** Ectopic pregnancy. *(A)* Note extrauterine gestational sac (calipers) containing a live embryo with cardiac activity and a heart rate of 154 beats per minute on M mode ultrasound image *(B)*. *(C)* Image of the pelvis reveals echogenic clotted blood *(arrow)* and anechoic free fluid (F) in the cul de sac. *(D)* Anechoic fluid consistent with acute hemoperitoneum *(arrow)* also is noted in the upper abdomen in Morrison's pouch, indicating a relatively large amount of intraperitoneal bleeding. *Abbreviation:* L, liver.

in the pelvis (usually in the adnexa or cul de sac), any adnexal mass (usually representing hematoma) or even hemorrhagic free fluid, must be considered highly suspicious (Fig. 48) [56–59]. Free fluid containing low-level echoes and amorphous, heterogeneous avascular echogenic masses representing clot are suggestive of hemoperitoneum, which occurs either from retrograde reflux from the open, fimbriated end of the fallopian tube, or from rupture of an EP (Fig. 47B, C). Because free intraperitoneal hemorrhage may accumulate in Morrison's pouch or in the subphrenic space, these areas always should be examined with transabdominal ultrasound in a clinical setting when there is concern for EP (see Fig. 47C) [60]. In a small percent of cases, the presence of hemorrhagic free fluid may be the only finding on initial ultrasound examination in a woman who has an EP. This finding, however, is nonspecific, and peritoneal fluid containing internal echoes may be seen in patients with intra-abdominal infection or hemorrhage from other causes such as ruptured hemorrhagic ovarian cysts or bleeding from liver metastases.

Implantation of the conceptus in the mural or interstitial portion of the fallopian tube as it courses through the myometrium may cause significant intraperitoneal hemorrhage, as interstitial ectopic pregnancies tend to rupture at a later gestational age when they are larger. Sonographic signs currently used to diagnose interstitial ectopic pregnancies include eccentric location of the gestational sac within the uterus, absence of myometrium around the outer margin of a gestational sac, and the interstitial line sign (Fig. 49) [57,61]. Akerman and colleagues [61] described the interstitial line sign as a thin echogenic line extending from (or representing a continuation of) the endometrial canal to the intramural gestational sac or mass. The interstitial line sign was found to be present in 92% of cases of interstitial pregnancies in this large retrospective review [61]. The presence of normal myometrium separating an intramural gestational sac or mass from the echogenic endometrial stripe, however, is believed to be even more specific (see Fig. 49).

Rupture of a hemorrhagic ovarian cyst also may result in hemoperitoneum and acute onset of severe

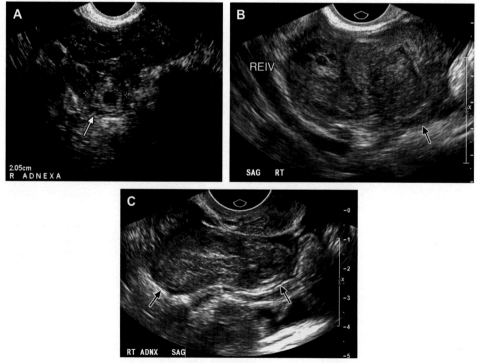

*Fig. 48.* Adnexal masses consistent with ectopic pregnancy in three different patients. *(A)* Note echogenic adnexal tubal ring separate from the ovary in a pregnant woman with a B-hCG greater than 4000 mIU/mL and no evidence of intrauterine gestational sac. *(B)* Note amorphous, heterogenous mass *(arrow)* in the right adnexa in a pregnant patient with right lower quadrant (RLQ) pain. *(C)* In this pregnant patient with RLQ pain, the right adnexal clot *(arrows)* is shaped like the fallopian tube. In the absence of an intrauterine pregnancy in a woman with a B-hCG greater than 2000 mIU/mL, these findings are most consistent with an adnexal hematoma caused by an ectopic pregnancy. *Abbreviation:* REIV, right external iliac vein.

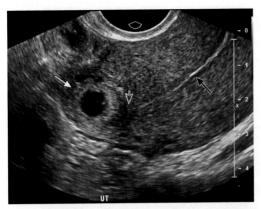

Fig. 49. Interstitial ectopic pregnancy. The echogenic tubal ring *(white arrow)* only partially surrounded by myometrium represents an ectopic pregnancy within the interstitial (myometrial) portion of the fallopian tube. The presence of normal myometrium *(open arrow)* separating the edge of the tubal ring from the endometrium *(black arrow)* has been described as the interstitial line sign.

pelvic and/or abdominal pain. On ultrasound examination, leaking hemorrhagic cysts typically contain low-level echoes and have a crenated configuration. Adjacent free fluid is noted commonly (Fig. 50). On occasion, blood loss may be so extensive that patients become hemodynamically unstable, requiring transfusion or even emergent surgery. Typically, when a ruptured ovarian cyst is the cause of massive hemoperitoneum, the ovary will be surrounded by a heterogenous mass of clot (Fig. 51). Occasionally, the vascular wall of the cyst will be demonstrable on color or power Doppler interrogation within the clotted blood. Clotted intraperitoneal blood may be difficult to differentiate from adjacent loops of bowel, as the echotexture will be similar. Bowel loops, however, will elongate on oblique imaging and will be

observed to peristalse. Rupture of an ovarian cyst with hemoperitoneum is one of the most common causes of a false-positive diagnosis of EP, particularly in early pregnancy (less than 4 to 5 weeks) before an intrauterine pregnancy (IUP) can be documented on ultrasound examination [62].

Although patients who have PID most often present with pelvic pain, vaginal discharge, cervical motion tenderness, and fever, they may present with acute abdominal pain caused by bacterial peritonitis and/or adhesions resulting in small bowel obstruction. Inflammation of the liver capsule may cause severe RUQ pain, termed Fitz Hugh-Curtis syndrome (Fig. 52). PID most commonly is caused by *Chlamydia trachomatis, Neisseria gonorrhea*, or mixed anaerobes and aerobes, and the clinical spectrum of PID ranges from cervicitis/endometritis to tubo–ovarian abscess (TOA). Ultrasound findings include an ill-defined, vascular endometrial stripe sometimes containing fluid or air, thickened fallopian tube, hydro- or pyosalpinx, echogenic pelvic fat, complex intraperitoneal fluid, and complex adnexal masses (TOAs), which are usually bilateral (see Fig. 52). An ill-defined hypoechoic rim of exudative fluid or pus surrounding the uterus occasionally can be seen, suggesting inflammation of the serosal surface uterus (see Fig. 52) [63].

Ovarian torsion may cause sudden onset of excruciating abdominal/pelvic pain. Occasionally, however, pain may be relatively mild and intermittent, likely caused by partial or intermittent torsion. Ovarian torsion is most common in younger women and adolescents, but it may occur in postmenopausal women also. Patients are typically afebrile and have a normal WBC count. Although relatively uncommon, it is important to make this diagnosis expeditiously, as prompt surgical intervention will result in salvage of the ovary. Ovarian torsion is more common on the right, and risk factors include pregnancy, ovarian mass or cyst (such

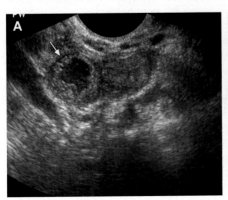
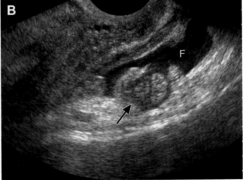

Fig. 50. Hemorrhagic corpus luteal cyst. (A) Ultrasound image of the right adnexa reveals a crenated ovarian cyst *(arrow)* containing low-level echoes consistent with hemorrhage. (B) Image of the cul de sac reveals echogenic free fluid (F), consistent with hemoperitoneum and focal clot *(arrow)*.

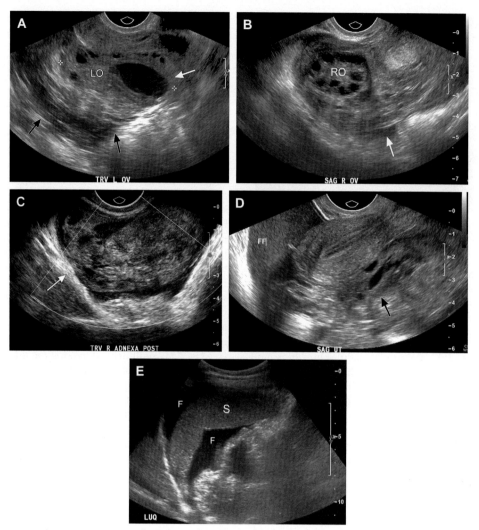

*Fig. 51.* Hemorrhagic corpus luteal cyst. *(A)* The left ovary (LO) contains a leaking, crenated cyst *(white arrow)* and is surrounded by a large amount of heterogeneous clot *(black arrow)*. *(B)* Similar findings are noted on the right. Adnexal hematoma *(arrow)*. *(C)* Color Doppler image of the cul de sac reveals no evidence of blood flow in the large amount of clotted blood *(arrow)*. *(D)* Sagittal view of the uterus demonstrates a large amount of hemorrhagic fluid in the anterior cul de sac (FF) and clotted blood *(arrow)* posteriorly. *(E)* Image of the left upper quadrant reveals a large amount of hemoperitoneum (F) around the spleen (S). This patient was hypotensive because of hemorrhage from this ovarian cyst and required emergent surgery. *Abbreviation:* RO, right ovary.

that the ovary is greater than 6 cm in diameter), tubal ligation, hydrosalpinx, and prior pelvic surgery [64–67]. Ultrasound findings depend upon the time course and presence or absence of an underlying ovarian mass [64]. Acutely, the ovary often will be enlarged, with loss of the normal ovarian sonographic architecture. The central stroma will become heterogeneous and expanded, displacing the follicles peripherally with hypoechoic areas due to edema from lymphatic obstruction and echogenic areas due to hemorrhage (Fig. 53). Adjacent free fluid may be present [64]. Over time, the ovary remains enlarged but becomes more complex and amorphous in appearance [64]. Color Doppler imaging may demonstrate a twisted pedicle of vessels and absent parenchymal blood flow (see Fig. 53C) [65,66]. Absence of venous flow, decreased diastolic arterial flow, and asymmetrically diminished peak systolic velocity in comparison to the normal contra-lateral ovary may be observed. Arterial and even venous flow, however, may be preserved early on [67,68]. Hence, in the appropriate clinical setting and in the presence of suggestive gray scale findings, the presence of blood flow on Doppler interrogation should not be used to exclude the diagnosis of ovarian torsion [67,68].

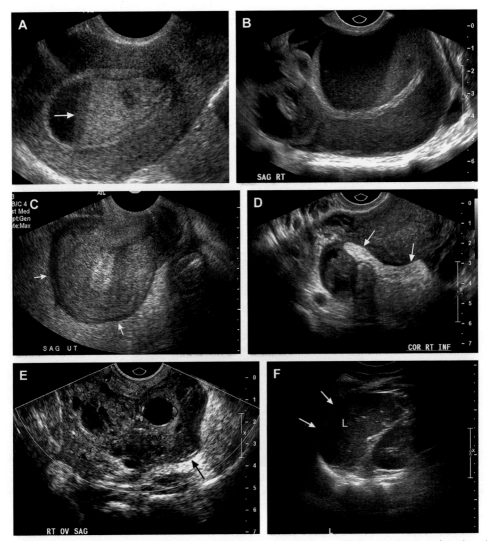

*Fig. 52.* Pelvic inflammatory disease (PID). Variable ultrasound findings. *(A)* Pyometria. Note layering debris *(arrow)* within the distended endometrial cavity. *(B)* Pyosalpinx. Note layering debris in the distended right fallopian tube. *(C)* Uterine serositis. Note hypoechoic material *(arrows)* outlining the uterus. This represents exudative purulent material coating the serosal surface of the uterus. *(D)* Echogenic adnexal fat. Note increased echogenicity of the pelvic fat under the uterus and right fallopian tube. The increased echogenicity indicates acute inflammation. *(E)* Tubo–ovarian abscess. Sagittal color Doppler image of the right adnexa demonstrates a large, complex mass engulfing the right ovary. *(F)* Note thin rim of fluid underneath the diaphragm above the liver in a patient with PID presenting with acute right upper quadrant pain radiating to the right shoulder, Fitz-Hugh-Curtis Syndrome.

## Miscellaneous causes of acute abdominal pain

Most patients who have acute intra-abdominal hemorrhage present with acute abdominal pain, peritoneal signs, and often an acute surgical abdomen. Overall, rupture from a hemorrhagic ovarian cyst is the most common cause of nontraumatic intraperitoneal bleeding to present with acute abdominal or pelvic pain. Other common causes include:

- Ruptured hemorrhagic ovarian cyst
- Ectopic pregnancy
- Trauma (including iatrogenic)
- Coagulopathy/anticoagulation therapy
- Splenic rupture
- Variceal or pseudoaneurysm rupture
- Hemorrhagic pancreatitis
- Rupture of abdominal aortic aneurysm

The presence of echoes within intra-abdominal fluid is suggestive of hemorrhage, although the

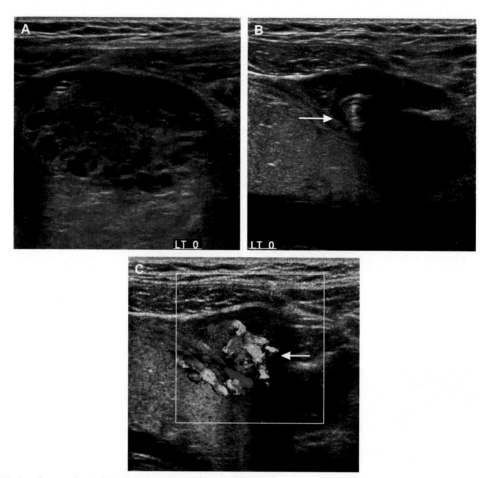

Fig. 53. Ovarian torsion. This 24-year-old woman presented with excruciating left lower quadrant pain. *(A)* The enlarged left ovary has numerous small peripheral cysts. The central ovarian stroma is markedly heterogeneous. *(B)* Gray scale image of the left adnexa demonstrates an echogenic mass *(arrow)* with concentric circular layers adjacent to the abnormal left ovary. This represents the twisted vascular pedicle, which is seen to better advantage *(arrow)* on the color Doppler image *(C)*.

findings are nonspecific and can be mimicked by infected peritoneal fluid and more rarely by debris in chronic ascites. The presence of clot suggests that bleeding is acute and extensive. Clot is typically of medium echogenicity and, therefore, can be difficult to recognize, as it may silhouette with fluid containing bowel. Clot, however, will remain rounded and irregular in contour, and stable on examination, while bowel will peristalse and elongate on a 90° imaging plane.

Acute hemorrhage into the rectus or psoas muscles also may be a cause of acute abdominal pain. The involved muscle will be asymmetrically enlarged compared with the contralateral side and heterogeneous in echotexture, with areas of increased and/or decreased echogenicity depending on the time since the hemorrhage (Fig. 54). Layering or an echogenic rind may be observed in more

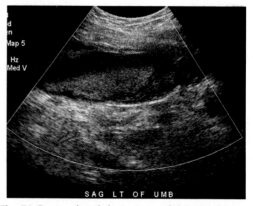

Fig. 54. Rectus sheath hematoma. *(A)* Sagittal image of the anterior abdominal wall reveals a layering hematoma *(arrow)* in the rectus muscle. This patient on coumadin had an elevated international normalized ratio (INR) and a spontaneous bleed.

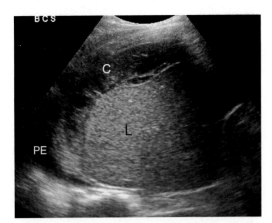

**Fig. 55.** Subdiaphragmatic abscess. Note complex collection (C) between the diaphragm and liver (L). There is a small associated pleural effusion (PE).

chronic hemorrhages as the red blood cells lyse and the hematoma becomes encapsulated.

Patients who have acute intra-abdominal infection/abscess also may present with acute abdominal pain. Although CT is considered the first-line imaging modality of choice for evaluation of such patients, ultrasound can be used to localize intra-abdominal collections for diagnosis and to provide guidance for drainage. Ultrasound is especially helpful in evaluation of pelvic or subdiaphragmatic collections, which will be visualized as complex fluid collections containing multiple septations and low-level echoes representing debris, hemorrhage, or pus (Fig. 55). An echogenic rind may be present if the abscess is chronic. Such ultrasound findings are nonspecific, however, and hematomas or lymphoceles may have a similar ultrasound appearance. Aspiration may be required for differentiation. Patients who have hemorrhagic or infected pleural effusions and/or pneumonia also

may present rarely with acute upper quadrant pain that may mask or exceed symptoms directly related to the lung condition because of irritation of the diaphragm. Ultrasound examination will demonstrate complex pleural fluid and collapsed echogenic lung that may look like the liver parenchyma, thereby mimicking mirror image artifact from the liver/diaphragmatic interface at first glance (Fig. 56). Occasionally, linear echogenic streaks with dirty shadowing indicative of air bronchograms within the collapsed lung or air within an empyema will be demonstrated.

## Summary

Ultrasound is an invaluable imaging technique for evaluating patients presenting with acute abdominal pain, and in experienced hands, it provides important diagnostic information that may not be obtainable by other imaging modalities. In particular, ultrasound remains the first-line imaging modality of choice for evaluating suspected biliary tract disease and gynecologic pathology. In children and pregnant women, ultrasound should be the first step in the work up of suspected appendicitis or renal calculi. In addition, ultrasound should be performed emergently at the bedside in the hemodynamically unstable elderly patient who has back pain to search for an abdominal aortic aneurysm. Furthermore, with careful attention to technique and more subtle ultrasound findings, the sonographer may identify clinically unsuspected pathology when ultrasound is performed to evaluate the patient who has nonspecific abdominal pain. Despite the advantages of ultrasound and the diagnostic utility detailed, however, there are distinct disadvantages. Evaluation of the obese patient is limited with ultrasound. The ultrasound

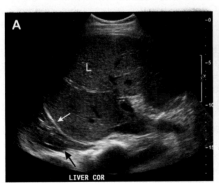

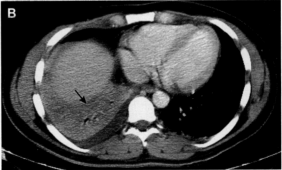

**Fig. 56.** Pneumonia. *(A)* Ultrasound of the right upper quadrant (RUQ) in a patient with acute RUQ pain, cough, and fever reveals consolidation of the right lower lobe of the lung *(black arrow)* above the echogenic diaphragm *(white arrow)*. Consolidation of the lung easily can be mistaken for mirror image artifact. Note, however, that although the echotexture of the material above and below the diaphragm is similar, the internal markings are quite different. *(B)* CT scan confirms the presence of right lower lobe pneumonia with air bronchograms *(arrow)*. Abbreviation: L, liver.

beam can penetrate neither bone nor gas. Lastly, ultrasound is the most operator-dependent abdominal imaging modality in current widespread use, and optimal examination requires thorough knowledge of the technical aspects of sonography and clinical expertise to focus the ultrasound examination. Thus, if initial ultrasound evaluation does not reveal the clinically anticipated abnormality, evaluation of the entire abdomen with CT should be considered as clinically indicated.

## References

[1] Dhillon S, Halligan S, Goh V, et al. The therapeutic impact of abdominal ultrasound in patients with acute abdominal symptoms. Clin Radiol 2002;57:268–71.

[2] Puylaert JBCM. Ultrasonography of the acute abdomen: lost art or future stethoscope? Eur Radiol 2003;13:1203–6.

[3] Ralls PW, Colletti PM, Lapin SA, et al. Real-time sonography in suspected acute cholecystitis: prospective evaluation of primary and secondary signs. Radiology 1985;155:767–71.

[4] Hanbidge AE, Buckler PM, O'Malley ME, et al. Imaging evaluation for acute pain in the right upper quadrant. Radiographics 2004;24:1117–35.

[5] Laing FC, Jeffrey RB, Wing VW. Improved visualization of choledocholithiasis by sonography. AJR Am J Roentgenol 1984;143:949–52.

[6] Behan M, Kazam E. Sonography of the common bile duct: value of the right anterior oblique view. AJR Am J Roentgenol 1978;130:701–9.

[7] Ralls PW. Focal inflammatory disease of the liver. Radiol Clin North Am 1998;36:377–89.

[8] McDonald AP, Howard RJ. Pyogenic liver abscess. World J Surg 1980;4:369–80.

[9] Mohsen AH, Green ST, Read RC, et al. Liver abscess in adults: ten years experience in a UK centre. QJM 2002;95:797–802.

[10] Grazioli L, Federle MP, Brancatelli G, et al. Hepatic adenomas: imaging and pathologic findings. Radiographics 2001;21:877–94.

[11] Primary liver cancer in Japan. Sixth report. The Liver Cancer Society Group of Japan. Cancer 1987;60:1400–11.

[12] Hotokezaka M, Kojima M, Nakmura K, et al. Traumatic rupture of hepatic hemangiomas. J Clin Gastroenterol 1996;23:69–71.

[13] Graham E, Cohen AW, Soulen M, et al. Symptomatic liver hemangiomas with intratumor hemorrhage treated by angiography and embolization during pregnancy. Obstet Gynecol 1993;81:813–6.

[14] Diehl AK, Holleman DR, Chapman JB, et al. Gallstone size and risk of pancreatitis. Arch Intern Med 1997;157:1674–8.

[15] Chang L, Lo S, Stabile BE, et al. Preoperative versus postoperative endoscopic retrograde cholangiopancreatography in mild-to-moderate gallstone pancreatitis: a prospective randomized trial. Ann Surg 2000;231:82–7.

[16] Folsch U, Nitche R, Lutdke R, et al. Early ERCP and papillotomy compared with conservative treatment for acute biliary pancreatitis. N Engl J Med 1997;336:237–42.

[17] Finstad TA, Tchelepi H, Ralls PW. Sonography of acute pancreatitis. Ultrasound Q 2005;21:95–104.

[18] Bennett GL, Hann LE. The pancreas revisited I: diagnosis, chronic pancreatitis. Surg Clin North Am 2001;81:259–81.

[19] Gottlieb RH, Luhmann K, Oates RP. Duplex ultrasound evaluation of normal kidneys and native kidneys with urinary obstruction. J Ultrasound Med 1989;8:609–11.

[20] Platt JF, Rubin JM, Ellis JH. Acute renal obstruction: evaluation with intrarenal duplex Doppler and conventional US. Radiology 1993;186:685–8.

[21] Campbell SC, Cullinan JA, Rubens DJ. Slow flow or no flow? Color and power Doppler US pitfalls in the abdomen and pelvis. Radiographics 2004;24:497–506.

[22] Burge HJ, Middleton WD, McClennan BL, et al. Ureteral jets in healthy subjects and in patients with unilateral ureteral calculi: comparison with color Doppler. Radiology 1991;180(2):437–42.

[23] Grayson DE, Abbott RM, Levy AD, et al. Emphysematous infections in the abdomen and pelvis: a pictorial review. Radiographics 2002;22:543–61.

[24] Patel NP, Lavengood RW, Ernande SM, et al. Gas-forming infection in the genitourinary tract. Urology 1992;39:341–5.

[25] Maresca G, Mirk P, De Gaetano A, et al. Sonographic patterns in splenic infarct. J Clin Ultrasound 1986;14:23–8.

[26] Goerg C, Schwerk WB, Goerg K. Splenic lesions: sonographic patterns, follow-up, differential diagnosis. Eur J Radiol 1991;13:59–66.

[27] Andrews MW. Ultrasound of the spleen. World J Surg 2000;24:183–7.

[28] Schuman WP, Hastrup W, Kohler TR, et al. Suspected leaking abdominal aortic aneurysm: use of sonography in the emergency room. Radiology 1988;168:117–9.

[29] Catalano O, Siani A. Ruptured aortic aneurysm. Categorization of sonographic findings and report of 3 new signs. J Ultrasound Med 2005;24:1077–83.

[30] Birnbaum BA, Wilson SR. Appendicitis at the millennium. Radiology 2000;215:337–48.

[31] Balthazar EJ, Rofsky NM, Zucker R. Appendicitis: the impact of computed tomography imaging on negative appendectomy and perforation rates. Am J Gastroenterol 1998;93:768–71.

[32] Schuler JG, Shortsleeve MJ, Goldenson RS, et al. Is there a role for abdominal computed tomographic scans in appendicitis? Arch Surg 1998;133:373–6.

[33] Jeffrey RB, Laing FC, Townsend RR. Acute appendicitis: sonographic criteria based on 250 cases. Radiology 1988;167:327–9.

[34] Kessler N, Cyteval C, Gallix B, et al. Appendicitis: evaluation of sensitivity, specificity, and predictive values of US, Doppler US, and laboratory findings. Radiology 2004;230:472–8.

[35] Jeffrey RB, Jain KA, Nghiem HV. Sonographic diagnosis of acute appendicitis: interpretive pitfalls. AJR Am J Roentgenol 1994;162:55–9.

[36] Quillin SP, Siegel MJ. Diagnosis of appendiceal abscess in children with acute appendicitis: value of color Doppler sonography. AJR Am J Roentgenol 1995;164:1251–4.

[37] Borushok KF, Jeffrey RB Jr, Laing FC, et al. Sonographic diagnosis of perforation in patients with acute appendicitis. AJR Am J Roentgenol 1990; 154:275–8.

[38] Jeffrey RB Jr, Laing FC, Lewis FR. Acute appendicitis: high resolution real-time US findings. Radiology 1987;163:11–4.

[39] Abu-Yousef MM, Bleicher JJ, Maher JW, et al. High-resolution sonography of acute appendicitis. AJR Am J Roentgenol 1987;149:53–8.

[40] Sivit CJ, Newman KD, Boenning DA, et al. Appendicitis: usefulness of US in diagnosis in a pediatric population. Radiology 1992;185: 549–52.

[41] Puylaert JBCM, Rutgers PH, Lalisang RI, et al. A prospective study of ultrasonography in the diagnosis of appendicitis. N Engl J Med 1987; 317:666–9.

[42] Wilson EB, Cole JC, Nipper ML, et al. Computed tomography and ultrasonography in the diagnosis of appendicitis: when are they indicated? Arch Surg 2001;136:670–5.

[43] Rao PM, Boland GW. Imaging of acute right lower abdominal quadrant pain. Clin Radiol 1998;53:639–49.

[44] Puylaert JBCM. Ultrasonography of the acute abdomen: gastrointestinal conditions. Radiol Clin North Am 2003;41:1227–42.

[45] Rioux M, Langis P. Primary epiploic appendagitis: clinical, US, and CT findings in 14 cases. Radiology 1994;191:523–6.

[46] Wilson SR. Gastrointestinal tract sonography. Abdom Imaging 1996;21:1–8.

[47] Pradel JA, Adell JF, Taourel P, et al. Acute colonic diverticulitis: prospective comparative evaluation with US and CT. Radiology 1997;205:503–12.

[48] O'Malley ME, Wilson SR. US of gastrointestinal tract abnormalities with CT correlation. Radiographics 2003;23:59–72.

[49] Wilson SR, Toi A. The value of sonography in the diagnosis of acute diverticulitis of the colon. AJR Am J Roentgenol 1990;154:1199–202.

[50] Zielke A, Hasse C, Nies C, et al. Prospective evaluation of ultrasonography in acute colonic diverticulitis. Br J Surg 1997;84:385–8.

[51] Sarrazin J, Wilson SR. Manifestations of Crohn's disease at US. Radiographics 1996;16:499–520.

[52] Maconi G, Radice E, Greco A, et al. Bowel ultrasound in Crohn's disease. Best Pract Res Clin Gastroenterol 2006;20:93–112.

[53] Swischuk LE, Hayden CK, Boulden T. Intussusception: indications for ultrasonography and an explanation of the doughnut and pseudokidney sign. Pediatr Radiol 1985;15:388–91.

[54] Lim HK, Bae SH, Lee KH, et al. Assessment of reducibility of ileocolic intussusception in children: usefulness of color Doppler sonography. Radiology 1994;191:781–5.

[55] Lam AH, Firman K. Value of sonography including color Doppler in the diagnosis and management of longstanding intussusception. Pediatr Radiol 1992;22:112–4.

[56] Frates MC, Laing FC. Sonographic evaluation of ectopic pregnancy: an update. AJR Am J Roentgenol 1995;165:251–9.

[57] Brown DL, Doubilet PM. Transvaginal sonography for diagnosing ectopic pregnancy: positivity criteria and performance characteristics. J Ultrasound Med 1994;13:259–66.

[58] Atri M, Leduc C, Gillett P, et al. Role of endovaginal sonography in the diagnosis and management of ectopic pregnancy. Radiographics 1996;16:755–74.

[59] Russell SA, Filly RA, Damato N. Sonographic diagnosis of ectopic pregnancy with endovaginal probes: what really has changed? J Ultrasound Med 1993;12:145–51.

[60] Nyberg DA, Hughes MP, Mack LA, et al. Extrauterine findings of ectopic pregnancy at transvaginal US: importance of echogenic fluid. Radiology 1991;178:823–6.

[61] Akerman TE, Levi CS, Dashefsky SM, et al. Interstitial line: sonographic finding in interstitial (cornual) ectopic pregnancy. Radiology 1993;189:83–7.

[62] Hertzberg B, Kliewer M, Bowie J. Adnexal ring sign and hemoperitoneum caused by hemorrhagic ovarian cyst: pitfall in the sonographic diagnosis of ectopic pregnancy. AJR Am J Roentgenol 1999;173:1301–2.

[63] Horrow M. Ultrasound of pelvic inflammatory disease. Ultrasound Q 2004;20:171–9.

[64] Albayram F, Hamper UM. Ovarian and adnexal torsion: spectrum of sonographic findings with pathologic correlation. J Ultrasound Med 2001; 20:1083–9.

[65] Lee EJ, Kwon HC, Joo HJ, et al. Diagnosis of ovarian torsion with color Doppler sonography: depiction of twisted vascular pedicle. J Ultrasound Med 1998;17:83–9.

[66] Vijayaraghavan SB. Sonographic whirlpool sign in ovarian torsion. J Ultrasound Med 2004;23: 1643–9.

[67] Peña JE, Ufberg A, Cooney N, et al. Usefulness of Doppler sonography in the diagnosis of ovarian torsion. Fertil Steril 2000;73(5):1047–50.

[68] Fleischer AC, Stein SM, Cullinan JA, et al. Color Doppler sonography of adnexal torsion. J Ultrasound Med 1995;14:523–8.

ULTRASOUND
CLINICS

Ultrasound Clin 2 (2007) 525–540

**ELSEVIER
SAUNDERS**

# Ultrasound in the Assessment of the Acute Abdomen in Children: Its Advantages and Its Limitations

Cindy R. Miller, MD

- Pathology unique to infants
- Pathology commonly presenting in infancy, but not limited to infancy
- Pathology most commonly limited to young children
- Other bowel associated pathology seen in the pediatric population
- Malignancy and its complications presenting as an acute abdomen
- Summary
- References

There is a wide spectrum of differential diagnoses to be considered in children presenting with acute abdominal pain. The entities that are most common vary depending on the age of the child. Some of the advantages of ultrasound when imaging children, such as the lack of ionizing radiation and the relatively short length of the exam obviating sedation, are obvious. This article outlines the diagnostic considerations within the different pediatric age groups, and considers the ways in which ultrasound can facilitate diagnosis, the cases in which ultrasound is limited in its ability to make a diagnosis, and the ways in which ultrasound can monitor the efficacy of treatment. As it would be beyond the scope of this article to consider each entity in detail, there is a focus on several diseases relatively unique to children. Attention is also paid to appendicitis, an entity seen in both children and adults, which continues to pose diagnostic challenges.

Just as children cannot be thought of as little adults, all children are not the same when trying to determine the differential diagnosis for the acute abdomen. The age of the child is critical, as certain diagnoses are much more common at particular ages. Within the first few months of life, congenital anomalies, including midgut malrotation and its complications and disease states related to prematurity, such as necrotizing enterocolitis, would be highest on the list of differential diagnoses. Shortly thereafter, but still within the first few years of life, intussusception and incarcerated inguinal hernias are important considerations. Rarely, complications of malignancy, such as rupture of a Wilms tumor, may present as an acute abdomen.

There is significant overlap between older children and adolescents in terms of the differential diagnosis of the acute abdomen, with very few entities being specific to one particular age group. The myriad possible etiologies include Meckel's diverticulum and its complications, Henoch-Schonlein purpura, hemolytic uremic syndrome, cholecystitis, appendicitis, mesenteric adenitis, testicular torsion, ovarian cysts and torsion, pelvic inflammatory disease, and ectopic pregnancy. Renal pathology, including pyelonephritis, acute hydronephrosis, and calculous disease may also occasionally present as an acute abdomen. In addition to there being a wide spectrum of pathology which may present with abdominal pain in adolescents, frequently it

Department of Diagnostic Radiology, Yale University School of Medicine, P.O. Box 208042 (CH-272B), New Haven, CT 06510-8042, USA
E-mail address: cindy.miller@yale.edu

1556-858X/07/$ – see front matter © 2007 Elsevier Inc. All rights reserved.
ultrasound.theclinics.com

doi:10.1016/j.cult.2007.08.010

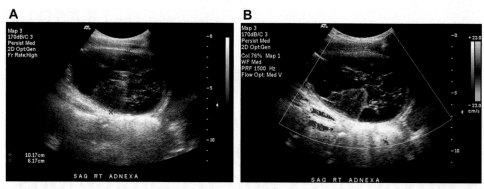

**Fig. 1.** Intermittent ovarian torsion. (*A*) This teenager, with a family history positive for renal calculi, presented with symptoms strongly suggestive of stones. Evaluation of the kidneys was unremarkable, but a large, complex septated lesion involving the right adnexa was discovered. (*B*) Color Doppler imaging revealed flow in a very focal area. At surgery, it was felt that there had been intermittent torsion of this ovary.

is difficult to localize the pain, even with a complete history and physical examination as in the patient depicted in (Fig. 1).

When considering a patient with an acute abdomen, it is critical to distinguish between a disease that will be treated medically and one which requires surgical intervention. Ultrasound can frequently make that distinction. As in adults, the utility of ultrasound in the pediatric population can be limited by large body habitus of the patient, by shadowing from adjacent bowel gas, and by the skill of the sonographer.

## Pathology unique to infants

Necrotizing enterocolitis (NEC) is relatively common in neonatal intensive care units, occurring in 1% to 2% [1] of infants. There is no single etiology of NEC; rather, it is felt to reflect a combination of prematurity, enteral nutrition, bacterial colonization of the gastrointestinal (GI) tract, and hypoxia. Plain radiographs have been the mainstay in imaging NEC, with attention given to the degree of bowel distention; the presence of pneumatosis intestinalis, portal venous gas, or free intraperitoneal air; and the presence of nonchanging loops of bowel over the course of a sequence of films. It has been reported that there is very high specificity for the findings on plain films of pneumatosis (100%), portal venous gas (100%), free air (92%), and a gasless abdomen (92%) for the diagnosis of NEC, but the sensitivity of these findings is significantly lower; for pneumatosis, the sensitivity is 44%, for portal venous gas 13%, for free air 52%, and for a gasless abdomen 32% [2]. Given the high mortality (20%–40%) of NEC [1] and its high morbidity if the infant survives, it has been recognized that there would be tremendous utility in identifying an imaging modality that could improve the sensitivity of plain X-rays and provide

information regarding bowel viability. To that end, numerous investigators [1,3–5] have assessed the role of ultrasound in not only making the diagnosis, but also in assessing the severity of disease.

Distention of the bowel is said to be the earliest plain film sign of NEC, but is a nonspecific finding as it may also be seen, for instance, in the setting of sepsis or in patients on continuous positive airway pressure [1]. Ultrasound has been shown to provide a greater degree of specificity to this finding if the bowel wall is noted to be echogenic. The increased echogenicity of the bowel wall is felt to reflect the presence of pneumatosis [1]. When making a diagnosis of pneumatosis ultrasonographically, it is important to avoid the pitfall of misdiagnosing pseudopneumatosis. This latter entity will only be present in the nondependent bowel wall in the superficial layer of the bowel wall. In addition, in patients with pseudopneumatosis, the pattern of echogenicity of the bowel wall will change with change in patient position or by varying the degree of compression applied to the abdominal wall by the transducer. Such changes in bowel wall echogenicity will not occur if pneumatosis is truly present [1]. Kim and colleagues [1] reported that in 40 infants with NEC, compared with age-matched asymptomatic controls, ultrasound was demonstrated to detect pneumatosis earlier than did plain films.

Ultrasound has also proven useful in establishing a diagnosis of NEC in infants with clinical findings, such as blood in the stool and abdominal distention, when plain radiographs were nondiagnostic. Specifically, it has been shown that portal venous gas can be diagnosed ultrasonographically in patients in whom it is not evident on plain films. In a study reported in 1986 by Lindley and colleagues [3] of 15 newborns with clinical NEC with nondiagnostic plain films, five were shown to have occult portal venous gas. Two of these infants required surgery and the other three were treated medically. Ultrasound has also been reported to be efficacious in the detection of occult bowel perforation.

In the study of Miller and colleagues [4], five infants had plain radiographs demonstrating a gasless abdomen and were experiencing clinical deterioration. Eighty percent of these children were shown to have an extraluminal fluid or debris level on ultrasound; all of these infants were proven to have had a perforation in the operating room. The infant whose ultrasound did not reveal a fluid or debris level experienced a clinical recovery. Other gray scale sonographic features that are assessed in patients with suspected NEC include the presence or absence of normal bowel wall signature, measurement of bowel wall thickness, and the demonstration of peristalsis, which is defined as the presence of contractions of the bowel occurring over a one minute period of observation [5]. Color Doppler using a low wall filter and a high gain setting is useful in assessing blood flow to the bowel. In the early stages of NEC, there will be inflammation of the bowel leading to increased blood flow. Later, a sequence of events occurs in which bacteria lead to cytokine expression and the complement cascade, which then leads to transmural inflammation and vascular compromise. The ultrasonographic correlates have been well described. Abnormal patterns of increased flow include a circular or rim pattern, a "Y" pattern reflecting flow in the distal superior mesenteric artery and subserosa, and a zebra pattern corresponding to flow within the valvulae conniventes. With more advanced disease, ultrasound has demonstrated an absence of flow, a sign with a sensitivity of 100% [5].

Although there has been an evolution in surgical practice in the treatment of NEC, for many years the only finding which would prompt immediate surgical intervention was the presence of free intraperitoneal air. As the presence of free air on plain films has a sensitivity of only 40% to 52% [2,5], it is evident that ultrasound, with its ability to visualize, for example, fluid or debris levels in the peritoneal cavity, offers a distinct advantage in imaging these infants. There are several factors which may be responsible for the fact that ultrasound is not done routinely in the assessment of children with NEC. The examination is time consuming, and the ability to visualize the bowel wall may be markedly compromised by the abundant intraluminal gas, which is often present. Its value in identifying findings which would lead to earlier surgical therapy is being increasingly recognized; nevertheless, ultrasound in the setting of NEC will likely remain a problem solving tool only, including the setting where NEC is being treated and there is lack of clinical improvement or a frank clinical deterioration (Fig. 2).

## Pathology commonly presenting in infancy, but not limited to infancy

Midgut malrotation is a relatively common entity, being present in 1 out of every 500 live births [6]. The majority of children who become symptomatic from malrotation and its complications present in the first month of life. Symptoms in infants include bilious vomiting and bright red blood per rectum, while episodic pain or failure to thrive are more common presentations in older children. In children with such symptoms who may indeed be malrotated, it is more important to exclude the possibility of malfixation, as it is in situations where there is a short mesentery with improper fixation that the midgut is prone to volvulize with subsequent vascular compromise. For many years, radiologists have advocated upper GI examination as the study of choice for this indication. The upper GI series has a sensitivity of 85% to 95%, and an even higher specificity.

Numerous studies [7–12] have been performed to evaluate whether ultrasound can replace the upper GI in making the diagnosis of malrotation. The majority of these studies evaluated the relative positions of the superior mesenteric artery (SMA) and vein (SMV), considering the position to be abnormal if the SMV was ventral or to the left of the SMA (Fig. 3). In the retrospective study reported by Weinberger and colleagues [7] of 337 infants with vomiting, referred for ultrasound to assess the pylorus, the relative locations of the SMA and SMV were evident in 249 (74%). An abnormal relationship was seen in nine infants. In 100% of those (five out of five) in whom the SMV was to the left of the SMA, malrotation was present, while in 25% (one out of four) the SMV ventral to the SMA were malrotated. Pracros and colleagues [8] used color Doppler to assess 24 patients with surgically proven malrotation, 18 of whom had volvulus. The whirlpool sign in which the SMV and associated mesentery are seen wrapped around the SMA was seen in 15 out of 18 (83%) (Fig. 4).

More recently, Orzech and colleagues [9] reported on 255 patients in whom a study was designed specifically to determine if ultrasound is a good screening test for malrotation. All of the patients had both upper GI and ultrasound. Of these subjects, 211 had concordance between their studies; in 62%, both studies were normal, and in 15%, both were abnormal. Forty-four subjects showed discordance in their results, with 21% having a false positive ultrasound (abnormal ultrasound, normal upper GI) and 2% having a false negative ultrasound (normal ultrasound, abnormal upper GI). Of these five latter patients, none had a short mesentery such that although all were

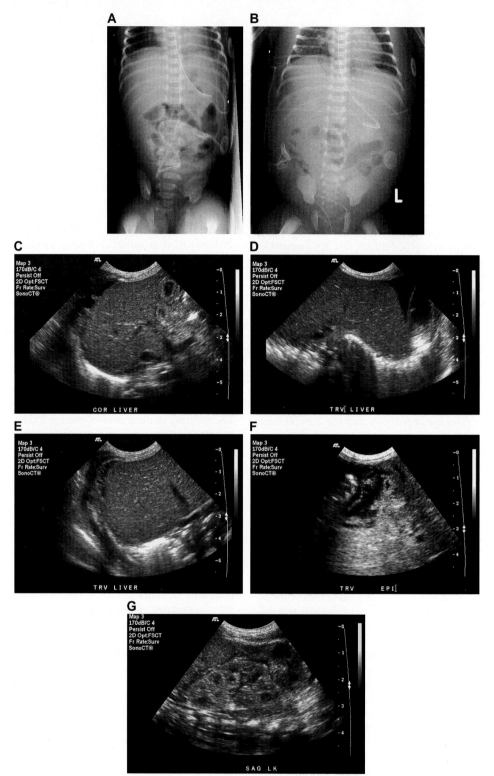

*Fig. 2.* (*A*) This preterm infant developed abdominal distention at 6 days of life. While her plain film demonstrated no pneumatosis, the disorganization of bowel loops, which were somewhat featureless in appearance, was abnormal. Additionally, a lucency was seen over the liver on two consecutive films, suggesting free intraperitoneal air. NEC was diagnosed, and a drain was placed. (*B*) An abdominal film, obtained several days after placement of the drain, demonstrated centralization of loops of bowel, suggesting ascites. As the patient was deteriorating clinically, an ultrasound was recommended. (*C-G*) Several days after the drain was placed, an ultrasound of the abdomen revealed multiple complex fluid collections that reflected the fact that there had been perforation of the bowel; none had features to definitely suggest abscess.

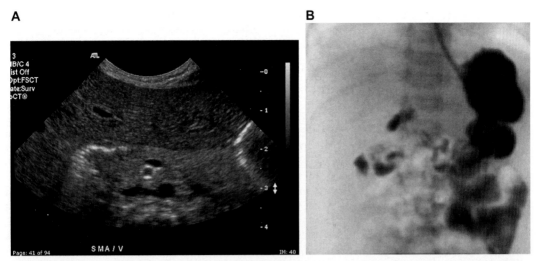

*Fig. 3.* (*A*) Ultrasound was performed in this infant with imperforate anus, as there was clinical suspicion of hepatomegaly. Incidentally, it was noted that the SMV was anterior to the SMA. (*B*) Upper GI examination confirmed that this patient was malrotated with the proximal loops of small bowel remaining to the right of the spine. (Contrast seen in loops to the left of the spine had been introduced one day earlier during an esophagram.)

malrotated, none was predisposed to volvulus. There were essentially three abnormalities that were considered on ultrasound: anterior-posterior relationship of the SMV to the SMA, inverted relationship of the vessels, or a whirlpool pattern. An inverted relationship had the greatest sensitivity for malrotation with a narrow mesentery (71.4%); the whirlpool sign had the greatest specificity (99%), positive predictive value (71.4%), and negative predictive value (97.1%). In total, 64%

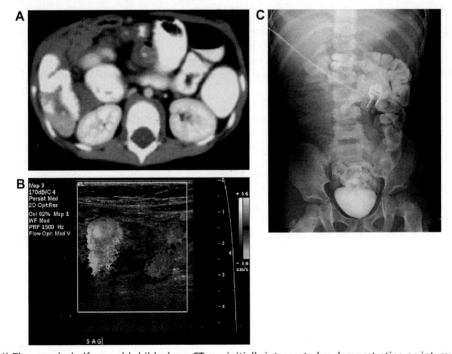

*Fig. 4.* (*A*) Three and a half year old child whose CT was initially interpreted as demonstrating an intussusception based on the appearance of concentric rings in the epigastrium. In the center of the ring were two foci of increased attenuation felt to represent mesenteric vessels. (*B*) Ultrasound did not demonstrate the concentric rings of intussusception, but instead showed a whirlpool pattern of malrotation. (*C*) Malrotation, in this case nonrotation of the bowel, was confirmed on plain radiograph obtained after the CT scan. There was no bowel obstruction.

of the subjects had a normal ultrasound and 36% had an abnormal ultrasound, as compared with 82.5% with normal upper GI and 17.5% with an abnormal upper GI. The sensitivity of ultrasound for malrotation was determined to be 86.5%, the specificity 74.7%, the positive predictive value 42.1%, and the negative predictive value 96.3% [9].

It is not only the finding of malrotation which is important, but the potential for volvulus which is critical. A small 3-year prospective study of 20 infants with inverted SMA and SMV and surgically proven malrotation was reported by Chao and colleagues [10], in which they sought to find sonographic features predictive of volvulus. There was high sensitivity (89%) and specificity (92%) for duodenal dilatation with tapering, a fixed midline loop of bowel, and the whirlpool sign. A dilated SMV had significantly lower sensitivity (56%) and specificity (73%) [10]. Note has also been made that it is a clockwise direction of the whirlpool sign which is diagnostic of volvulus [11]. In the study of Shimanuki and colleagues [11] of 160 children between the ages of 1 day and 14 years, 16 demonstrated a whirlpool sign. Of the 13 whose whirlpool ran clockwise, 12 had surgically proven volvulus; none of those whose whirlpool progressed counterclockwise had volvulus. The utility of the whirlpool sign was further stressed by Patino and Munden [12] in a study of children between the ages of 1 day and $5\frac{1}{2}$ years who presented with symptoms that would not typically be associated with malrotation, including nonbilious vomiting, colicky pain suggesting intussusception, right lower quadrant pain suggesting appendicitis, a palpable mass, and chronic diarrhea.

Despite its seeming promise, ultrasound has a couple of important limitations. There are a significant number (ranging from 16%–77% in various studies) [7,9] of patients in whom the superior mesenteric artery and vein are obscured by bowel gas, such that their relationship to one another cannot be assessed on ultrasound examination. Furthermore, ultrasound cannot reliably estimate the length of the mesentery, the feature that is most critical in determining the potential for volvulus [9].

## Pathology most commonly limited to young children

This section considers inguinal hernia (which may or may not contain bowel) and intussusception. The parietal peritoneum extends through the internal inguinal ring to form the processus vaginalis in the fetus. Between 28- and 40-weeks gestational age, the processus vaginalis attaches to the testes as they descend, and remains in close contiguity as the

tunica vaginalis. In 20% of the cases, the processus vaginalis remains open, but typically the boys are asymptomatic [13]. However, a hydrocele or indirect hernia may occur. Given the inaccuracy of clinical signs, ultrasound has been explored as a means to evaluate the likelihood of a contralateral inguinal hernia by assessment of the processus vaginalis and by noting the presence or absence of intra-abdominal organs within the inguinal canal [14]. Patients are divided into five categories: I (intra-abdominal organs seen); II (cyst-like appearance, measuring 20 mm); III (widens with increased intra-abdominal pressure with a length greater than 20 mm); IV (does not widen, but contains fluid); V (widens with increased intra-abdominal pressure, but does not measure 20 mm). As children who have anatomy type III or IV do not present with inguinal bulging on physical exam, ultrasound has been considered a useful tool in predicting the development of hernias. It has been observed that 71% of boys with symptomatic inguinal hernias had type III anatomy, and 50% of girls with symptomatic hernias had type II anatomy [14]. Ultrasound has relatively limited utility in girls over the age of 2 years because of the difficulty in finding the internal inguinal ring on ultrasound examination.

Seventy percent of irreducible hernias occur in children under the age of 1 year, with a slight increased incidence in girls [15]. In addition to the signs and symptoms suggestive of an acute abdomen, including pain, vomiting, and irritability, a groin mass is frequently detected (Fig. 5). Hernias may contain bowel, omentum, or ovaries [16]. The majority (70%) of girls whose hernias contain fallopian tubes or ovaries are seen under the age of 5 years [17]. It is not infrequent that ovaries contained within a hernia will undergo torsion, such that the assessment of an inguinal hernia for the presence of ovaries is critical. Even upon return to the peritoneal cavity, previously torsed ovaries often have impaired function [15].

Intussusception, in which a more proximal loop of bowel becomes telescoped into more distal bowel, is said to be the most common cause for the acute abdomen in infancy. The majority (75%) occurs under the age of 2 years, is slightly more common in males than in females, and has an increased incidence in the spring and fall. The classic clinical triad of colicky abdominal pain, bloody stool, and a palpable mass is present in only about 50%. The preponderance (90%) of cases are idiopathic, in which it is felt that hypertrophied lymphatic tissues serve as a lead point [17].

For many years the imaging of possible intussusception had relied on plain films, although the limited sensitivity and lack of specificity of findings

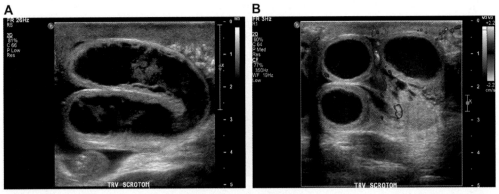

*Fig. 5.* (*A, B*) This 2-week-old patient had had a history of meconium peritonitis and large bilateral hydroceles containing on the first day of life. Multiple thick walled loops of bowel are seen within the scrotum. Note the calcified meconium in the upper right hand corner of image A.

was well recognized. Plain films are felt to be diagnostic in only about 50% of cases. Nonspecific signs on plain films include soft tissue obscuring the liver tip, absence of gas in the right lower quadrant of the abdomen, and small bowel obstruction. A meniscus sign in which air in the intussuscipiens outlines the apex of the intussusceptum is seen in a minority (30%) of patients, while a target sign in which a soft tissue mass with surrounding lucency corresponding to the mesenteric fat wrapping around the intussusceptum is seen in as many as 63% of patients [17]. It is this latter sign which has the well-described ultrasound correlate of a donut sign, a hypoechoic rim corresponding to the edematous muscularis of the bowel wall surrounding an echogenic center, which corresponds to mesenteric fat (Figs. 6–8). Similarly, the target sign, in which there is an anechoic center representing fluid, has been described. Other descriptors of the ultrasonographic appearance of an intussusception include "pseudokidney," the "sandwich sign" (hypoechoic bands separated by linear echogenic bands of mesenteric fat), and a "hayfork." The ultrasound diagnosis of intussusception is highly sensitive (98%–100%) and slightly less specific (88%)

and has a negative predictive value of 100% [17]. Similar appearances may be seen in other entities with bowel wall thickening, including Crohn's disease and Henoch-Schonlein purpura.

Certain ultrasonographic features are predictive of a decreased success rate of nonsurgical reduction. These include absence of flow to the bowel wall and the presence of anechoic rings, alternating with the hypoechoic rings of the muscularis and the echogenic rings of mesenteric fat [17]. The anechoic rings reflect fluid trapped between the serosal layers of the intussuscepted bowel. Another feature, which when present connotes a decreased rate of success with attempts at reduction, is the presence of lymph nodes [16].

Ultrasound also has a role in determining if there is a pathologic lead point. Navarro and colleagues [18] assessed 43 cases of intussusception caused by pathologic lead points (PLPs) in which 23 PLPs were seen by ultrasound, and in 11 of whom ultrasound was able to make a specific diagnosis. Although there may be a history of recurrent intussusceptions when there is a PLP, the majority will have only a single event. Intussusceptions caused by PLPs may be associated with weight loss and

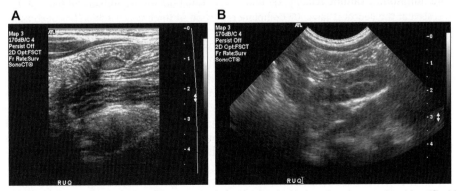

*Fig. 6.* (*A, B*) This 15-month-old child with crampy abdominal pain had an intussusception identified by ultrasound in the right upper quadrant. Ovoid structures compatible with lymph nodes were contained within.

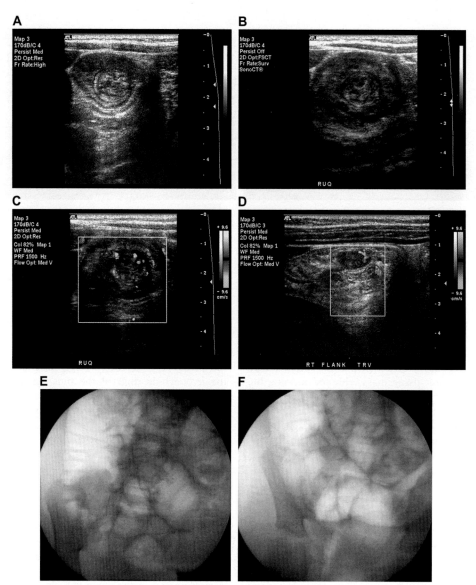

*Fig. 7.* (*A*) This 2-year-old patient's intussusception also included lymph nodes. (*B, C*) It was successfully reduced and then recurred one day later. Color Doppler revealed that the bowel was viable, and it was again reduced pneumatically. (*D*) Nearly 2 years later, there was another recurrence and again lymph nodes were seen associated with the intussusception. (*E*) As previously, pneumatic reduction was attempted. On this image, the intussusceptum is seen at the ileocecal valve. (*F*) Complete reduction of the intussusception has been achieved, and the intussusceptum is no longer seen.

can be in a variety of locations, while idiopathic intussusceptions tend to present acutely and are most commonly ileocolic. Navarro and colleagues [19] noted that approximately 26% with recurrent intussusception had a pathologic lead point, compared with 5.3% with a single episode. They further determined that ultrasound was able to determine an exact diagnosis in 60% with a focal lead point. Ultrasound can depict the relatively specific appearance of an inverted Meckel's diverticulum functioning as a pathologic lead point. The tip of the

diverticulum and its artery are surrounded by fat, which is brought into the center as the diverticulum inverts. The fat surrounding a Meckel's diverticulum will reflect the typical bulbous or tear drop shape of the diverticulum, in contrast to the crescentic shape on transverse images of mesenteric fat surrounding the distal ileum, for example, in an idiopathic intussusception [20]. Ultrasound can also be used to assess the success of nonsurgical reduction or to guide such reductions, as in the case of saline enemas, which have efficacy between 76.5% and 95.5%

A   B

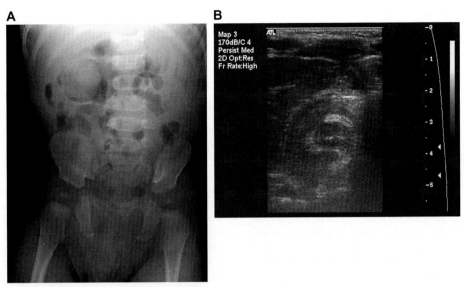

*Fig. 8.* (*A*) This patient presented with vomiting. A plain film showed the soft tissue mass of the intussusceptum inside the lumen of the intussuscipiens at the hepatic flexure. (*B*) Ultrasound revealed the classic concentric rings of an intussusception, reflecting the hypoechoic muscularis of the intussuscipiens surrounding an echogenic ring, consisting of the mucosa of the intussuscipiens and mesenteric fat surrounding the hypoechoic muscularis of the intussusceptum surrounding the echogenic mucosa of the intussusceptum.

[21]. Additionally it can be used during the performance of pneumatic reduction [22]; in that situation, the pitfall in which air enters the terminal ileum before reduction can be avoided. However one pitfall that may be encountered is the identification of a persistent donut sign; even if reduction has been successful, a donut appearance of edematous bowel may still be seen.

## Other bowel associated pathology seen in the pediatric population

Hemolytic uremic syndrome (HUS) is comprised of a triad of hemolytic anemia, thrombocytopenia, and decreased renal function [23]. It is often associated with the 0157 strain of *E coli*, which elaborates a verotoxin that has affinity for and is toxic to the endothelial cells of vessels, particularly those of the renal microvasculature where there is a high receptor density for the endotoxin [23]. HUS is quite similar clinically to thrombotic thrombocytopenic purpura (TTP). Frequently the two entities are distinguished based on clinical manifestations, such that when neurologic manifestations predominate, a diagnosis of TTP is made, and when renal dysfunction predominates, a diagnosis of HUS is made. HUS may be seen with or without a diarrheal prodrome. When associated with diarrhea, it is often referred to as the epidemic form; this is the form of HUS that is most commonly seen in children. Not only is it associated with the ingestion of undercooked meat, unpasteurized milk, and

certain fruits and vegetables, but person to person transmission has also been described in the setting of day care centers and nursing homes [24]. There are a variety of bowel pathologies that may account for abdominal pain and bloody diarrhea in these patients, including colitis, intussusception, necrosis, and perforation. There have been very few reports of the use of ultrasound in its diagnosis, however. Friedland and colleagues [25] did describe color Doppler findings of an avascular, thick-walled colon that was felt to be helpful in distinguishing the GI prodrome of HUS from other hemorrhagic colitides. The utility of ultrasound in the diagnosis of intussusception has already been discussed elsewhere in this article and will be considered further in the discussion of Henoch-Schonlein purpura.

Henoch-Schonlein purpura (HSP) is an IgA mediated inflammation affecting small blood vessels. The Michel criteria for the diagnosis include palpable purpura, history of bowel angina, gastrointestinal bleeding, hematuria, age less than 20 years at time of diagnosis, and absence of medications before the onset of symptoms [26]. Despite the fact that one of the Michel criteria is age less than 20 years, HSP can also occur in adults. The GI symptoms are similar in both children and adults, whereas renal manifestations are increased in severity in adults [26]. Complaints referable to the abdomen are quite common in pediatric patients with HSP, being seen in approximately 60% in one study of 261 patients [27]. About one third of these patients had GI bleeding, in seven of whom it was grossly bloody, one had an acute intussusception, and one had a bowel perforation.

Numerous studies [28–32] have investigated the utility of ultrasound in the setting of children with HSP and abdominal pain. The findings most often described were those of hypoechoic, asymmetric thickening of the bowel wall, bowel dilatation, free fluid, and hypomotility [29,31,32]. Intussusception and evidence of perforation were less common [29,30]. In the study of Connolly and O'Halpin [31] of 44 children with HSP, 15 underwent ultrasound examination. All showed bowel wall thickening, 67% had free fluid, 50% had dilated bowel, and 33% showed intussusception, including two patients who had recurrent intussusceptions (Fig. 9). Approximately half of the intussusceptions were described as being "loose," denoting the fact that there was fluid between the intussusceptum and the intussuscipiens. Repeat ultrasounds were performed in 12 of 15 children; all demonstrated resolution of abnormal findings. Couture and colleagues [30] report on the evaluation of abdominal pain in HSP with high frequency ultrasound assessed bowel wall thickening more specifically. An abnormally thickened wall measured between 3 mm and 11 mm. Involvement was noted to be diffuse in 6 of 14 and focal in the remainder, in whom it was most common that the duodenum was involved. Three children were demonstrated to have intussusceptions by ultrasound.

Because of their relatively small size, most children are well suited to be evaluated with ultrasound when appendicitis is being considered. Ultrasound has been demonstrated to have high sensitivity (94%) and specificity (89%) [33]. The findings considered to be indicative of appendicitis are the same in children as in adults: an appendix measuring more than 6 mm from outer wall to outer wall which does not compress (Figs. 10 and 11).

Other ultrasonographic findings reported by Vignault and colleagues [33] in children with appendicitis included free fluid in 40% (in relatively equal numbers of those with and without perforation at surgery), lymph nodes measuring more than 4 mm (19%), and a fecalith in 14% (not seen on plain film in three out of five in whom it was identified on ultrasound) (Fig. 12). Amongst those with a dilated, noncompressible appendix, three different patterns were seen: (1) in those with the least advanced disease, there were three concentric circles: a central hypoechoic ring representing pus, an echogenic ring of submucosa, and a hypoechoic outer ring of muscularis; (2) with more advanced disease, the echogenic submucosal line was not present, suggesting ulceration or disruption of the mucosa; (3) a diffusely hypoechoic tubular structure with increased through transmission was felt to reflect a pus filled appendix. Other studies have compared the sensitivity and specificity of ultrasound and CT in making the diagnosis of appendicitis [34,35]. In one study of 270 children [34], the sensitivity of ultrasound was considerably lower (74%) than in Vignault's study, while in another study of 600 children, the sensitivity of ultrasound was 86%, more nearly approximating Vignault's study.

Although there is a relatively long list of entities that can mimic appendicitis clinically, including inflammatory bowel disease, intussusception, Meckel's diverticulitis, omental infarction, and renal and ovarian pathologies [36], the entity which is most commonly present when appendicitis is not diagnosed is mesenteric adenitis. In fact, it has been said that the most common medical cause of acute abdominal pain in children is mesenteric adenitis [37]. Because of the frequent association of enlarged lymph nodes with inflammation of the bowel, mesenteric adenitis and terminal ileitis are often thought of as a constellation of findings

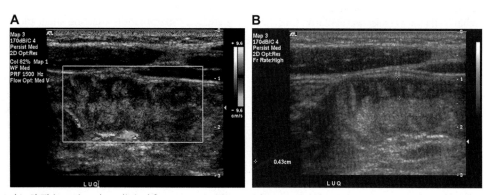

Fig. 9. (*A*, *B*) This patient has clinical features consistent with Henoch-Schonlein purpura and had complained of abdominal pain. The question of a small bowel intussusception was raised. None was seen, but several loops of edematous, hyperemic bowel were seen on ultrasound examination.

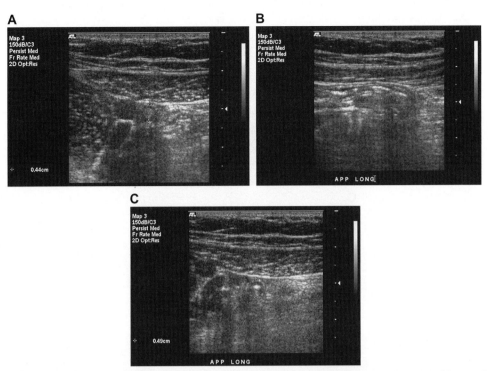

*Fig. 10.* There is debate regarding how often the normal appendix can be seen with certainty. In this case, it was easily identifiable (*A*), measuring .44 cm and compressed (*B*) with graded compression on this longitudinal image. The focus of increased echogenicity seen on this image (*C*) does not shadow as would an appendicolith; it represents air in the appendiceal lumen.

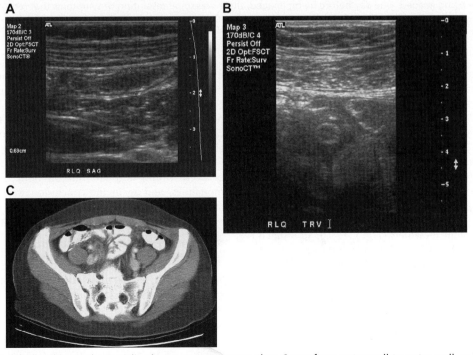

*Fig. 11.* (*A*) The abnormal appendix always measures more than 6 mm from outer wall to outer wall, as in the longitudinal image of the appendix seen here, which measures 6.9 mm and did not compress. No hyperemia was noted. (*B*) In this young woman, there was difficulty distinguishing ovarian and appendiceal pathology. (*C*) While somewhat difficult to identify, it appeared that there was a noncompressible tubular structure measuring 1.01 cm. CT verified that the appendix was abnormal, but demonstrated no additional findings of appendicitis.

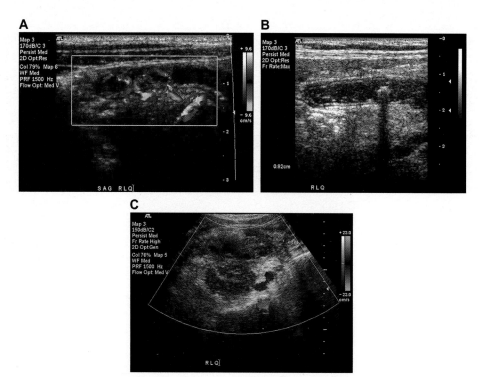

*Fig. 12.* (*A*) This appendix was not only thickened and noncompressible, but also demonstrated marked hyperemia. (*B*) In this case of appendicitis, in addition to dilation and noncompressibility, there was an echogenic, shadowing focus compatible with an appendicolith. The mesenteric fat was felt to be of increased echogenicity as well. (*C*) This patient with a markedly elevated white blood cell count (> 20,000) had initially presented 3 days before being imaged. One day before being imaged, there was some resolution of symptoms that returned on the day of imaging. The appendix itself was not seen, but the heterogeneous collection seen was felt to represent a phlegmon or developing abscess.

rather than as separate entities. Lymph nodes felt to be pathologic by imaging criteria measure more than 4 mm in antereo-posterior dimension, are more numerous, less echogenic, more sharply defined, and more commonly spherical in their shape than nonpathologic nodes [38]. Additional imaging findings in the mesenteric adenitis/terminal ileitis constellation include nodularity of small bowel folds, circumferential mucosal thickening, foci of hypoechogenicity within the submucosa reflecting hypertrophied Peyer's patches, and thickening of the mesentery (Fig. 13) [39]. Although it is tempting to assign a diagnosis of mesenteric adenitis to all children with abdominal pain who have enlarged lymph nodes on ultrasound examination, this opinion is not without controversy. In the study of Sivit and colleagues [40], which compared symptomatic with asymptomatic children, enlarged nodes were identified in 14% of those with symptoms and 4% of those without (Fig. 14). Forty six percent of the symptomatic group did have a specific diagnosis established, most commonly appendicitis. The investigators concluded that the presence of enlarged lymph nodes was a nonspecific

finding and not one that would allow a diagnosis to be rendered. In a study performed by Rathaus and colleagues [41], the frequency of mesenteric lymph nodes was assessed on ultrasound and CT in children being imaged for reasons other than acute abdominal pain. Approximately 29% of children were noted to have lymph nodes measuring between 4 mm and 20 mm on both imaging modalities, and again the conclusion was drawn that these nodes were not of significance.

## Malignancy and its complications presenting as an acute abdomen

Wilms tumor is the most common malignancy affecting the kidney in children, and is also one of the most common pediatric intra-abdominal malignancies. If unilateral, the peak age at diagnosis is 41.5 months in males and 46.9 months in females; the peak age at diagnosis is considerably lower in those in whom the tumor is bilateral, 29.5 months in males and 32.6 months in females [42]. Ultrasound has been an important part of the diagnostic armamentarium in children with

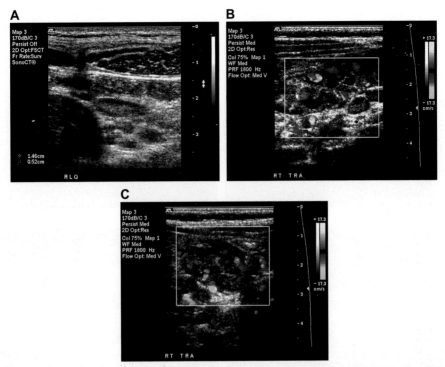

**Fig. 13.** (A) Frequently patients with suspected appendicitis do not have sonographic evidence of the disease, but do show enlarged lymph nodes as seen here, where the largest measured 1.5 cm by 0.5 cm. There is much controversy regarding whether this truly represents an entity of mesenteric adenitis. (B, C) In other cases of suspected appendicitis, enlarged lymph nodes are seen in association with thick walled terminal ileum. Many investigators believe this to represent a constellation of findings representing terminal ileitis/mesenteric adenitis.

abdominal masses because of its ability to distinguish solid from cystic masses, the absence of radiation, and the relatively short examination time, obviating sedation. A limitation has been the inability to assess the organ of origin of a large mass with certainty, something that can be more easily done using the multiplanar capabilities of CT and MR imaging. On the other hand, ultrasound's advantage over CT in assessing invasion of the renal vein and inferior vena cava has been recognized.

Children with Wilms tumor most commonly present with a nontender flank mass. A minority will have symptoms referred to the kidney, such as hematuria, dysuria, or hypertension, or may have constitutional symptoms of malaise, weight loss, or anemia. Rarely, a child with Wilms tumor will present with a left-sided hydrocele caused by obstruction of the left spermatic vein by the tumor. In addition, children with Wilms tumor may present with abdominal pain. In fact, when the 250 patients treated at the Children's Hospital of Philadelphia between 1970 and 1995 were reviewed [43], it was determined that 14% had presented with a chief complaint of abdominal pain.

Amongst these patients, 50% had presented with peritoneal signs. Those who presented with abdominal pain were noted to have higher grade tumors (stage I 6%, stage II 23%, stage III 52%, stage IV 20%) as compared with those who presented with other symptoms (stage I 47%, stage II 15%, stage III 23%, stage IV 15%) and tended to be older (mean age of 5.5 years versus 3.8 years). It is believed that in cases where there has been intraperitoneal rupture, abdominal pain is secondary to peritoneal irritation by blood products or tumor [44]. In those cases where there has been no rupture, it is surmised that abdominal pain results from stretching of the renal capsule because of bleeding into the tumor. If a renal tumor is discovered when imaging a child with abdominal pain, it is important to remember to do a thorough assessment of the contralateral kidney, as well as a Doppler evaluation of the ipsilateral renal vein and inferior vena cava. Although vascular invasion will not upstage the tumor, it will dictate the surgical approach. In those cases in which there has been intraperitoneal rupture, there will be ascites with echogenic material as a component. Preoperative rupture of the tumor will lead to its stage being

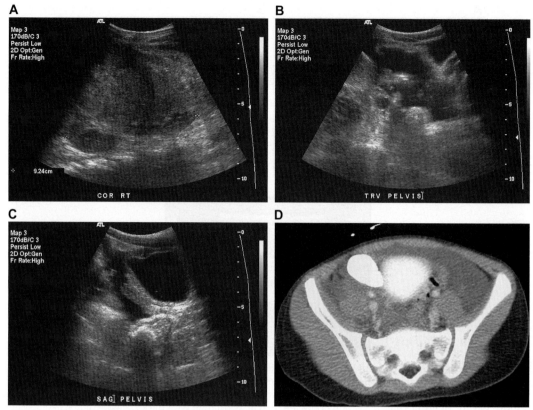

**Fig. 14.** (A) This 5-year-old patient presented with diffuse abdominal pain and a right flank mass on physical exam. Ultrasound showed a slightly heterogeneous mass that appeared to emanate from the right kidney. (B, C) Images of the pelvis revealed free fluid with echogenic, layering debris. (D) CT confirmed that the right kidney was the organ of origin of the mass and demonstrated that free fluid secondary to rupture of the mass was present throughout the abdomen and pelvis.

changed from II to III, even if the kidney can be entirely resected, just as intraoperative rupture will lead to upgrading of the tumor.

## Summary

There are many challenges when faced with a child with an acute abdomen. The difficulties in diagnosis can be reduced by considering the age of the child and any associated symptoms, such as rash or renal insufficiency. Significant challenges will remain for a variety of reasons, including young age and inability to verbalize the exact location of pain, and the inevitable confusion that ovarian pathology can create in the adolescent female with lower abdominal pain. There are multiple ways in which ultrasound can be used in the assessment of these children. It can direct the physician to the organ of origin of the patient's symptoms and can be useful in separating out conditions which need to be treated surgically from those which need to be treated medically. Color Doppler flow imaging can provide additional useful diagnostic and prognostic information.

## References

[1] Kim W-Y, Kim SK, Kim J-O, et al. Sonographic evaluation of neonates with early stage necrotizing enterocolitis. Pediatr Radiol 2005;35:1056–61.

[2] Tam AL, Cambreros A, Applebaum H. Surgical decision making in NEC and focal intestinal perforation: predictive value of radiologic findings. J Pediatr Surg 2002;37(912):1688–91.

[3] Lindley S, Mollett DL, Seibert JJ, et al. Portal vein ultrasonography in the early diagnosis of necrotizing enterocolitis. J Pediatr Surg 1986;21(6): 530–2.

[4] Miller SF, Seibert JJ, Kinder DL, et al. Use of ultrasound in the detection of occult bowel perforation in neonates. J Ultrasound Med 1993; 12(9):531–5.

[5] Fangold R, Daneman A, Tomlinson G, et al. Necrotizing enterocolitis: assessment of bowel viability with color Doppler ultrasound. Radiology 2005;235:587–94.

[6] Strouse P. Disorders of intestinal rotation and fixation ("malrotation"). Pediatr Radiol 2004; 34:837–51.

[7] Weinberger E, Winters WD, Liddell RM, et al. Sonographic diagnosis of intestinal malrotation in infants: importance of relative positions of SMV and SMA. AJR Am J Roentgenol 1992;159(4):825–8.

[8] Pracros JP, Sann L, Genin G, et al. Ultrasound diagnosis of midgut volvulus: the "whirlpool" sign. Pediatr Radiol 1992;22(1):18–20.

[9] Orzech N, Navarro O, Langer J. Is ultrasonography a good screening test for intestinal malrotation? J Pediatr Surg 2006;41(5):1005–9.

[10] Chao HC, Kong MS, Chen JY, et al. Sonographic features related to volvulus in neonatal intestinal malrotation. J Ultrasound Med 2000;19(6):371–6.

[11] Shimanuki Y, Aikara T, Takano H, et al. Clockwise whirlpool sign at color Doppler US: an objective and definite sign of midgut volvulus. Radiology 1996;199(1):261–4.

[12] Patino MO, Munden MM. Utility of sonographic whirlpool sign in diagnosing midgut volvulus in patients with atypical clinical presentations. J Ultrasound Med 2004;23(3):397–401.

[13] Rathaus V, Konen O, Shapiro M, et al. Ultrasound features of spermatic cord hydrocele in children. British J of Radiology 2001;74:818–20.

[14] Tobi A, Watanabe Y, Sasaki K, et al. Ultrasonographic diagnosis for potential contralateral inguinal hernia in children. J Pediatr Surg 2003; 39:224–6.

[15] Merriman TE, Auldist AW. Ovarian torsion in inguinal hernias. Pediatr Surg Int 2000; 16(5–6):383–5.

[16] Babcock D. Sonography of the acute abdomen in the pediatric patient. J Ultrasound Med 2002; 21(8):887–99.

[17] Fowler C. Sliding indirect hernia containing both ovaries. J Pediatr Surg 2005;40(9):e13–4.

[18] Navarro O, Dugougeat F, Kornecki A, et al. The impact of imaging in the management of intussusception owing to pathologic lead points in children: a review of 43 cases. Pediatr Radiol 2000;30:594–603.

[19] Navarro O, Daneman A, Chae A. The use of delayed repeated reduction attempts and the management of pathologic lead points in pediatric patients. AJR Am J Roentgenol 2004;182:1169–76.

[20] Daneman A, Myers M, Shuckett B, et al. Sonographic appearances of inverted Meckel diverticulum with intussusception. Pediatr Radiol 1997; 27:295–8.

[21] Sorantin E, Lindbichler F. Management of Intussusception. Eur Radiol 2004;(Suppl 4):L146–54.

[22] Lee JH, Choi SH, Jeong YK, et al. Intermittent sonographic guidance in air enema for reduction of childhood intussusception. J Ultrasound Med 2006;25(9):1125–30.

[23] Lin J, Hutzler M, Li C, et al. Thrombotic thrombocytopenic purpura (TTP) and hemolytic uremic syndrome (HUS): the new thinking. J Thromb Thrombolysis 2001;11(3):261–72.

[24] Amirlak I, Amirlak B. Hemolytic uraemic syndrome: an overview. Nephrology 2006; 11(3):213–8.

[25] Friedland JA, Herman TE, Siegel MJ. Escherichia coli 0157:H7—associated hemolytic uremic syndrome: value of colonic Doppler sonography. Pediatr Radiol 1995;25(Suppl 1):565–7.

[26] Garcia-Porrua C, Calvino MC, Llorca J, et al. Henoch-Schonlein purpura in children and adults: clinical differences in a defined population. Semin Arthritis Rheum 2002;32(3):149–56.

[27] Chang WL, Yang YH, Lin TY, et al. GI manifestations in HSP: a review of 261 patients. Acta Paediatr 2004;93(11):1127–31.

[28] Hu SC, Feeney MS, McNicholas M, et al. Ultrasonography to diagnose and exclude intussusception in Henoch-Schonlein purpura. Arch Dis Child 1991;66(9):1065–7.

[29] Bomelburg T, Claasen U, von Lengerke HJ. Intestinal ultrasonographic findings in Schonlein-Henoch purpura. Eur J Pediatr 1991;150(3):158–60.

[30] Couture A, Veyrac C, Baud C, et al. Evaluation of abdominal pain in Henoch-Schonlein syndrome by high frequency ultrasound. Pediatr Radiol 1992;22(1):12–7.

[31] Connolly B, O'Halpin D. Sonographic evaluation of the abdomen in Henoch Schonlein purpura. Clin Radiol 1994;49(5):320–3.

[32] Ozdemir H, Isik S, Buyan N, et al. Sonographic demonstration of intestinal involvement in Henoch-Schonlein syndrome. Eur J Radiol 1995;20(1):32–4.

[33] Vignault F, Filiatrault D, Brandt ML, et al. Acute appendicitis in children: evaluation with ultrasound. Radiology 1990;176(2):501–4.

[34] Karakas SP, Gulfquat M, Leonidas JC, et al. Acute appendicitis in children: comparison of clinical diagnosis with ultrasound and CT imaging. Pediatr Radiol 2000;30(2):94–8.

[35] Kaiser S, Jorulf H, Soderman E, et al. Impact of radiologic imaging on the surgical decision making process in suspected appendicitis in children. Acad Radiol 2004;11(9):971–9.

[36] Sung T, Callahan M, Taylor GA. Clinical and imaging mimickers of acute appendicitis in the pediatric population. AJR Am J Roentgenol 2006;186(1):167–74.

[37] Alamduran A, Hirafar M, Zandi B, et al. Diagnostic value of ultrasound findings in mesenteric lymphadenitis in children with acute abdominal pain. Iran J Radiol 2005;2:137–40.

[38] Puylaert J. Mesenteric adenitis and acute terminal ileitis: ultrasound evaluation using graded compression. Radiology 1986;161:691–5.

[39] Swischuk LE, John SD, Tschoepe EJ. Mesenteric adenitis—acute ileitis: a constellation of findings identifiable with ultrasound. Emerg Radiol 1998; 5(4):210–8.

[40] Sivit CJ, Newman KD, Chandra RS. Visualization of enlarged mesenteric lymph nodes at US examination: clinical significance. Pediatr Radiol 1993;23:471–5.

[41] Rathaus V, Shapiro M, Grunebaum M, et al. Enlarged mesenteric lymph nodes in asymptomatic children: the value of the finding in various imaging modalities. Br J Radiol 2005;78(925): 30–3.

[42] Green DM, D'Angio GJ, Beckwith JB, et al. Wilms tumor. CA Cancer J Clinic 1996;46(1):46–63.

[43] Davidoff AM, Soutter AD, Shochat SJ. Wilms tumor presenting with abdominal pain: a special subgroup of patients. Ann Surg Oncol 1998; 5(3):213–5.

[44] Kosloske AM, McIver WJ, Duncan MH. Intraperitoneal rupture of a Wilms' tumor. West J Med 1985;142(5):694–6.

ELSEVIER
SAUNDERS

ULTRASOUND
CLINICS

Ultrasound Clin 2 (2007) 541–559

# Ultrasound Evaluation of Pediatric Abdominal Masses

Sarah Sarvis Milla, MD[a],*, Edward Y. Lee, MD, MPH[b],
Carlo Buonomo, MD[b], Robert T. Bramson, MD[b]

- Diagnostic algorithm
  *Neonatal abdominal masses (younger
  than 12 months of age)*
  *Abdominal masses in the older infant and
  child (greater than 12 months of age)*
- Summary
- Acknowledgment
- References

Ultrasound is a noninvasive imaging modality that aids in diagnosis without the potentially damaging effects of ionizing radiation, a particularly important consideration in the evaluation of pediatric patients. Ultrasound is widely available, easy to use, and reliable; it is therefore the imaging method of choice in evaluating most known or suspected abdominal masses in neonates or older children. This article focuses on the clinical and sonographic features of selected common abdominal masses in infants and children. The authors highlight the important clinical characteristics of these abdominal masses and specific sonographic imaging features that allow clinicians to differentiate among the common abdominal masses in pediatric patients.

## Diagnostic algorithm

When an abdominal mass is suspected by physical examination or plain film radiography, ultrasound is typically the initial imaging modality of choice in infants and children. Often a focused differential diagnosis can be formed from the sonographic imaging characteristics. This allows for an appropriate

discussion of clinical management and recommendation for any further imaging the patient may need.

During the ultrasound examination there are certain characteristics of the mass that should be noted, including echogenicity and vascularity, which help define the internal characteristics and may aid in determining the organ of origin. The larger the abdominal mass, the more difficult it may be to discern the organ of origin. Continuity of the mass with a specific organ and any displacement or mass effect on the organ's internal vascularity may also point to the correct etiology of an abdominal mass. In addition to pinpointing the organ of origin, all other organs and adjacent structures should be closely scrutinized for evidence of direct or indirect involvement, such as invasion of adjacent solid organs, vascular invasion or thrombosis, lymphadenopathy, or involvement of other organs to suggest metastatic disease.

When abdominal masses are imaged by ultrasound, the sonographer should use the optimal transducer, which provides the best image quality (highest possible frequency) while maintaining

[a] Department of Radiology, New York University, 560 First Avenue, New York, NY 10016, USA
[b] Department of Radiology, Children's Hospital Boston and Harvard Medical School, 300 Longwood Avenue, Boston, MA 02115, USA
* Corresponding author.
*E-mail address:* sarahsarvismilla@gmail.com (S.S. Milla).

doi:10.1016/j.cult.2007.08.002

appropriate soft-tissue penetration. Curved array or linear array transducers may be used, depending on patient body habitus. Multiple imaging planes and positions are often required. Fluid intake during the examination may also help in some cases to distinguish bowel from the organ or mass being evaluated or to provide an improved acoustic window.

One of the most important considerations in formulating a differential diagnosis is the patient's age. For example, the most commonly found abdominal masses in neonates rarely present in older children and vice versa. Once the respective pathologic entities are understood, a narrow and accurate list of differential diagnoses can be made by considering sonographic characteristics and patient demographics, such as age and sex. After an appropriate discussion of the differential diagnoses, recommendations for any necessary additional imaging can be made.

## Neonatal abdominal masses (younger than 12 months of age)

### Kidneys

Approximately two thirds of neonatal abdominal masses are renal in origin, most of benign etiology [1]. Hydronephrosis and cystic renal pathology in the neonate account for most of these renal masses. The differential diagnosis for a solid renal mass in the neonate is limited, however, led by mesoblastic nephroma and distantly followed by Wilms tumor.

The increased use of prenatal ultrasound has resulted in the diagnosis of many abnormalities in utero, alerting clinicians to potential problems later in gestational age or following delivery. Once fetal defects have been identified, additional abdominal imaging typically takes places early in the neonatal period. Approximately 1% of all fetal ultrasounds reveal a significant abnormality. Among fetal abnormalities, those affecting genitourinary organs and systems are second in prevalence only to cardiac anomalies, with hydronephrosis being the most common genitourinary abnormality [2,3]. Common causes of neonatal hydronephrosis include ureteropelvic obstruction, vesicoureteral reflux, ureterovesicular junction obstruction (ie, primary megaureter), and the presence of posterior urethral valves.

The most common cause of neonatal hydronephrosis is ureteropelvic junction obstruction (UPJO), with an incidence of 1 in every 1000 births. Typically unilateral and more commonly presenting in boys, UPJO is reported to be the cause of approximately 50% of cases of prenatally diagnosed hydronephrosis [4–8]. Etiologies of UPJO include an adynamic short segment of proximal ureter, a remnant fold within the ureteral lumen resulting in backup of urine in the collecting system, and a vessel that crosses the UPJ that results in occasional obstruction and flank pain in older patients. The sonographic findings of UPJO are typically limited to dilation of the renal pelvis without ureteral or bladder abnormalities (Fig. 1). UPJO can also be associated with other renal abnormalities, however, such as vesicoureteral reflux, or it can be part of a duplicated collecting system, which can make the diagnosis more difficult to make by sonography. The treatment for UPJO is somewhat controversial and varies slightly, depending on the etiology of the UPJO and the individual practices of the urologist managing the patient [9,10]. Treatment may begin with watchful waiting and prophylactic antibiotics. Differential renal function, change in

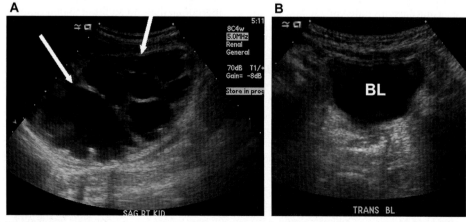

**Fig. 1.** Newborn who had a ureteropelvic junction obstruction. (*A*) Longitudinal image of the kidney demonstrates severe hydronephrosis without dilation of the ureter. Marked renal cortical thinning is seen (*arrows* indicate thinned cortex). (*B*) Transverse image of the bladder (*BL*) demonstrates the absence of dilated distal ureters.

the clinical picture, or change in imaging characteristics, however, may ultimately result in surgical intervention [9,10].

Posterior urethral valves (PUV) are caused by a malformation in the posterior urethra of boys, with an incidence reported from 1 in 5000 to 1 in 8000 male births [11]. PUV is the cause of 10% of all fetal hydronephrosis, but with increased prenatal screening this defect is now detected and treated earlier. Sonography of patients who have PUV demonstrates a trabeculated, thick-walled bladder, often with diverticula. Occasionally a dilated posterior urethra can be visualized, particularly if using a transperineal approach [12]. Vesicoureteral reflux is common in these boys, seen in approximately 30% of patients [13]. The presence of reflux allows the pressure and urine to decompress into the ureters and renal collecting systems, often causing significant enlargement of the ureters and resulting in pelvocaliectasis that is typically easily detected on sonography. Renal cortical thinning and increased cortical echogenicity can also be seen. If the pressure has further decompressed by rupture of a fornix and pyelosinus extravasation, a urinoma may be visualized (Fig. 2). The obstructed valve is cleared by surgical excision or fulguration.

Vesicoureteral reflux (VUR) is a common condition, with an estimated incidence of greater than 10% [14]. Primary VUR is caused by an abnormal insertion of the distal ureter into the bladder. The severity scale typically used refers to the amount of retrograde flow and any secondary dilation of the ureter and renal collecting system. In many mild cases of reflux, and less frequently in moderate or severe cases, there may be no sonographic findings in neonates who have VUR. In the more moderate to severe cases, hydroureteronephrosis is usually seen with a normal-appearing bladder.

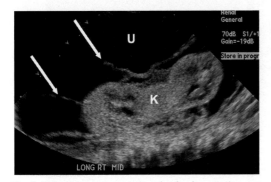

*Fig. 2.* Urinoma in a neonate who had posterior urethral valves. Longitudinal imaging demonstrates absence of significant hydronephrosis in the right kidney (*K*), which is surrounded by a hypoechoic collection with septae (*arrows*). This collection was a urinoma (*U*) caused by caliceal rupture owing to high collecting system pressures.

Focal or diffuse renal cortical thinning and increased cortical echogenicity can be seen, indicating long-standing reflux with scarring. Uroendothelial thickening can sometimes be seen sonographically as focal nodular or diffuse echogenic thickening of the collecting system and ureter.

The diagnosis is generally made on voiding cystourethrography (VCUG) or by a radionuclide cystogram (RNC). Although VCUG delivers a higher radiation dose and has slightly lower sensitivity, it offers finer detail and can demonstrate important findings, such as an ectopic insertion site; hence, it is the study of choice when evaluating a neonate who has a history of urinary tract infections and fever. Because of strong familial patterns of reflux (approximately 27% in siblings), siblings are screened, often by RNC [14]. Treatment of VUR depends on the grade of reflux, the clinical situation, and the degree of renal function [15]. In lower grades of reflux, the ureteral insertion angle often normalizes with bladder growth. More severe grades of reflux, however, frequently require surgical ureteral reimplantation to avoid continued reflux with resultant renal scarring and permanent renal damage.

Another cause of neonatal hydronephrosis is ureterovesicular junction obstruction (UVJO). This entity is also known as primary obstructing megaureter. Bilateral involvement is present in approximately 20% of patients who have UVJO, with left-sided predominance in unilateral disease. Primary obstructed megaureter is three to four times more likely to occur in male than in female infants [14,16]. Primary obstructing megaureter is caused by an aperistaltic segment of ureter at the ureterovesical junction. Sonographic findings of UVJO include a dilated distal ureter, and to a lesser extent, dilation of the proximal ureter and renal collecting system (Fig. 3). If reflux is concurrently present, a VCUG often demonstrates a short segment of normal caliber distal ureter at the UVJ. In the differential for primary obstructive megaureter is severe VUR. The treatment for UVJO has typically been resection of the aperistaltic segment of ureter with tapering and reimplantation. In recent years, however, nonoperative management with prophylactic antibiotics and close follow-up is often attempted first [17].

A completely duplicated collecting system is seen in 1 of 500 individuals, and by definition these individuals have at least one ectopically inserted distal ureter [18]. The Weigert-Meyer rule states that the upper pole duplicated system typically has an ectopic inferomedially inserted ureter that often becomes obstructed, causing dilation of the upper pole collecting system. This upper pole ureter can insert into the bladder neck, proximal urethra, or, in girls, into the vagina. The rule also states that the lower pole, which can also be ectopically

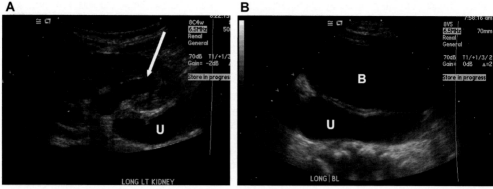

**Fig. 3.** Newborn who had primary megaureter. (*A*) Longitudinal image of the left kidney demonstrates mild to moderate hydronephrosis (*arrow*) and a moderately to severely dilated proximal ureter (*U*). (*B*) Longitudinal view of the bladder (*B*), slightly to the left of midline, demonstrating a moderately to severely dilated distal left ureter (*U*).

inserted, often demonstrates reflux. On ultrasound the duplex kidney is larger than a single-system kidney and has separate upper and lower renal collecting systems. If these collecting systems are not dilated, this can be a subtle finding. Often, however, one collecting system is more dilated than the other, which may suggest the presence of the anomaly. When scanning in a transverse orientation, the appearance of the interpolar region of the kidney lacks a visualized collecting system, the sonographic correlate to the so-called "faceless kidney" on CT imaging of duplex kidneys. At least one of the ureters is often dilated and can be visualized sonographically. The upper pole ureter can form a ureterocele at its bladder insertion site, seen as a round anechoic structure with a thin echogenic rim within the bladder (Fig. 4A).

VCUG can demonstrate a ureterocele on early filling images (Fig. 4B), document reflux, and suggest duplication by an abnormal angulation or smaller-than-expected size of the contrast-filled lower pole collecting system. Management for these patients is similar to that for other neonates who have hydronephrosis. Specifically, to avoid or minimize renal damage in these patients, the insertion sites of ectopically positioned ureters are typically surgically repaired, particularly if causing ureteral obstruction or vesicoureteral reflux or in a significantly ectopic position (eg, the vaginal ureteral insertion site).

Multicystic dysplastic kidney (MCDK) is another condition that typically presents in the antenatal period, with renal cystic abnormalities first identified on prenatal screening. MCDK has a unilateral

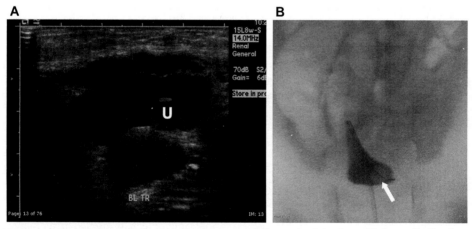

**Fig. 4.** Ureterocele in a 21-day-old infant who had a prenatal diagnosis of duplicated left renal collecting system. (*A*) Transverse image through the bladder demonstrates a round, thin-walled, anechoic structure (*U*) seen within the bladder to the left of midline representing a ureterocele. The ureterocele is the distal portion of the ectopically inserted upper pole ureter. (*B*) Early filling images of the same patient's VCUG demonstrate a filling defect representing the ureterocele (*arrow*). Subsequent images from the VCUG demonstrate reflux into the left lower pole system. The bladder catheter seen is a neonatal feeding tube.

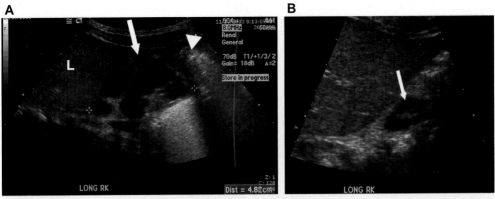

*Fig. 5.* Multicystic dysplastic kidney in a neonate. (*A*) Longitudinal imaging of the right kidney demonstrates multiple cystic areas within the kidney (*arrow*) that do not communicate with the renal pelvis. The liver is seen superiorly (*L*) and echogenic bowel loops are seen inferiorly (*arrowhead*). (*B*) Eight months later the multicystic dysplastic kidney (*arrow*) is much smaller. Continued follow-up (not shown) showed regression of the dysplastic kidney.

incidence of 1 in 2500 to 1 in 4200 children, and a bilateral incidence of 1 in 25,000, with a male predominance in unilateral disease and female predominance in bilateral disease [19–21]. Patients who have unilateral disease often have a contralateral abnormality, with UPJO in 3% to 12% and reflux in 18% to 43% [20]. The fetuses diagnosed with bilateral disease, however, do not usually survive long after birth owing to the most serious sequela of oligohydramnios, lung hypoplasia. MCDK is believed to occur secondary to high-grade stenosis at the UPJ. Many investigators believe it is the extreme end of the UPJO spectrum. On sonography, multiple round anechoic structures of varying sizes are seen within the dysplastic kidney; however, the overall total size of the dysplastic kidney at birth can be enlarged. No ureter or collecting system is typically visualized in this condition, excepting the rare incidence of an MCDK in one pole of a duplicated collecting system. In this case, the cystic, dysplastic pole (typically occurring in the upper pole moiety) does not demonstrate a focal collecting system or ureter. The appearance of MCDK is classic, and most patients are followed by ultrasound to demonstrate involution of the MCDK (Fig. 5) [22]. There have been a few reports of Wilms tumors developing in multicystic dysplastic kidneys, which have lent support to arguments for prophylactic nephrectomy. This, however, is not considered standard of care and is controversial [21].

Autosomal recessive polycystic kidney disease (ARPKD), a genetic condition often imaged in the perinatal period because it is most commonly detected by an abnormal prenatal renal sonogram, is also classified in the cystic renal disease category. ARPKD results from ectasia, dilation, and elongation of the renal tubules. Patients with ARPKD

often have biliary ductal ectasia also; the severity is typically inversely proportional to the renal involvement. That is, severe renal involvement typically presents with mild hepatic disease and vice versa [23]. ARPKD kidneys can have a variable phenotypic and sonographic appearance. If presenting in the neonatal period, the disease is typically severe and sonography demonstrates enlarged and echogenic kidneys with poor corticomedullary differentiation caused by dilated collecting ducts causing multiple acoustic interfaces with the ultrasound beam (Fig. 6) [24,25]. Treatment for ARPKD patients is supportive, with close renal and hepatic monitoring. Dialysis and renal transplant are end-stage treatments available to those who have severe disease resulting in renal failure.

Congenital mesoblastic nephroma (CMN) is the most common abdominal neoplasm in the neonate

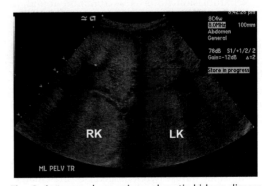

*Fig. 6.* Autosomal recessive polycystic kidney disease in a neonate who had a distended abdomen. Transverse imaging of the pelvis reveals enlarged right (*RK*) and left (*LK*) kidneys with tiny peripheral, round, anechoic spaces and loss of corticomedullary differentiation.

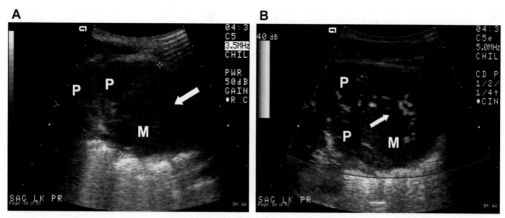

**Fig. 7.** Mesoblastic nephroma in a 1-day-old infant who had a renal abnormality seen on prenatal ultrasound. (*A*) Longitudinal gray-scale image demonstrates normal hypoechoic medullary pyramids (*P*) in the upper pole of the left kidney and a mass (*M*) in the lower pole of the left kidney, with mild heterogeneity and central hypoechogenicity (*arrow*). (*B*) Longitudinal Doppler image demonstrates normal hypoechoic medullary pyramids (*P*) in the upper pole of the left kidney and a mass (*M*) in the lower pole of the left kidney, with mild heterogeneity, vascularity, and central hypoechogenicity (*arrow*).

(Fig. 7) [1,26]. CMN can be detected prenatally, but it typically presents in children at a mean age of 3 months as a palpable abdominal mass. CMN is believed to be a generally benign lesion with some malignant potential that warrants nephrectomy and complete resection. Sonographic findings of CMN include a large solid renal mass with heterogeneous or low echogenicity. Color Doppler demonstrates internal flow. A central hypoechoic area representing necrosis can be seen centrally. The tumor may extend beyond the capsule, but does not typically involve the renal vein [27]. Further evaluation of the mass and adjacent structures should be done by CT or MR imaging to exclude metastasis, because these may rarely occur in the case of cellular type pathology. CMN can have a similar appearance to Wilms tumor, but Wilms tumor is statistically less likely given its rare incidence in neonates.

Nephroblastomatosis is a condition found in 25% of patients who have unilateral Wilms tumor and 99% to 100% of patients who have bilateral Wilms tumors [28]. Nephroblastomatosis is defined as the histologic presence of multiple persisting embryonic nephrogenic rests. There are two types of nephrogenic rests: (1) the more common perilobar type, which has a predilection for subcapsular and peripheral locations, and (2) the rarer intralobar type, which has a more random occurrence throughout the parenchyma. Corresponding to diffuse, multifocal, or focal involvement, sonography can demonstrate diffuse hypoechogenicity and enlargement of the kidney with poor corticomedullary differentiation or spherical areas of abnormal echogenicity that are typically hypoechoic, but occasionally iso-, or hyperechoic (Fig. 8) [29]. These patients are considered to be at high risk for developing

Wilms tumor and are generally screened by ultrasound every 3 months for any change in size or appearance and by CT or MR imaging at yearly intervals or whenever there are any suspicious sonographic changes.

### Adrenal gland

The incidence of neuroblastoma (NB) is approximately 1 in 10,000. Neonatal NB represents 30% of all newly diagnosed NB [30]. Prenatal ultrasound has increased the perinatal suspicion for NB. Most patients diagnosed with NB in the perinatal period have a high 5-year survival rate, up to 95%. In a small number of infants, NB presents with a localized primary tumor and metastatic disease confined to the liver, skin, and bone marrow (stage 4S), although these infants have a much better prognosis as opposed to older patients presenting with stage 4

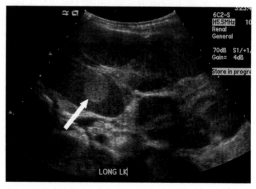

**Fig. 8.** Nephroblastomatosis in a 1-year-old girl. Longitudinal sonogram of the left kidney demonstrates enlargement, with a thickened, lobulated cortex and a focal echogenic nodule (*arrow*).

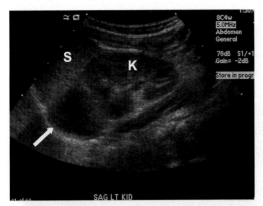

**Fig. 9.** Neuroblastoma in a 6-week-old infant evaluated for pyloric stenosis. Longitudinal sonogram demonstrates a fairly homogeneous mass (*arrow*) located superior to the left kidney (*K*) and inferior to the spleen (*S*).

disease. Regardless of age, all patients whose *MYCN* gene has amplified within the tumor tend to have tumor progression and a poor prognosis.

Sonographic findings in NB vary slightly with stage. Lower stage abdominal NB may present as a mass with homogeneous or slightly heterogeneous echotexture replacing the adrenal gland (Fig. 9). In more advanced stages, the mass is heterogeneous in echotexture, often with echogenic areas caused by calcification and vessels within the mass. These tumors can be large, and it may be difficult to define the tumor as distinctly adrenal. Staging NB depends on whether the tumor extends across the midline and has nodal or distant metastases. All patients who have NB should receive staging CT examinations for evaluation of the extent of disease. MR imaging is often used for additional

imaging, especially if extension into the neural foramina or spinal canal is suspected. Radiolabeled metaiodobenzylguanidine (MIBG) scans are also used to evaluate NB involvement, including cortical bone and bone marrow disease. Treatment for neonatal NB depends on staging. Case studies suggest close monitoring without chemotherapy or radiation for localized disease and stage 4S in neonatal NB, because spontaneous regression has been seen in some cases [31,32]. In the rarer cases of neonatal NB with an intermediate to poor prognosis, adjuvant chemotherapy, surgery, and radiotherapy are performed [33].

Adrenal hemorrhage rarely presents clinically as a mass, but has been detected by ultrasound at a rate of 1.9 cases per 1000 live births. When detected in an acute setting, the sonographic findings include unilateral or bilateral homogeneous masses in the adrenal glands. If imaging is performed in a chronic setting, rim-calcification may be seen as thin, curvilinear echogenicity with shadowing (Fig. 10). No vascularity is demonstrated within the lesion [34]. In neonates, close sonographic follow-up is recommended to assure resolution. There is no definite role for CT or MR imaging unless the diagnosis is unclear. If this is the case, urine catecholamines and nuclear imaging may be helpful.

### Liver

Although primary hepatic neoplasms account for only between 0.5% and 2.0% of all pediatric neoplasms, they are clinically significant, because two thirds of them are malignant [35]. Neonatal hepatic tumors are extremely rare. Hepatic hemangioendothelioma is the most commonly diagnosed symptomatic tumor in infants younger than 6 months [36,37] and represents approximately 12% of all

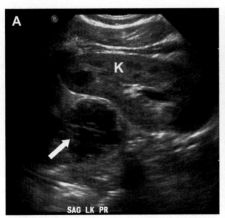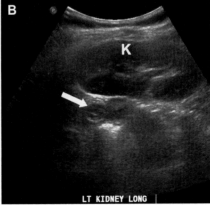

**Fig. 10.** Adrenal hemorrhage in a neonate. (*A*) Longitudinal sonogram demonstrates a round heterogeneous mass (*arrow*) superior to the left kidney (*K*). The mass did not have internal vascularity (not shown). (*B*) Three months later the mass (*arrow*) above the kidney (*K*) had decreased in size and now has an echogenic rim, representing rim calcifications.

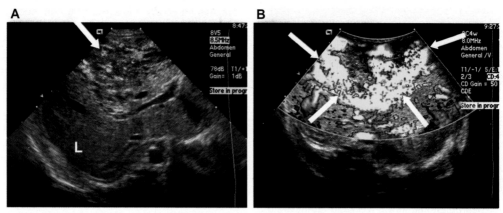

**Fig. 11.** Hemangioendothelioma in a neonate who had thrombocytopenia and coagulopathy. (*A*) Transverse sonography of the liver (*L*) demonstrates a large, heterogeneous mass (*arrow*). (*B*) Power Doppler imaging demonstrates significant blood flow within the mass (*arrows*). Follow-up imaging (not shown) demonstrated interval resolution of the mass.

pediatric hepatic neoplasms. Eighty-five percent of patients are diagnosed in the first 6 months of life. Hepatic hemangioendotheliomas typically present with one or more of the following: a palpable mass, congestive heart failure from vascular shunting, thrombocytopenia caused by platelet trapping (Kasabach-Meritt syndrome), jaundice, and hemoperitoneum from rupture of a superficial hemangioendothelioma.

Sonographically, hemangioendotheliomas typically appear as complex solid hepatic lesions with a heterogeneous echotexture, but predominantly hypoechoic [37]. Doppler color flow is seen within the tumor and can be marked, depending on the amount of AV shunting (Fig. 11). During involution, the mass can increase in echogenicity as it decreases in size. Complex ascites can be present, representing hemoperitoneum. Multiple hemangioendotheliomas can be present within the liver, and if present denote an unfavorable prognosis.

Spontaneous regression is usually seen in patients who have a single hepatic hemangioendothelioma, and long-term survival is approximately 70% [36]. Various pharmacotherapies may be used to achieve regression. Embolization and surgery are reserved for patients who have severe complications and for whom regression has failed, despite appropriate therapies.

### Biliary/gallbladder

Choledochal cysts are congenital malformations of the biliary system believed to be secondary to an abnormal configuration of the insertion of the common bile duct into the pancreatic duct. Although the occurrence of choledochal cysts is somewhat common in Asia, particularly in Japan where it occurs in 1 in 1000 births, it is rare in the United States,

where the occurrence rate is 1 in 100,000 to 1 in 1,000,000. The Todani classification separates these biliary abnormalities into five types, depending on the presence of intra- or extrahepatic involvement and fusiform or saccular changes. The fifth type, Caroli disease, is characterized by dilation of only the intrahepatic ducts [38]. The initial diagnosis is usually made by sonography, which can demonstrate dilation of the intra- or extrahepatic ducts. Specifically this diagnosis is suggested by the presence of a cystic structure near the porta hepatis and is established with certainty if the structure is shown to be continuous with the biliary system (Fig. 12). Choledochal cysts are treated surgically, with transplantation indicated for patients who have intrahepatic involvement. Patients who have choledochal cysts are at risk for developing cholangiocarcinoma, and those who have chronic cholestasis may eventually

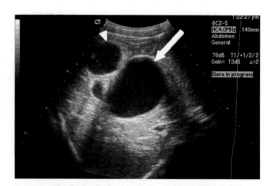

**Fig. 12.** Choledochal cyst in a 9-year-old child who had abnormal liver function tests and right upper quadrant fullness. Transverse sonography of the right upper quadrant demonstrates the gallbladder (*arrowhead*) and a separate cystic structure (*arrow*). At surgery the separate cystic structure was confirmed to be a choledochal cyst.

succumb to the disease. Despite surgical treatment, patients remain at risk for cholangiocarcinoma and are regularly screened following excision of the choledochal cyst.

## Pancreas

Pancreatic masses are rarely seen in infants, but when they are identified, pancreatoblastoma should be considered. Approximately 50% of the cases reported are in patients of Asian descent. Congenital pancreatoblastoma has been identified in patients who have Beckwith Wiedemann syndrome and have been described as predominantly cystic in nature. In the older infant and young child, most pancreatoblastomas appear sonographically as well circumscribed masses with solid and cystic components. Hyperechoic septa can be seen within the hypoechoic cystic portions. CT and MR imaging can help determine the extent of local disease and any evidence of metastatic disease. Pancreatoblastoma can metastasize to several organs, most commonly to the lymph nodes and liver. Surgical resection is the primary treatment, with chemotherapy and radiation indicated for metastatic disease [39,40].

## Pelvis

Hydrocolpos and hydrometrocolpos are conditions in which blood or fluid are contained in a dilated proximal vagina because of a distal vaginal obstruction. This can present from the neonatal period up through early adolescence. In the neonate, this is caused by maternal estrogens, hCG, and FSH stimulating ovarian and endometrial activity. Often the cause is an imperforate hymen; however, vaginal and cervical atresias are in the differential. The diagnosis of hydrometrocolpos can be made by ultrasound if a dilated fluid- or debris-filled structure is visualized posterior to the bladder in apparent continuity with a distended and fluid-filled uterine cavity (Fig. 13) [40]. If the diagnosis is unclear, then MRI can be obtained for further visualization of the pelvic anatomy.

Neonatal ovarian cysts are common, likely because of in utero exposure to maternal hormones. The likelihood that an individual child has an ovarian cyst seems to depend on hCG levels and placental permeability. The incidence is higher in premature infants and in girls who have diabetic mothers and Rh immunization [41]. With increased use of fetal sonography, there has been a corresponding increase in the detection of ovarian cysts [42]. Infants who have ovarian cysts may present symptomatically with pain, vomiting, fever, and abdominal distension from ovarian torsion or cyst rupture or hemorrhage. On sonography many of these cysts demonstrate characteristics of a simple cyst with increased through transmission, absence

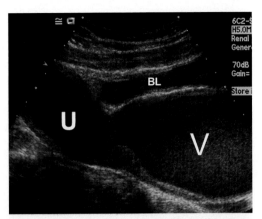

*Fig. 13.* Hydrometrocolpos. Longitudinal image demonstrates a dilated uterine cavity (*U*) and vagina (*V*) caused by an imperforate hymen. The bladder (*BL*) is seen anteriorly.

of internal echoes, and a thin wall without internal septations. If there has been torsion or internal hemorrhage, a fluid–debris level, retractile clot, septations, and echogenic walls from dystrophic calcifications are seen [41]. A rare occurrence is ascites or hemoperitoneum from rupture of the cyst or peritonitis from torsion. CT or MR imaging are occasionally performed, particularly if the cyst is complex and alternate diagnoses are questioned. Treatment for large ovarian cysts is often surgical, especially if there is presence of torsion. If the cyst is simple in appearance, some may elect to follow until resolution [43].

Sacrococcygeal teratomas (ST) are often diagnosed prenatally because of the typical exophytic component protruding from the fetal buttock. The prevalence is 1 in 40,000 live births with a female predilection of at least 3:1. ST are classified by the presence or absence of internal (presacral) or external components. Serum alpha fetal protein (AFP) levels are typically elevated with ST. Sonographically, teratomas demonstrate variable patterns of solid and cystic areas, typically with echogenic foci from calcification and fat, and hypoechoic portions from cystic or necrotic portions (Fig. 14). Fluid–fluid levels are less common than they are in ovarian teratomas. The imaging appearance of ST cannot definitively be used to predict histology; however, it has been reported that benign tumors are more likely to be cystic and malignant tumors are more likely to be solid [44]. Surgical excision is the recommended treatment, with the addition of chemotherapy in cases in which malignancy is determined.

## Bowel

A meconium pseudocyst results from perforation of the intestines during fetal life, which causes

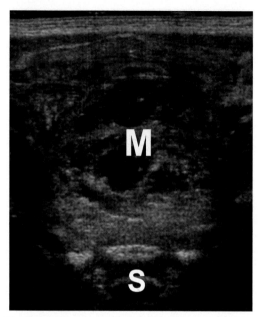

Fig. 14. Sacrococcygeal teratoma. Transverse images through the pelvis demonstrate a large pelvic mass (*M*) anteriorly along the sacrum (*S*).

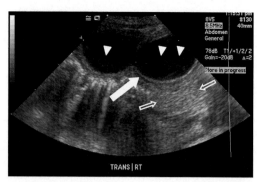

*Fig. 15.* Gastric duplication cyst. Transverse sonography demonstrates a bilobed cystic structure that demonstrates alternating inner echogenic and outer hypoechoic rims (*arrow*), considered to be the sonographic signature of bowel. Low-level internal echoes (*arrowheads*) within the cyst and posterior acoustic enhancement (*open arrows*) are also present.

a chemical peritonitis. The inflammatory reaction causes the perforation to seal, and a pseudocyst can form as the released peritoneal meconium walls off. Granulomatous changes cause peritoneal and cyst wall calcifications [45]. Ultrasound findings include a mass with heterogeneous internal echoes, often with increased through transmission. The presence of calcifications can cause the rim to be echogenic with shadowing [46]. This condition can often be suspected on plain radiographs by the identification of areas of calcification in the peritoneum and, in infant boys, within the scrotum.

Enteric duplication cysts can occur anywhere along the bowel on the mesenteric side, but are most common in the small intestine (ileum, jejunum, and duodenum, respectively) [47]. Duplication cysts can act as the lead point for an intussusception, which may be the cause of the patient's presentation. Sonographically an enteric duplication cyst appears as a hypoechoic or anechoic structure, but the wall of the cyst often demonstrates an echogenic inner mucosal layer and a hypoechoic outer muscular layer. Layering debris can occasionally be seen (**Fig. 15**) [48,49]. If uncomplicated by intussusception, enteric contrast studies or CT may demonstrate the cyst as a submucosal structure with mass effect protruding into the lumen of the gastrointestinal tract.

A mesenteric cyst is also in the differential for a cystic mass in the abdomen. Ultrasound demonstrates a thin-walled hypo- or anechoic structure with posterior acoustic enhancement, possibly with thin internal septations or internal echoes from debris, hemorrhage, or infection [50]. An abdominal lymphangioma can have a similar appearance. CT or MR imaging can be used for further evaluation in defining extent of the lesion and proximity to vessels but is typically performed to fully characterize a cystic mass of uncertain etiology.

## Abdominal masses in the older infant and child (greater than 12 months of age)

### Kidneys

**Malignant** Wilms tumor is the most common renal malignancy in children, with a peak incidence between 1 and 5 years of age [29]. Pathologically it is a sharply circumscribed tumor, which usually contains areas of necrosis, hemorrhage, and cystic degeneration. Wilms tumor spreads by way of contiguous invasion of adjacent organs or by extension into the renal vein and inferior vena cava. Distant spread is most commonly to the lung and liver. The typical clinical presentation is as an asymptomatic abdominal mass. An increased incidence of Wilms tumor is seen in association with Beckwith-Wiedemann syndrome, sporadic aniridia, hemihypertrophy, and the Drash syndrome (male pseudohermaphroditism and glomerular disease) [51]. Patients who have Beckwith-Wiedemann or hemihypertrophy syndrome should be screened by sonography every few months because of their increased risk for abdominal tumors, such as Wilms tumor [52].

On sonography Wilms tumors are echogenic intrarenal masses that may contain cystic areas [29,53] reflecting varying degrees of hemorrhage and necrosis (**Fig. 16**). Rarely Wilms tumor contains focal areas of fat or calcifications. The tumor

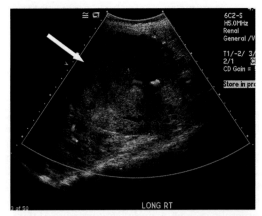

**Fig. 16.** Wilms tumor in a 3-year-old child who had a palpable abdominal mass. Color Doppler imaging demonstrates vascularity within the mass in the lower pole of the right kidney.

may invade the perinephric space, inferior vena cava, and even extend into the right atrium. Retroperitoneal adenopathy, synchronous tumor in the contralateral kidney, and hepatic metastases also may be noted. Increased tumoral vascularity is noted on color Doppler sonography. CT is preferred over sonography for staging to precisely assess extrarenal extension and to show lung metastases.

Renal cell carcinoma (RCC), although extremely rare in the young infant, increases in incidence with age. RCC accounts for only 2% to 6% of all primary renal neoplasms in children. Although RCC represents only 1.4% of all renal tumors in patients younger than 4 years, it accounts for 15.2% in patients aged 5 to 9 years, and 52.6% in patients aged 10 to 15 years [54]. The most common presentations include abdominal pain or hematuria, and less commonly a palpable mass [55].

Sonography of RCC often demonstrates a mass of heterogeneous echotexture, not only from calcifications (in up to 28% of RCC), but also from tumor necrosis and hemorrhage. It can be difficult to radiologically differentiate between RCC and Wilms tumors. Nephron-sparing surgery may be attempted in cases in which the tumor is small. Many patients present with more advanced disease, however, and nephrectomy is typically necessary [56].

Clear cell sarcoma of the kidney (CCSK) is a rare tumor, and unlike Wilms tumor, it is not associated with intralobar nephrogenic rests. Also in contrast to Wilms tumor, CCSK has a propensity to metastasize to bone following nodal involvement. Sonographic imaging features of CCSK, however, are similar to Wilms tumor, typically depicted as a large heterogeneous mass extending from the kidney, sometimes with extension into the renal vein. Treatment usually involves radical nephrectomy with

chemotherapy and radiation. CCSK is said to have a less favorable prognosis than Wilms; however, the 8-year relapse-free survival rate for localized CCSK stages I to III is 88% [57,58].

One of the most aggressive and lethal pediatric tumors is the rhabdoid tumor of the kidney. The median age of presentation is approximately 15 months of age. Abdominal mass, hypertension, fever, and hematuria are common presentations. Following initial diagnosis, the central nervous system (CNS) should be evaluated, because approximately 15% of patients who have rhabdoid tumor of the kidney have synchronous or metachronous CNS lesions. Rhabdoid tumors can occur in any organ; however, the kidney is the most common. Sonographic findings include a large heterogeneous renal mass that can have internal echogenic foci from calcifications and hypoechoic subcapsular areas of fluid density (Fig. 17). Although calcifications and subcapsular fluid densities are findings more common in rhabdoid tumors than in Wilms tumors, rhabdoid tumors are so rare that these findings do not necessarily result in a definitive diagnosis [59,60]. Surgery, chemotherapy, and radiation are generally recommended; however, the survival rate for rhabdoid tumor of the kidney is only 20% to 25%, with most patients succumbing to the disease within a year.

Renal lymphoma usually develops secondary to extranodal spread of lymphoma; it is much less likely to occur as primary disease, presenting more frequently in immunocompromised patients than in the general pediatric population. Though up to one third of patients who have lymphoma have some renal involvement on histopathology, less

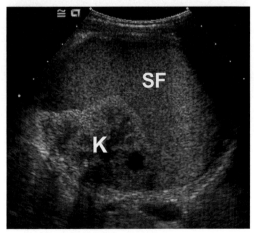

**Fig. 17.** Rhabdoid tumor of the kidney. Axial image of the kidney (*K*) demonstrates hypoechoic subcapsular fluid (*SF*). A discrete tumor mass is not shown on this image.

than 10% have involvement demonstrated on imaging. The sonographic appearance can be subtle, with only heterogeneity of the renal parenchyma noted, or there can be one or more focal hypoechoic regions within the parenchyma. Sonography is not as sensitive as CT and MR imaging, and if renal involvement is suspected, those modalities are recommended [61]. In general, renal lymphoma is successfully treated with chemotherapy.

**Benign** Multilocular cystic renal tumor (MCRT), as the name suggests, is a septated, cystic tumor of the kidney that typically presents as a large mass in children between 3 months and 2 years of age, with a slight male predominance. Histologically two subtypes are described: cystic nephroma (lacking blastemal or other embryonal elements) and cystic partially differentiated nephroblastoma (blastema present). Radiologically the two have identical appearances. On ultrasound MCRT typically appears as a mass with multiple anechoic spaces with thin septations. On occasion, because the cysts can be small, the MCRT can appear as a complex, echogenic mass because of the multiple acoustic interfaces of the cysts. MCRT can herniate into the renal collecting system, which may be demonstrated on imaging (Fig. 18) [62]. CT and MR imaging can be performed to confirm the imaging findings and diagnosis. Surgical excision is the definitive treatment for symptoms towing to mass effect and pathologic confirmation.

Angiomyolipomas (AML) are benign neoplasms with fat, vascular, and smooth muscle tissue. They are common in patients who have tuberous sclerosis (TS), occurring in approximately 80% of all pediatric TS patients [63]. Patients who have neurofibromatosis and von Hippel–Lindau syndrome also have increased incidence of angiomyolipomas [53]. In the general pediatric population, however, they are much rarer. Although histologically benign, lesion necrosis takes place secondary to the vascular components, which can form aneurysms and hemorrhage. Sonographic findings demonstrate highly echogenic non-shadowing foci, representing the fatty components, with variable heterogeneity and vascularity within the rest of the lesion (Fig. 19). These masses can range in size from tiny, punctuate lesions to large lesions. Lesions larger than 4 cm in diameter are more likely to spontaneously hemorrhage and are pre-emptively surgically excised. Actively hemorrhaging AML can often be temporarily treated by interventional embolozation until the patient can have a partial or total nephrectomy.

### Adrenal gland

If an adrenal mass is found incidentally in a pediatric patient and does not show signs of regression, it is generally recommended that it should be surgically removed. Many incidentally found pediatric adrenal tumors prove to be malignant on pathologic examination; this is especially true with NB, particularly in the younger child [64]. NB, while also discussed in the neonatal section, is common in the young child also. Approximately 40% of patients are younger than 1 year of age when diagnosed; 35% are between 1 and 2 years of age; 25% are between 2 and 5 years of age; and after age 10 years, the disease is rarely seen. Although the imaging features are similar regardless of the age of diagnosis, the prognosis for older patients is not as favorable as it is for younger patients.

Adrenocortical adenoma (ACA) and adrenocortical carcinoma (ACC) are rare entities in children. Of the adrenocortical tumors in children, ACC is

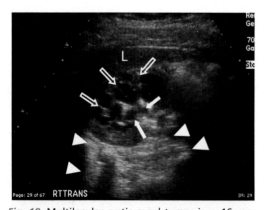

*Fig. 18.* Multilocular cystic renal tumor in a 16-year-old girl. Transverse image of the right kidney demonstrates a septated cystic mass in the mid to lower pole with projection (*solid arrows*) into the renal pelvic fat. Posterior acoustic enhancement (*arrowheads*) and thin septations (*empty arrows*) are noted. The liver (*L*) is seen anteriorly.

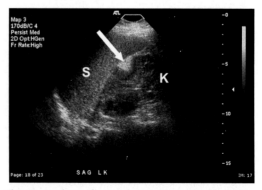

*Fig. 19.* Angiomyolipoma in a patient who had tuberous sclerosis. Longitudinal sonography of the left kidney (*K*) demonstrates an echogenic renal cortical mass (*arrow*). The spleen is seen superiorly (*S*).

reported to be more common than ACA [65]. Patients who have adrenocortical tumors often present with virilization and less often with Cushing syndrome symptoms [65,66]. Some tumors, typically ACCs, have no hormonal function and present when a palpable mass is incidentally identified. ACC can be associated with certain syndromes (eg, Li-Fraumeni complex, Beckwith-Wiedemann syndrome, Carney complex, multiple endocrine neoplasia type I, and hemihypertrophy syndrome) and a P53 deletion. ACAs most often are small, limited to the adrenal gland, and can be homogeneous or heterogeneous on sonography. The sonographic characteristics of ACC depend on the stage, but the lesions usually appear as large, heterogeneous, well-defined suprarenal tumors, containing echogenic areas with shadowing, representing calcifications. The presence of a thin tumor capsule, a stellate central zone of necrosis, hormonal function, and the presence of lung metastases can help distinguish ACC from NB by imaging [67]. Treatment for ACA is surgical excision and is considered curative.

### Liver

Hepatoblastoma (HB) is the most common liver tumor in children. Patients typically present between the ages of 1 and 3 years with a palpable abdominal mass. Serum AFP levels are elevated in children who have hepatoblastoma, and, although not a specific sign, is a sensitive marker for response to therapy, disease progression, and detection of recurrent disease. Children who have Beckwith-Wiedemann and familial adenomatous polyposis are at increased risk for HB. Lung and porta hepatis involvement are the most common sites of metastasis. Sonographic evaluation is used for visualization of the heterogeneous tumor and for evaluating vascular involvement. The tumor is often well delineated, with septations and heterogeneous echotexture caused by internal cysts, necrosis, and calcification (Fig. 20) [68]. High-frequency (>7 MHz) linear array transducers can be helpful in evaluating the portal and hepatic venous systems; color imaging and pulse Doppler waveform analysis can assist with assessing intravascular tumor extension. Tumor extension into the portal venous system can cause disruption of the normal hyperechoic stripe of the vein wall [69]. Echogenic material in the lumen of the vein may represent thrombus or extension of tumor. If there is Doppler evidence of arterial blood flow within the intraluminal material, then venous invasion must be considered [70].

Although there is widespread discussion about various treatment approaches for hepatoblastoma, surgery still prevails as the gold standard. In the United States, surgical resection with postoperative chemotherapy is standard, with preoperative

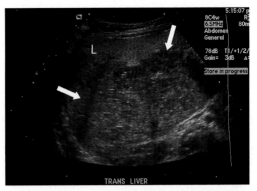

**Fig. 20.** Hepatoblastoma in a 5-month-old boy who had an abdominal mass on physical examination. Axial sonography through the liver (*L*) demonstrates a large heterogeneous mass within and extending from the liver (*arrows*).

chemotherapy recommended for patients who have initially unresectable disease. In patients who have unresectable disease, liver transplant is performed. Overall, 5-year survival rates are more than 70%, with greater than 90% survival in early-stage patients who have had complete resection and adjuvant chemotherapy [71].

Hepatocellular carcinoma (HCC) is the second most common hepatic malignancy in children, accounting for 20% of primary hepatic tumors; it is more often encountered in older children, with the median age of onset at 12 years. Certain infectious and congenital conditions increase an individual's risk, such as hepatitis B, glycogen storage disorders, and hereditary tyrosinemia. The serum AFP level is elevated in most patients.

On sonography, HCCs are typically hypoechoic and sometimes isoechoic with a thin hypoechoic halo representing the tumor capsule. A diffuse form of HCC, however, causes a more subtle abnormality of the normal hepatic echotexture, with anechoic areas resulting from necrosis. As with HB, tumor location and degree of vascular involvement must be documented in advance of surgical planning. CT and MR imaging are used to further evaluate the tumor and to assess for local and metastatic disease [72]. Although treatment is surgical excision, many patients do not have resectable disease and only 18% to 36% are completely resectable [73]. Chemotherapy, embolization, radiofrequency ablation, and ethanol injection can be used for tumor shrinkage in hopes of subsequent resection or for palliative care.

Mesenchymal hamartoma (MH) are benign hepatic tumors often presenting as large abdominal masses; they account for approximately 6% to 8% of all hepatic tumors in childhood. MH can present from birth to 10 years of age, with its peak incidence occurring between 15 and 20 months. The histopathology of the tumor demonstrates its origin from the mesenchyma of the periportal tracts, and the tumor can have cystic and stromal components.

Sonography demonstrates a range of appearances from a mostly anechoic mass with septations indicating predominately cystic composition to a complex solid mass, corresponding to a stromal predominance (Fig. 21) [68–74]. CT and MR imaging confirm its cystic and solid nature, demonstrating mild enhancement within the solid portions of the tumor. The tumor does not metastasize, and surgical resection is curative.

Embryonal sarcoma (ES) is a rare tumor of the liver, occurring in older children. Typically serum AFP levels are normal, and patients present with a palpable abdominal mass, with or without constitutional symptoms, such as pain, fever, or jaundice. Histopathologic findings include a fibrous capsule and myxoid stroma.

Sonographic findings can also be variable, with areas of solid and cystic components. Echogenic foci representing calcifications can be seen within the solid components. CT and MR imaging may be helpful following contrast administration, demonstrating an enhancing fibrous capsule and thick septations [75]. The combination of adjuvant chemotherapy and surgical resection has a reported 4-year survival of 70% to 83% [76].

## Pancreas

Pancreatic pseudocysts develop as a sequela from an episode of pancreatitis. Pancreatitis may be congenital or induced by medication or may develop following trauma. There is no specific age range

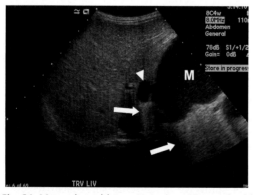

*Fig. 21.* Mesenchymal hamartoma in a 15-month-old girl who had abdominal distention. Transverse image of the liver demonstrates a large cystic mass (*M*) extending from the left hepatic lobe. Internal echoes within the large cyst and increased through transmission (*arrows*) from the large cyst and from a smaller cystic component (*arrowhead*) can be seen.

for pancreatitis, and the diagnosis is generally made clinically by elevation of the serum amylase and lipase levels or by an appropriate history. Pseudocysts develop as an inflammatory response to the pancreatic enzymes released into the adjacent tissues. Pseudocysts can be uni- or multilocular, and a patient can have multiple separate pseudocysts within the abdomen. Sonographic images typically demonstrate an anechoic structure with thin walls. There may be internal septations or debris if there has been internal hemorrhage or superinfection [77]. CT or MR imaging demonstrates the position of the pseudocyst, its relationship to adjacent structures, and any internal debris or superinfection. Other complications of pancreatitis, such as arterial pseudoaneurysm formation and venous thrombosis, can also be imaged.

Solid pseudopapillary tumor, also known as solid and pseudopapillary epithelial neoplasm (SPEN), is a tumor of low malignant potential, most commonly affecting adolescent girls and young women. On sonography, SPEN tumors are typically large, well circumscribed, and can have a variable appearance, with areas of hypo- and hyperechogenicity, representing areas of necrosis and calcification [40]. Fluid–fluid levels are occasionally seen within the cystic portions. CT and MR imaging are used to evaluate local disease and any possible metastasis. Metastases are extremely rare in young children who have SPEN, and, if present, are often single hepatic lesions, amenable to resection.

## Pelvic

Rhabdomyosarcoma (RMS) is one of the most common malignant solid tumors of childhood, ranking fourth behind CNS neoplasms, NB, and Wilms tumor [78]. The genitourinary tract is the second most common site of RMS, behind the head and neck. The median age of presentation is approximately 7 years, with variability in patient presentation secondary to the different sites of origin within the genitourinary tract (including bladder, prostate, testes and paratesticular region, penis, vagina, perineum, and uterus). Ten percent to 20% of all patients who have RMS have metastases at the time of diagnosis, with lungs, cortical bone, and lymph nodes the most common sites of spread.

Sonography can help define the normal pelvic structures in attempt to determine the organ of origin of the primary RMS. Although the sonographic appearance of the tumor may be variable, tumors are mostly solid and can be hyper-, mixed, or hypoechoic (Fig. 22). Hemorrhage and necrosis can also cause hypoechoic areas within the largely solid tumor. Sonographic evaluation should include the entire genitourinary tract and the remaining

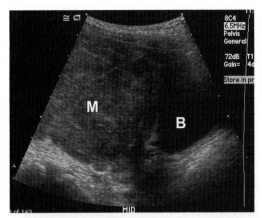

**Fig. 22.** Bladder rhabdomyosarcoma in a 7-year-old girl who had 2 weeks of abdominal pain. Longitudinal imaging of the pelvis reveals a heterogeneous solid mass (*M*) inseparable from the superior aspect of the bladder (*B*).

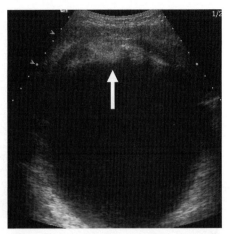

**Fig. 23.** Ovarian dermoid. Transverse image through the adnexa demonstrates a large cystic mass with echogenic material (*arrow*) anteriorly, which represents fat within the dermoid.

abdominal organs. Treatment is surgical excision. Often adjuvant chemotherapy is used to reduce primary tumor size to help obtain an adequate gross total resection. The survival rates for children who have RMS vary by stage and site of the primary tumor and probability of recurrence. Survival rates are as high as 89%, with 3-year survival in paratesticular RMS to 17%, and 2-year survival reported in patients who have recurrent disease [78,79].

Ovarian teratomas and dermoid cysts account for approximately two thirds of pediatric ovarian tumors. Many present with palpable abdominal or pelvic masses and some present with ovarian torsion. Although mostly unilateral, bilateral teratomas are present in 10% of patients [80]. Ovarian teratomas have a variable sonographic appearance because of their complex internal architecture and components such as hair, fat, mucus, and calcium (Fig. 23). In postpubertal girls, the most common sonographic findings are echogenic foci with acoustic shadowing and mural nodules within a cystic lesion, though these findings are slightly less common in prepubertal girls [81]. Areas of linear hyperechogenicity, described as the dermoid mesh sign, are sometimes seen within teratomas. Doppler vascularity can be used to demonstrate flow within the involved ovary. Occasionally teratoma is diagnosed incidentally by CT or MR imaging. As a rule, teratomas are surgically excised because of the increased risk for ovarian torsion and rupture.

When adolescent girls present with pelvic pain, pelvic sonography is often performed to evaluate for ovarian torsion (Fig. 24). A torsed ovary is classically enlarged and globular, sometimes five to six times as large as the normal contralateral ovary, with multiple, small peripheral cysts or follicles [82]. These characteristics are well demonstrated by sonography. The torsed ovary is often displaced out of the lateral true pelvis into the midline or lower abdomen. The whirlpool sign representing the twisted pedicle may be visualized on gray-scale or color Doppler imaging adjacent to the torsed ovary. Otherwise Doppler imaging has limited use in the evaluation of patients suspected of having ovarian torsion. It has been shown that the presence of blood flow in the ovarian parenchyma using color or pulse Doppler interrogation is not a reliable method of excluding ovarian torsion, with one series demonstrating blood flow within the ovarian parenchyma in almost 50% of proven torsed ovaries [83]. Large cysts and ovarian neoplasms (>5–6 cm) can predispose the ovaries to torsion, acting like a fulcrum. The younger the patient who has ovarian torsion, the more likely there is an underlying pathologic adnexal lesion. Sixty-five percent of neonates and infants who have torsion have pathologic lesions, whereas only 10% of postpubertal girls have pathologic lesions [84]. The most common predisposing factor for ovarian torsion in young girls is believed to be excessive mobility of the ovary caused by laxity of the mesosalpinx. The viability of the ovary depends on the timeliness of diagnosis and surgical treatment.

*Bowel*

Often the clinical picture of colicky abdominal pain in a young child, especially if there is blood in the stools, suggests to the clinician the possibility of an intussusception (Fig. 25). Intussusceptions occur in younger children, typically 5 months to 2 years of age [85]. Most often there is no pathologic lead point, and the intussusception begins at the terminal ileum and extends into the ascending

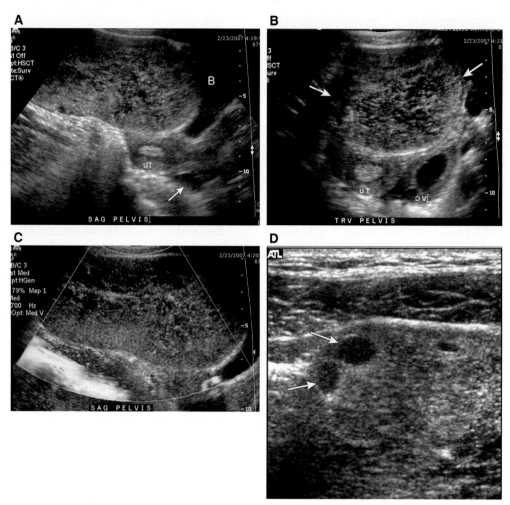

**Fig. 24.** Ovarian torsion. (*A*) Sagittal gray-scale image of the pelvis in a 15-year-old girl presenting with severe, acute pelvic pain demonstrates a large, heterogenous midline pelvic mass separate from the uterus (*UT*), left ovary (*arrow*), and bladder (*B*). (*B*) Transverse image depicting the midline mass (*arrows*). There is a small simple cyst in the left ovary (*OV*); uterus (*UT*). (*C*) There is no blood flow in the mass on this sagittal power Doppler image. (*D*) Image obtained with a higher resolution linear array transducer reveals several small peripheral cysts in the near field (*arrows*). The presence of the small peripheral cysts in a large midline mass with central heterogeneity in a girl who had acute onset of pelvic pain and lack of visualization of one of the ovaries is a classic presentation for ovarian torsion. (*Courtesy of* T. Robin Goodman, MD, New Haven, CT.)

colon (ileocolic). Pathologic lead points, however, should be suspected in older children who have intussusception. Certain conditions like Henoch-Schönlein purpura, lymphoma, familial polyposis syndromes, Meckel diverticulum, and enteric duplication cysts predispose patients to develop intussusceptions.

Plain films can demonstrate a paucity of right lower quadrant bowel gas and lateralization of the terminal ileum. Occasionally a soft-tissue mass can be seen representing the intussusceptum (proximal intussuscepting loop of bowel) within the intussuscipiens. Sonography is often used for diagnosis, and a technique of graded compression is used, typically with a linear high-resolution probe, imaging in longitudinal and transverse planes. The involved bowel demonstrates alternating hypoechoic and echogenic bands, which in the transverse plane can appear as multiple concentric rings like a target. This appearance is considered diagnostic of intussusception. When imaged longitudinally or obliquely, the alternating hypoechoic and echogenic layers may have a "pseudokidney" appearance. Variable color Doppler signals can be seen, depending on the length of time since the intussusception occurred. Reduction of the intussusceptum can be attempted by air or contrast enema, in the absence of free air or other signs of

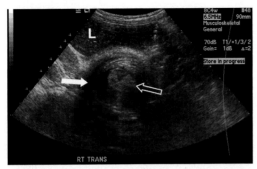

Fig. 25. Intussusception. Transverse image through the right midabdomen demonstrates hypoechoic and hyperechoic concentric rings, correlating to the intussusceptum and mesenteric fat and vessels (*open arrow*) within the intussuscipiens (*white arrow*). The liver (*L*) is seen anteriorly.

perforation [86]. If unsuccessful, surgical reduction is performed, with resection of any necrotic bowel.

Intestinal tumors are rare in children, with the most common being lymphoma. The most common extranodal site of lymphoma is within the bowel [87]. Lymphoma is usually best imaged by CT to evaluate for lymphadenopathy, parenchymal organ involvement, and for assessment of the entire bowel. If imaged sonographically, lobular solid masses can be seen within and extending from the bowel wall. These masses may involve the bowel wall circumferentially and may demonstrate internal vascularity. Post-transplant patients can develop a post-transplant lymphoproliferative disorder (PTLD) caused by Epstein-Barr virus infection that can appear radiographically identical to primary lymphoma. PTLD usually occurs within the first 1 to 2 years post-transplantation.

## Summary

With its noninvasiveness, wide availability, and ease of use without the risks associated with ionizing radiation exposure, ultrasound is an excellent imaging modality for initial evaluation of a suspected pediatric abdominal mass. When a mass is present, the sonographic features and the clinical presentation and age of the patient can lead to a focused differential diagnosis in most cases. In some cases, ultrasound may even facilitate a definitive diagnosis without the necessity of additional imaging studies.

## Acknowledgment

The authors acknowledge the editorial assistance of Nancy Drinan.

## References

[1] Pinto E, Guinard JP. Renal masses in the neonate. Biol Neonate 1995;68:175–84.

[2] Grisoni ER, Gauderer MWL, Wolfson RN, et al. Antenatal ultrasonography: the experience in a high risk perinatal center. J Pediatr Surg 1986; 21:358–61.

[3] Elder JS. Antenatal hydronephrosis: fetal and neonatal management. Pediatr Clin North Am 1997;44:1299–321.

[4] Reznick VM, Budorick NE. Prenatal detection of congenital renal disease. Urol Clin North Am 1995;22:21–30.

[5] Brown T, Mandell J, Lebowitz RL. Neonatal hydronephrosis in the era of sonography. AJR Am J Roentgenol 1987;148:959–63.

[6] DiSandro MJ, Kogan BA. Neonatal management of ureteropelvic junction obstruction: role for early intervention. Urol Clin North Am 1998; 25:187–97.

[7] Johnston JH, Evans JP, Glassberg KI, et al. Pelvic hydronephrosis in children: a review of 219 personal cases. J Urol 1977;117:97–101.

[8] Corteville JE, Gray DL, Crane JP. Congenital hydronephrosis: correlation of fetal ultrasonographic findings with infant outcome. Am J Obstet Gynecol 1991;165:384–8.

[9] Ransley PG, Dhillon HK, Gordon I, et al. The postnatal management of hydronephrosis diagnosed by prenatal ultrasound. J Urol 1990;144: 584–7.

[10] Woodward JR. Hydronephrosis in the neonate. Urology 1993;42(6):620–1.

[11] Thomas DF, Gordon AC. Management of prenatally diagnosed uropathies. Arch Dis Child 1989; 64:58–63.

[12] Cohen HL, Susman M, Haller JO, et al. Posterior urethral valve: transperineal US for imaging and diagnosis in male infants. Radiology 1994;192: 261–4.

[13] Pereira PL, Espinosa L, Urrutina MJM, et al. Posterior urethral valves: prognostic factors. BJU Int 2003;91(7):687–90.

[14] Atala A, Keating MA. Vesicoureteral reflux and megaureter. In: Walsh PC, Retik AB, Vaughan ED, et al, editors. Campbell's urology. 7th edition. Philadelphia: WB Saunders Co; 2002. p. 2053–116.

[15] Hsieh MH, Swana HS, Baskin LS, et al. Utility analysis of treatment algorithms for moderate grade vesicoureteral reflux using Markov models. J Urol 2007;177:703–9.

[16] Williams DI, Hulme-Moir I. Primary obstructive mega-ureter. Br J Urol 1970;42:140–9.

[17] Meyer JS, Lebowitz RL. Primary megaureter in infants and children: a review. Urol Radiol 1992; 14:296–305.

[18] Decter RM. Renal duplication and fusion anomalies. Pediatr Clin North Am 1999;44:1323–41.

[19] Zerres K, Volpel MC, Weiss H. Cystic kidneys. Genetics, pathologic anatomy, clinical picture,

and prenatal diagnosis. Hum Genet 1984;68: 104–35.

[20] Rudnik-Schoneborn S, John U, Deget F, et al. Clinical features of unilateral multicystic renal dysplasia in children. Eur J Pediatr 1998;157: 666–72.

[21] Glassberg K. Renal dysgenesis and cystic disease of the kidney. In: Walsh PC, Retik AB, Vaughan ED, et al, editors. Campbell's urology. 7th edition. Philadelphia: WB Saunders Co; 2002. p. 1925–94.

[22] Strife JL, Souza AS, Kirks DR, et al. Multicystic dysplastic kidney in children: US followup. Radiology 1993;186:785–8.

[23] Siegel MJ. Urinary tract. In: Siegel MJ, editor. Pediatric sonography. Philadelphia: Lippincott Williams & Wilkins; 2001. p. 411–5.

[24] Avni FE, Guissard G, Hall M, et al. Hereditary polycystic kidney diseases in children: changing sonographic patterns through childhood. Pediatr Radiol 2002;32(3):169–74.

[25] Lonergan GJ, Rice RR, Suarez ES. Autosomal recessive polycystic kidney disease: radiologic-pathologic correlation. Radiographics 2000;20: 837–55.

[26] Marsden HB, Lawler W. Primary renal tumors in the first year of life. A population-based review. Virchows Arch A Pathol Anat Histopathol 1983;399:1–9.

[27] Riccabona M. Imaging of renal tumours in infancy and childhood. Eur Radiol 2003;13(Suppl 4):L116–29.

[28] Beckwith JB, Kiviat NB, Bonadio JF. Nephrogenic rests, nephroblastomatosis, and the pathogenesis of Wilms' tumor. Pediatr Pathol 1990;10: 1–36.

[29] Lonergan GJ, Martinez Leom MI, Agrons GA, et al. Nephrogenic rests, nephroblastomatosis, and associated lesions of the kidneys. Radiographics 1998;18:947–68.

[30] Gurney JG, Severson RK, Davis S, et al. Incidence of cancer in children in the United States. Sex-, race-, and 1-year age-specific rates by histologic type. Cancer 1995;75:2186–95.

[31] Nuchtern JG. Perinatal neuroblastoma. Semin Pediatr Surg 2006;15(1):10–6.

[32] Schmidt ML, Lukens JN, Seeger RC, et al. Biological factors determine prognosis in infants with stage IV neuroblastoma: a prospective children's cancer group study. J Clin Oncol 2000;18(6): 1260–8.

[33] Kim S, Chung DH. Pediatric solid malignancies: neuroblastoma and Wilms' tumor. Surg Clin North Am 2006;86(2):469–87.

[34] Kawashima A, Sandler C, Ernst R, et al. Imaging of nontraumatic hemorrhage of the adrenal gland. Radiographics 1999;19:949–63.

[35] Emre S, McKenna GJ. Liver tumors in children. Pediatr Transplant 2004;8(6):632–8.

[36] Selby DM, Stocker JT, Waclawiw MA, et al. Infantile hemangioendothelioma of the liver. Hepatology 1994;20:39–45.

[37] Roos JE, Pfiffner R, Stallmacj T, et al. Infantile hemangioendothelioma. Radiographics 2003;23: 1649–55.

[38] Todani T, Urushihara N, Morotomi Y, et al. Characteristics of choledochal cysts in neonates and early infants. Eur J Pediatr Surg 1995;5(3): 143–5.

[39] Montemarano H, Lonergan G, Bulas D, et al. Pancreatoblastoma: imaging findings in 10 patients and review of the literature. Radiology 2000;214:476–82.

[40] Chung E, Travis M, Conran R. Pancreatic tumors in children: radiologic–pathologic correlation. Radiographics 2006;26:1211–38.

[41] Schmahmann S, Haller J. Neonatal ovarian cysts: pathogenesis, diagnosis, and management. Pediatr Radiol 1997;27:101–5.

[42] Nussbaum AR, Sanders RC, Hartman DS, et al. Neonatal ovarian cysts: sonographic–pathologic correlation. Radiology 1988;168:817–21.

[43] Mirk P, Pintus C, Speca S. Ultrasound diagnosis of hydrocolpos: prenatal findings and postnatal follow-up. J Clin Ultrasound 1994;22: 55–8.

[44] Keslar PJ, Buck JL, Suarez ES. Germ cell tumors of the sacrococcygeal region: radiologic pathologic correlation. Radiographics 1994;14:607–20.

[45] Silverbach S. Antenatal real-time identification of meconium cyst. J Clin Ultrasound 1983;11: 455–7.

[46] Carroll BA, Moskowitz PS. Sonographic diagnosis of neonatal meconium cyst. Am J Roentgenol 1981;137(6):1262–4.

[47] Tong S, Pitman M, Anupindi SA. Ileocecal enteric duplication cyst: radiologic–pathologic correlation. Radiographics 2002;22:1217–22.

[48] Barr LL, Hayden CK Jr, Stansberry SD, et al. Enteric duplication cysts in children: are their ultrasonographic wall characteristics diagnostic? Pediatr Radiol 1990;20(5):326–8.

[49] Macpherson R. Gastrointestinal tract duplications: clinical, pathologic, etiologic, and radiologic considerations. Radiographics 1993;13: 1063–80.

[50] Bliss DP Jr, Coffin CM, Bower RJ, et al. Mesenteric cysts in children. Surgery 1994;115(5): 571–7.

[51] Geller E, Smergel EM, Lowry PA. Renal neoplasms of childhood. Radiol Clin North Am 1997;35(6):1391–413.

[52] Choyke PL, Siegel MJ, Craft AW, et al. Screening for Wilms' tumor in children with Beckwith-Wiedemann syndrome or idiopathic hemihypertrophy. Med Pediatr Oncol 1999;32: 196–200.

[53] Lowe LH, Isuani BH, Heller RM, et al. Pediatric renal masses: Wilms tumor and beyond. Radiographics 2000;20(6):1585–603.

[54] Uchiyama M, Iwafuchi M, Yagi M, et al. Treatment of childhood renal cell carcinoma with lymph node metastasis: two cases and a review of literature. J Surg Oncol 2000;75:266–9.

[55] Estrada C, Suthar A, Eaton S, et al. Renal cell carcinoma: Children's Hospital Boston experience. Urology 2005;20:1296–300.

[56] Cook A, Lorenzo AJ, Salle JL, et al. Pediatric renal cell carcinoma: single institution 25-year case series and initial experience with partial nephrectomy. J Urol 2006;175(4):1456–60.

[57] Argani P, Perlman EJ, Breslow NE, et al. Clear cell sarcoma of the kidney: a review of 351 cases from the National Wilms Tumor Study Group Pathology Center. Am J Surg Pathol 2000;24(1):4–18.

[58] Seibel NL, Li S, Breslow NE, et al. Effect of duration of treatment on treatment outcome for patients with clear-cell sarcoma of the kidney: a report from the National Wilms' Tumor Study Group. J Clin Oncol 2004;22(3):468–73.

[59] Winger DI, Buyuk A, Bohrer S, et al. Radiology–Pathology Conference: rhabdoid tumor of the kidney. Clin Imaging 2006;30(2):132–6.

[60] Agrons GA, Kingsman KD, Wagner BJ, et al. Rhabdoid tumor of the kidney in children: a comparative study of 21 cases. AJR Am J Roentgenol 1997;168(2):447–51.

[61] Sheth S, Syed A, Fishman E. Imaging of renal lymphoma: patterns of disease with pathologic correlation. Radiographics 2006;26:1151–68.

[62] Agrons G, Wagner B, Davidson A, et al. Multilocular cystic renal tumor in children: radiologic–pathologic correlation. Radiographics 1995;15:653–69.

[63] Ewalt DH, Sheffield E, Sparagana SP, et al. Renal lesion growth in children with tuberous sclerosis complex. J Urol 1998;160:141–5.

[64] Masiakos PT, Gerstle JT, Cheang T, et al. Is surgery necessary for incidentally discovered adrenal masses in children? J Pediatr Surg 2004;39(5):754–8.

[65] Michalkiewicz E, Sandrini R, Figueiredo B, et al. Clinical and outcome characteristics of children with adrenocortical tumors: a report from the International Pediatric Adrenocortical Tumor Registry. J Clin Oncol 2004;22(5):838–45.

[66] Ciftci AO, Tanyel FC, Senocak ME, et al. Adrenocortical tumors in children. J Pediatr Surg 2001;36(4):549–54.

[67] Ribeiro J, Ribeiro RC, Fletcher BD. Imaging findings in pediatric adrenocortical carcinoma. Pediatr Radiol 2000;30(1):45–51.

[68] Helmberger TK, Ros PR, Mergo PJ, et al. Pediatric liver neoplasms: a radiologic–pathologic correlation. Eur Radiol 1999;9(7):1339–47.

[69] Sato M, Ishida H, Konno K, et al. Liver tumors in children and young patients: sonographic and color Doppler findings. Abdom Imaging 2000;25:596–601.

[70] Ohtsuka Y, Takahashi H, Ohnuma N, et al. Detection of tumor thrombus in children using color Doppler ultrasonography. J Pediatr Surg 1997;32:1507–10.

[71] Roebuck DJ, Perilongo G. Hepatoblastoma: an oncological review. Pediatr Radiol 2006;36(3):183–6.

[72] Miller JH, Greenspan BS. Integrated imaging of hepatic tumors in childhood. Part I. Malignant lesions (primary and metastatic). Radiology 1985;154:83–90.

[73] Chen JC, Chen CC, Chen WJ, et al. Hepatocellular carcinoma in children: clinical review and comparison with adult cases. J Pediatr Surg 1998;33:1350–4.

[74] Bejvan SM, Winter TC, Shields LE, et al. Prenatal evaluation of mesenchymal hamartoma of the liver: gray scale and power Doppler sonographic imaging. J Ultrasound Med 1997;16:227–9.

[75] Ros PR, Olmsted WW, Dachman AH, et al. Undifferentiated (embryonal) sarcoma of the liver: radiologic–pathologic correlation. Radiology 1986;161:141–5.

[76] Kim DY, Kim KH, Jung SE, et al. Undifferentiated embryonal sarcoma of the liver: combination treatment with surgery and chemotherapy. J Pediatr Surg 2002;37:1419–23.

[77] Lawson TL. Acute pancreatitis and its complications. Computed tomography and sonography. Radiol Clin North Am 1983;21(3):495–513.

[78] Agrons GA, Wagner BJ, Lonergan GJ, et al. Genitourinary rhabdomyosarcoma in children: radiologic–pathologic correlation. Radiographics 1997;17:919–37.

[79] Maurer HM, Beltangady M, Gehan EA, et al. The Intergroup Rhabdomyosarcoma Study I: a final report. Cancer 1988;61:209–20.

[80] Laing FC, van Dalsan VF, Marks WM, et al. Dermoid cysts of the ovary: their ultrasonographic appearances. Obstet Gynecol 1981;57:99–104.

[81] Sisler CL, Siegel MJ. Ovarian teratomas: a comparison of the sonographic appearance in prepubertal and postpubertal girls. AJR Am J Roentgenol 1990;154:139–41.

[82] States L, Bellah R. Imaging the pediatric female pelvis. Semin Roentgenol 1996;31(4):312–9.

[83] Stark JE, Siegel MJ. Ovarian torsion in prepubertal and pubertal girls: sonographic findings. AJR Am J Roentgenol 1994;163:1479–82.

[84] Siegel MJ. Female pelvis. In: Siegel MJ, editor. Pediatric sonography. Philadelphia: Lippincott Williams & Wilkins; 2001. p. 529–77.

[85] Vasavada P. Ultrasound evaluation of acute abdominal emergencies in infants and children. Radiol Clin North Am 2004;42(2):445–56.

[86] Bisset GS III, Kirks DR. Intussusception in infants and children: diagnosis and therapy. Radiology 1988;168(1):141–5.

[87] Ladd AP, Grosfeld JL. Gastrointestinal tumors in children and adolescents. Semin Pediatr Surg 2006;15(1):37–47.

# ULTRASOUND CLINICS

Ultrasound Clin 2 (2007) 561–567

# Index

*Note:* Page numbers of article titles are in **boldface** type.

doi:10.1016/S1556-858X(07)00100-4